Diabetic Retinopathy: *The Essentials*

Diabetic Retinopathy: *The Essentials*

Gloria Wu, MD

Adjunct Clinical Instructor
Department of Ophthalmology
Stanford University School of Medicine

Clinical Associate Professor
Department of Ophthalmology
Tufts University School of Medicine

Wolters Kluwer Health | Lippincott Williams & Wilkins

Philadelphia • Baltimore • New York • London
Buenos Aires • Hong Kong • Sydney • Tokyo

Senior Executive Editor: Jonathan W. Pine, Jr.
Senior Product Manager: Emilie Moyer
Senior Manufacturing Manager: Benjamin Rivera
Marketing Manager: Lisa Lawrence
Design Coordinator: Teresa Mallon
Production Service: SPi Technologies

Two Commerce Square
2001 Market Street
Philadelphia, PA 19103 USA
LWW.com

Printed in China

Library of Congress Cataloging-in-Publication Data
Wu, Gloria.
Diabetic retinopathy : the essentials / Gloria Wu.
p. ; cm.
Includes bibliographical references and index.
ISBN 978-1-60547-662-9 (alk. paper)
1. Diabetic retinopathy. I. Title.
[DNLM: 1. Diabetic Retinopathy. WK 835 W959d 2010]

RE661.D5W8 2010
617.7'35—dc22

2010001230

---

10 9 8 7 6 5 4 3 2 1

CCS0310

CONTENTS

PREFACE

In 2008, the World Health Organization estimated that more than 180 million people worldwide had diabetes and that by 2030, this number would double. Thus, diabetes has become epidemic in the world at large. China and India both have increasing rates of diabetes in their populations. Thus, diabetic retinopathy has become a more common problem in physicians' offices. In California, where our patients come from all over the globe, we have seen diabetic retinopathy in all stages of severity. In fact, many of the patients present with decreased vision and diabetic retinopathy but do not yet know that they have diabetes since they have never had the appropriate laboratory testing.

I wrote this book for the ophthalmology resident-in-training, the general ophthalmologist or optometrist, the family practitioner, the diabetologist, and the general internist. I wanted to answer their questions about diabetic retinopathy.

The first three chapters deal with the background of diabetes and diabetic retinopathy. These chapters serve to bridge our background as retinal specialists to our colleagues'. Chapter 4 describes our diagnostic testing and what we, as retinal specialists, use for the examination of a diabetic patient. Chapter 5 specifically goes through our ophthalmic examination using the slit lamp. Chapter 6 summarizes the new treatment modalities of this past decade including the anti-VEGF treatments. Chapters 7 through 9 have clinical correlations with photographs and case reports. These chapters would be useful for all clinicians, especially ophthalmologists and optometrists. The photographs would be interesting for our internal medicine and family practice colleagues. Chapter 10 is a summary of surgical techniques for diabetic retinopathy and vitreous hemorrhages. This might be useful for our internal medicine colleagues. Chapter 11 is for our colleagues who see pregnant diabetic patients. Chapter 12 is about complications of medical and surgical treatment. Chapter 13 is about diabetes and neovascular glaucoma, a common complication of diabetes. Chapter 14 is about informed consent and how it applies to all of us as clinicians. In this chapter, cross-cultural concerns are discussed. Chapter 15 gives guidelines for nurses and office assistants. In this chapter, specific telephone scripts addressing cross-cultural considerations are given. Appendix A is entirely devoted to the visual image of diabetic retinopathy as can be seen in a modern retina-vitreous practice. There are scans using Optical Coherent Tomography to show the retina in cross section. Appendix B lists medical equipment companies and supplies. This appendix also provides web addresses for patient information. This is useful to all clinicians who want to provide reading materials for their patients. Appendix C is a short diabetic cookbook which can be shared with our patients.

I hope that this book proves to be useful. I look forward to your emails if you have additional questions.

Gloria Wu, MD
email: gloria_wumd@sbcglobal.net

ACKNOWLEDGMENTS

I thank my patients who have inspired me to think deeply about diabetes and diabetic retinopathy. Their questions have motivated all of us, as physicians, to further our quest for solutions. I thank Jonathan Pine, my editor, for his continuing support of this project. We have had an email correspondence spanning 3,000 miles that resulted in the production of this book.

I am especially indebted to my teachers in ophthalmology and retina. Beginning with Dr. Myles Behrens, who taught me the importance of research and inquiry when I was a fourth-year medical student at Columbia University College of Physicians and Surgeons, with whom I wrote my first paper, a case report, "Hyphema in the Newborn." Dr. D. Jackson Coleman, Dr. Harvey Lincoff, and Dr. Stanley Chang were outstanding role models and teachers to me. Dr. Coleman taught me ultrasound along with the art of medicine. It was with Dr. Lincoff that I found my first retinal hole. Dr. Chang and his fellows taught by example: in the operating rooms of Cornell University Medical Center, the techniques of vitreous surgery leading to the complex reattachment of diabetic traction detachments and proliferative vitreoretinopathy. To Dr. Charles Schepens, Dr. J. Wallace McMeel, Dr. Hal Freeman, Dr. Clement Trempe, Dr. Ronald Pruett, Dr. Felipe Tolentino, Dr. Tatsuo Hirose, Dr. John Weiter, Dr. Sheldon Buzney, and Dr. Alexandre Jalkh, I say earnest and sincere thanks for the transformative role that they played in my professional life. In my fellowship days at the Massachusetts Eye and Ear Infirmary, I had the opportunity to learn from Dr. Evangelos Gragoudas and his fluorescein conferences and from Dr. Claes Dohlman in his grand rounds for the residents and fellows. My formative years in Boston were made memorable by my time at the Joslin Diabetes Center, under the skillful and watchful guidance of Dr. Lloyd M. Aiello and Dr. Lawrence I. Rand. The Joslin Diabetes Center and its approach to diabetes have informed my practice patterns to this day. I thank Dr. Joseph Googe, Dr. Lory Snady-McCoy, Dr. Aaron Appiah, Dr. Sal Melgen, Dr. Jerry Sebag, and Dr. Susan Elner, my co-fellows at the Schepens Retina Associates; and Dr. David Lee, Dr. Joan Miller, Dr. Joan O'Brien, Dr. Robert Bhisitkul, and Dr. Lucy Young, my fellow residents and fellows at the Massachusetts Eye and Ear Infirmary, for their friendship for the past 20 years. A special word of thanks goes to Dr. Jay Duker who has supported my professional collaboration with Tufts University School of Medicine.

A word of appreciation goes to Dr. Mark Blumenkranz, chairman of the Department of Ophthalmology at Stanford University School of Medicine, who provided an academic home for me when I moved to California. I also thank Dr. Brian Ward, Dr. Patrick Monahan, Dr. Howard Chen, Dr. Amr Dessouki, Dr. Keshav Narain, Dr. Sonia Ghosh, Dr. Edwin Boldrey, Dr. James Palmer, Dr. Luis Borillo, Dr. Mark Wieland, Dr. Steven Sanislo, and Dr. Darius Moshfeghi, my California retina colleagues, who welcomed me into their world. I am indebted to Dr. James Liu, Dr. Tony Andrews, Dr. Krikor Barsoumian, Dr. Donald Lesser, Dr. Timothy Parsons, Dr. Arthur Basham, Dr. Martin Fishman, and Dr. Christopher Engelman, my ophthalmology colleagues in the San Jose area, who befriended me as a new colleague.

I would like to gratefully acknowledge the organizational skills of Janet Trang, Lesley Hughes, Allison Walewski, Alan Wei, Brian Ha, Quoc Nguyen, and Rona Lee, who compiled the manuscript.

Finally, I would like to thank my family, my husband Paul and my daughters Margaret and Catherine, for their patience, encouragement, and good humor as I wrote late into the night.

CHAPTER 1

Epidemiology

SCOPE OF THE PROBLEM

In 2007, the Center for Disease Control in the United States estimated that diabetes affects approximately 23.6 million children and adults or 8% of the US population. An estimated one third is unaware that they have the disease. An additional 57 million people who are prediabetic will become diabetic if they do not change their eating habits.[1] Diabetes is the fifth most common cause of death in America. In one study, 18% of the hospital admissions were found to have unrecognized and probable diabetes by the criteria of elevated HbA1c (>6.1).[2]

From 1990 to 2005, the prevalence of diabetes increased from 4.5 to 26.4 per 1,000 people, a sixfold increase. Researchers postulated that this increase was due to the increase in obesity during 1990–2005.[3] One study shows that currently 4% of obese white adolescents have diabetes and an additional 21% have abnormal glucose tolerance.[4]

In 2007, the economic cost of diabetes was estimated to be $174 billion.[1] Health care and medical expenditures related to diabetes totaled $116 billion (Table 1-1). Of that amount, $27 billion was for diabetes care, $31 billion for extra general medical costs, and $58 billion for chronic diabetic complications. People with diabetes had medical expenses that were 2.3 times higher than those for people without diabetes. Diagnosed diabetic patients accounted for 5.8% of the total US population. Inpatient hospital care accounted for $58.3 billion. For physician office visits, $9.9 billion was spent in 2007. Diabetes accounted for 24.3 million days of hospitalizations in 2007, whereas in 2002, that figure was 16.9 million days. In 2007, average cost for a hospital inpatient day due to diabetes was $1853 and $2281 due to diabetes-related chronic complications including neurological, peripheral-vascular, cardiovascular, renal, metabolic, and ophthalmic complications.

The indirect costs were estimated to $58 billion in 2007.[1] In 2007, diabetes accounted for 15 million work days of absence, 120 million work days with reduced performance, 6 million reduced productivity days for those not in the workforce, and an additional 107 million work days lost due to unemployment disability attributed to diabetes. Diabetes costs 445,000 cases of unemployment disability in 2007. The value of lost productivity due to premature death related to diabetes was $26.9 billion.

The increase in cost due to diabetes is related to (a) the growth of diabetes prevalence, (b) medical costs rising faster than general inflation, and (c) improvements made in the methods and data sources influencing cost estimates. The national burden of diabetes likely exceeds the $174 billion estimate because it omits the social cost of intangibles such as pain and suffering, care provided by nonpaid caregivers, excess medical costs associated with undiagnosed diabetes, and diabetes-attributed costs for health care expenditures categories not studied.[1]

Thus, the indirect cost of $58 billion dollars is from increased absenteeism, reduced productivity, disease-related unemployment disability, and loss of workplace productivity.[1] This $58 billion cost in 2007 eclipsed the $16 billion for the same problems in 2002. The reason for the increase is due to the obesity epidemic among teens. One out of every five health care dollars is spent caring for a diabetic patient, whereas 1 in 19 health care dollars is spent for the treatment of diabetes and its complications.[5]

TABLE 1.1 Cost of Diabetes ($174 Billion)

Medical cost $116 billion
$27 billion for diabetes care
$58 billion for chronic diabetes-related complications
$31 billion for related medical costs

Indirect cost $58 billion
15 million work days absent
120 million work days with reduced performance
6 million reduced productivity for those not in the workforce
107 million work days lost to unemployment disability
445,000 cases of unemployment disability

LIFETIME RISK FOR DIABETES MELLITUS IN THE UNITED STATES

Data from the National Health Interview Survey (1984–2000) show that the estimated lifetime risk of developing diabetes for individuals born in 2000 is 32.8% for males and 38.5% for females. Females have the higher residual lifetime risks for all age groups. The highest estimated lifetime risk for diabetes is among Hispanics (males 45.4% and females 52.5%). Individuals diagnosed as having diabetes have a large reduction in life expectancy. If a person is diagnosed at age 40, men will lose 11.6 life years and 18.6 quality-adjusted life years and women will lose 14.3 life years and 22.0 quality-adjusted life years. Thus, primary prevention of diabetes and its complications is an important public health priority.[6]

MEDICAL CARE FOR DIABETIC PATIENTS

In the 1989 National Health Interview Survey, 84,572 adults 18 years and older were studied. From this group, a subgroup of diabetic patients, 2,405 respondents, were queried about their diabetes care. More than 90% of the diabetic adults had one physician for the usual care of their diabetes, but 32% made fewer than four visits to the physician each year. Most physician visits by diabetic patients were not made to diabetes specialists. The visit rate to nonprimary care physicians such as other health care professionals such as ophthalmologists, podiatrists, nutritionists, was low. About half of the insulin-treated diabetic subjects used multiple daily insulin injections. Forty percent of patients with insulin-dependent diabetes and 26% with non–insulin-dependent diabetes mellitus (NIDDM) took insulin, and 5% of NIDDM patients not taking insulin monitored their blood glucose daily. Diabetes patient education classes were attended by 35% of diabetic adults. Thus, there is a need for specialists who treat diabetic patients.[7]

RACE AND ETHNIC DIFFERENCES

The association between impaired glucose tolerance (IGT) and the risk of Type 2 diabetes has been documented in a wide range of racial and ethnic groups (Table 1-2). In the San Antonio Heart Study, the relative risk of developing Type 2 diabetes conferred by IGT ranges from 4.3 to 7 depending upon race and gender.[8]

Native Americans

The 2005 Indian Health Service User population database indicated that 14.2% of American Indians and Alaskan Natives (AI/AN) aged 20 or older were diabetic. Rates varied from 6.0% in Alaska Native adults to 29.3% among American Indian adults in

TABLE 1.2 Clinical Interpretations of Plasma Glucose Concentrations

Fasting (mg/dL)
<100 within reference range
100–125 impaired fasting glucose/prediabetes mellitus
≥126 overt diabetes mellitus
2-hour post challenge load (75 g oral glucose tolerance test)
<140 within reference range
140–199 IGT
≥200 overt diabetes mellitus

Source: Diabetic Retinopathy Study Research Group. DRS report no. 3. Four risk factors for severe visual loss in diabetic retinopathy. *Arch Ophthalmol.* 1979;97:654–655.

Southern Arizona. In this study, diabetes occurred in 6.6% non-Hispanic whites, 7.5% Asian Americans, 10.4% Hispanics, and 11.8% non-Hispanic blacks.[9] In another study, American and Alaskan Native children (<15 years), adolescents (15–19 years), and young adults (20–34 years) had a 71% increase in diagnosis of diabetes. Diabetes prevalence increased by 46% from 1990 to 1998 in the above three groups.[10]

African Americans

In 1993, 1.3 million African Americans were known to have diabetes. This figure is almost three times the number of African Americans with diabetes in 1963. The actual number of diabetic African Americans is probably higher since there are many undiagnosed with the disease than reported. It is thought that for every African American diagnosed with diabetes, there is another African American yet to be diagnosed or who does not know that he or she has the disease. From 1980 to 2005, the age-adjusted prevalence of diagnosed diabetes doubled among black males and increased 69% among black females. However, of all groups observed, black females had the highest overall prevalence.[11]

After the 2000 census, it is known that 11% or 2.7 million of African Americans, aged 20 or older, have diabetes. One third of these do not even know that they have the disease. African Americans are 1.6 times more likely than white Americans to get diabetes.

One out of every four African American women is diabetic if they are 55 years or older. Twenty-five percent of blacks between the ages of 65 and 74 have diabetes.[12] Of note, African Americans are twice as likely to develop diabetic retinopathy than their white counterparts.[13]

In 1993, for the age group of 65 to 74 years, 17.4% of blacks were diabetic versus 9.5% of white Americans.[13] African Americans had a greater incidence of Type 2 diabetes. In fact, prevalence of Type 1 diabetes in white American children aged 15 and younger was nearly twice as that in African American children of the same age.[13] At age 45 and older, the prevalence of diabetes was 1.4 to 2.3 times as frequent in blacks as in whites. Within the age group of 65 to 74 years, 17.4% of blacks had diagnosed diabetes versus 9.5% of whites.

While gestational diabetes, which affects 2% to 5% of all pregnant women, usually resolves after childbirth, African American women have a higher rate of gestational diabetes. An Illinois study has shown an 80% higher incidence of gestational diabetes in black women as compared to their white counterparts. Experts estimate that about half of the women with gestational diabetes develop Type 2 diabetes within 20 years of pregnancy, regardless of race.[13]

African Americans may have a hemoglobin variant. Thus, the HbA1c of African Americans may not be accurate, falsely low or high, thus, it is important to check with the clinical laboratory to correlate the hemoglobin A1c with the patient's hemoglobin variant. African Americans have hemoglobin variants such as Hemoglobin S, Hemoglobin C, or Hemoglobin E.[14]

Latino Americans

Two in five Hispanics born in the year 2000 face a risk for diabetes. Compared to whites, Hispanics are more than two times as likely to have diabetes. From 1997 to 2005, the age-adjusted prevalence among Hispanics increased 16% among males and 21% among females.

In one study, the Hispanic population, which is the second largest and fastest growing minority in the United States, shares genetic markers with Americans, the Spanish, and Africans. The high frequency of Native American–derived genes in the contemporary Hispanic population predicts a higher frequency of NIDDM. The genetic markers, taken from 1,000 randomly selected Mexican Americans from Starr County, Texas, are used as a representative sample of the Mexican American population. For Mexican Americans, 31% of the contemporary gene pool is estimated to be Native American derived whereas 61% and 8% are Spanish and African derived, respectively. In Puerto Rico, the percentage of contributions of Spanish, Native American, and African mixture to the population are 15%, 18%, and 37%, respectively. In Cuba, the parallel estimates are 62%, 18%, and 20%. The high frequency of Native American-derived genes in contemporary Hispanic population predicts a higher frequency of NIDDM under the assumption that NIDDM may have genetic markers.[15]

Two million Latinos, aged 20 or older, have Type 1 or Type 2 diabetes. Latinos are 1.5 times more likely than non-Hispanic whites to have Type 2 diabetes, but Latinos are 2 times more likely than non-Hispanic whites to have any type of diabetes, Type 1 or Type 2. Specifically, Mexican Americans are 1.7 times more likely and Puerto Ricans are 1.8 times more likely to develop Type 2 diabetes than whites. Twenty-five percent to thirty percent of Hispanics older than age 50 have diabetes. Latinos are the fastest growing minority group in the United States. However, they have the lowest rates of insurance coverage and without regular and proper health, health care, and health care follow-up, diabetes can progress to blindness. Nearly half of the Latino children born in 2000 are likely to develop diabetes in their lifetime.[16]

Asian Americans

Diabetes is rising faster in Asian Americans than Caucasians. The rate among Asian Americans is 10% to 15% versus 6% to 8% in Caucasians.[9] These rates are similar to that found in Hong Kong.[16] The International Diabetes Federation predicts that diabetic rate in Asia are expected to rise to 160 million by 2025. India and China would account for 120 million by 2025.[16]

Top five countries with largest number of people affected by diabetes in 2003:

India—35.5 million
China—23.8 million
United States—16 million (by 2008, 21 to 23 million)
Russia—9.7 million
Japan—6.7 million

Ninety to ninety-five percent of Asians with diabetes have Type 2 diabetes. The rate of diabetes in Chinese Americans is notably higher than the rate of Chinese population in rural China. Thus, there are environmental factors that play a role in the development of diabetes in Chinese Americans in the United States. Indo-Asian women in America have the highest gestational diabetes rate in the country, with a prevalence of 56.1 per 100,000.[17] Native Hawaiians are 2.5 times likely to have diabetes than their white counterparts.[18] When Asians immigrate to the United States, their risk of developing diabetes increases significantly. This is most probably due to a change in lifestyle, diet, and exercise.[19]

Native Americans

AI/AN are people who have origins in any of the original peoples of North and South America including Central America and who maintain a tribal affiliation or community attachment. According to the 2000 US Census, those who identify as AI/AN constitute 0.9% of the US population or 2.5 million individuals. The greatest concentration of AI/AN populations are in the West, Southwest, and Midwest, especially in Alaska, Arizona,

TABLE 1.3 Risk Factors for Prediabetes and Diabetes Mellitus

Family history
Cardiovascular disease
Overweight or obese state
Sedentary lifestyle
Latino/Hispanic, non-Hispanic black, Asian American, Native American, or Pacific Islander ethnicity
Previously identified IGT or impaired fasting glucose
Hypertension
Increased levels of triglycerides, low concentrations of high-density lipoprotein cholesterol or both
History of gestational diabetes
History of delivery of infant with a birth weight greater than 9 lb
Polycystic ovary syndrome

Montana, New Mexico, Oklahoma, and South Dakota. There are 569 federally recognized AI/AN tribes, plus an unknown number of tribes that are not federally recognized. Each tribe has its own culture, beliefs, and practices. Among people younger than age 20, American Indians aged 10 to 19 years have the highest prevalence of Type 2 diabetes.[20] Gestational diabetes occurs more frequently among American Indians who are thought to have a high incidence of obesity during pregnancy. The risk factors for gestational diabetes include obesity and women with a family history of diabetes (Table 1-3).

TEEN OBESITY

In 2002–2003, SEARCH for Diabetes in Youth Study reported that 15,000 US children under the age of 20 years are diagnosed annually with Type 1 diabetes and 37,000 are newly diagnosed with Type 2 diabetes. While Type 2 diabetes is rare in children younger than 10 years of age, regardless of race and ethnicity, it becomes increasingly common in minority groups older than 10 years of age:

14.9% of new diabetes in Caucasians (non-Hispanic white)
46.1% Hispanic Youth
57.8% African Americans
69.7% in Asian and Pacific Islanders
86.2% in American Indian Youth

Results from the 2005–2006 National Health and Nutrition Examination Survey, using measured heights and weights, indicate that an estimated 16% to 17% of children and adolescents aged 2 to 19 had a BMI greater than or equal to 95th percentile of the age-and sex-specific BMI, about double the number of two decades ago.[21] Obesity in youth contributes to the increasing numbers of young people with Type 2 diabetes.[22]

GENETICS

Researchers suggest that African Americans and recent African immigrants to America have inherited a "thrifty" gene from their African ancestors. The presence of this gene has enabled Africans during "feast and famine" cycles to use food energy more efficiently when food was scarce. Today, with fewer "feast and famine" cycles, the thrifty gene that developed for survival may instead make weight control more difficult. This genetic predisposition with IGT occurs together with the genetic tendency of high blood pressure.[23]

EPIDEMIOLOGY OF DIABETIC RETINOPATHY

Diabetic retinopathy is the leading cause of blindness in working-age Americans, between 21 and 64 years of age. Diabetic retinopathy affects up to 16 million Americans, contributing to 14% of new blindness cases each year. It is estimated that 85% of the diabetics

TABLE 1.4 Eye Examination Schedule

Time of onset of DM	Recommended time of first exam	Routine minimum follow-up
≤30 y of age	5 y after onset	Annually
>30 y	At time of dx	Annually
Before pregnancy	Before or soon after conception	At least q 3 months

do not know that they have diabetic retinopathy. Twenty thousand people become legally blind each year from diabetes.

When diabetic retinopathy is appropriately handled, the 5-year risk of blindness for patients with proliferative diabetic retinopathy is reduced by 90% and the risk of visual loss from macular edema is reduced by 50%.[24] However, only 50% of diabetic patients receive regular dilated fundus examinations and many patients become legally blind without treatment.[25,26] The value of screening eye examinations has been known[27] (Table 1-4). The follow-up of patients with diabetic retinopathy depends on their presenting status of retinopathy (Table 1-5).

Diabetic retinopathy, a potential cause of irreversible vision loss, can cause a decrease in workplace productivity and a loss of income and productivity. Unfortunately, many diabetic patients are not aware of the possibility of early diagnosis and intervention which could save a lifetime of visual impairment.

Approximately 500,000 people in America have macular edema, which can be a harbinger of future acceleration of diabetic retinopathy. Seven hundred thousand Americans have proliferative diabetic retinopathy, and 65,000 new cases of proliferative diabetic retinopathy occur each year.

In one study evaluating diabetic retinopathy using a nonmydriatic fundus camera, the authors find that prevalence of any diabetic retinopathy in people with diagnosed diabetes is 46% higher in non-Hispanic blacks and 84% higher in Mexican Americans, compared with non-Hispanic whites. Blacks and Mexican Americans have higher rates of moderate and severe retinopathy and high levels of the risk factors of retinopathy. However, blacks have lower diabetic retinopathy prevalence among those with undiagnosed diabetes. Retinopathy in those with diagnosed diabetes is associated with diabetes severity, for example, duration of diabetes, severity, HbA1c, treatment with insulin and oral agents, and systolic blood pressure. Despite adjustment of these factors, the risk of retinopathy in Mexican Americans is twice that of non-Hispanic whites. Non-Hispanic blacks are not at a higher risk for retinopathy. The excess risk in Mexican Americans is unexplained by these researchers.[28]

NONPROLIFERATIVE DIABETIC RETINOPATHY: BACKGROUND DIABETIC RETINOPATHY

Nonproliferative Diabetic Retinopathy (NPDR) is a common yet underdiagnosed form of diabetic retinopathy. It is also known in the nonophthalmic, medical literature as "background diabetic retinopathy." The earliest form of NPDR is the appearance of microaneurysms or dot blot hemorrhages. These are outpouchings of the vessel walls and can be

TABLE 1.5 Follow-up Schedule

Recommended follow-up schedule	Follow-up in months
NDR or microaneurysms only	12
Mild/mod NPDR without DME	6–12
Mild/mod NPDR, + macular edema but not clinically significant	4–6
Mild/mod NPDR, + CSME	3–4
Severe/very severe NPDR	3–4

TABLE 1.6 Signs and Symptoms of Diabetic Retinopathy

Symptoms	Signs
Floaters, black lines	Vitreous hemorrhage
Cobwebs	
Loss of vision	Vitreous hemorrhage or retinal detachment
Loss of near vision	Macular edema
Transient loss of vision	TIA, emboli, vitreous hemorrhage, hypoglycemia, or hyperglycemia

50 μm in diameter or 100 μm in diameter. These are best seen upon slit lamp biomicroscopy with a 90 D or 60 D lens. Or, they can be photographed with a fundus camera. These abnormalities usually do not involve the macula and thus, there are no visual symptoms (Table 1-6).

CLINICAL CORRELATIONS

Patient complaints: Routine exam or mild visual loss on near vision or Amsler grid changes. Some patients might notice a smudge in central vision at near. Patients may present with the chief complaint of "I see a smudge when I read my book or when I use the computer."

Or suddenly, "I feel that I see better and do not need my glasses," denoting new diabetic cataracts from a recent diagnosis of diabetes.

Caveats: Many patients do not seek ophthalmic care or optometric care unless they experience a loss of vision. There may be a lack of health literacy and health education about diabetes. These patients do not understand the need for a dilated funduscopic examination yearly if they have diabetes.

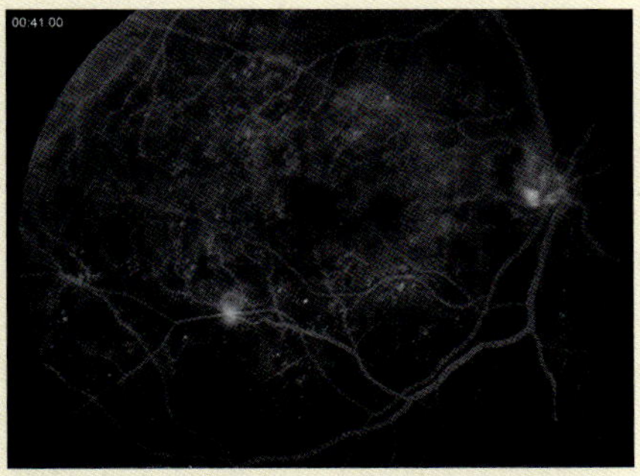

FIGURE 1-1. Background diabetic retinopathy.

Case Study (Fig. 1-1)

9–23–08: EG, is a 43-year-old Filipino male who presented with a new diagnosis with Type 2 diabetes and was referred to our office for a baseline evaluation.

Laboratory evaluation: HbA1c = 6.5%, Fasting blood sugar = 128 mg/dL, Cholesterol = 255 mg/dL (nL = 240), Triglycerides = 251 mg/dL (nL = 150).

V 20/15
20/15
Slit lamp examination
Cornea: Clear OU
Anterior chamber: D-deep and quiet OU
Iris: Normal, no rubeosis OU
Lens: Clear OU
Applanation tonometry = 18/18 mm Hg (2:30 PM)
Gonioscopy: No rubeosis OU for 360 degrees, angles open for 360 degrees OU.

Dilated funduscopic examination:

Right eye: Small hard exudates found in the macular region, 1:00 from the foveal avascular zone.

Left eye: No microaneurysms seen in the macular region. However, with Goldmann three-mirror examination, there are a few microaneurysms seen in the far equatorial region.

TABLE 1.7 "Moderate-to-Severe" Nonproliferative Retinopathy

Cotton-wool spots
Intraretinal hemorrhages: mild to moderate in four quadrants
Venous beading
IRMA

MODERATE NONPROLIFERATIVE DIABETIC RETINOPATHY

The ophthalmologist should look for venous beading and intraretinal microvascular abnormalities (IRMA) in the equator to the periphery. Cotton-wool spots are also present in these cases. These can be missed by the nonophthalmologist because of the difficulty in examining the fundus in some patients or the lack of seven standard photographic fields (Table 1-7).

Cotton-wool spots or areas of retinal ischemia can occur outside of the arcades, outside of the macula. Once cotton-wool spots are seen, the patient is in the moderate to severe category of NPDR. With increasing number of the cotton-wool spots and increasing involvement of the number of photographic fields, the patient may fall into the severe category of NPDR. If no photographic fields are available, the patient can be categorized by examining the optic nerve area, macula, temporal to the macula, superotemporal area, inferotemporal area, superonasal area, and inferonasal area to assess the involvement of the number of cotton-wool spots, venous beading, and venous abnormalities.

CLINICAL CORRELATIONS

Patient complaints: Some decrease in vision is noted on physical examination, usually 20/25 visual acuity or worse vision. Patients have more vague and more frequent complaints of vision loss.

Caveats: Is there loss to medical follow-up because of inadequate health literacy or denial? The patient may have cross-cultural needs in that his or her diabetic diet has to be tailored to his or her preferred diet patterns.

Case Study (Fig. 1-2)

4–10–09: DC, a 61-year-old unemployed male engineer, presents to our office for decreased vision for six months. He was last seen by a physician 10 years earlier and was lost to follow-up. He was referred by a local optometrist who noted decreased vision. At the time, he brought no laboratory records with him.

Laboratory evaluation: HbA1c = 12%, Fasting blood sugar = 256 mg/dL, Cholesterol 400 mg/dL (nL = 200), Triglycerides 399 mg/dL (nL = 150).

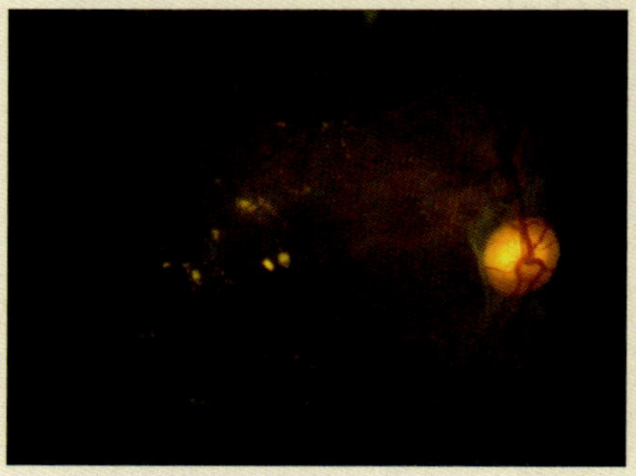

FIGURE 1-2. Macular edema and nonproliferative diabetic retinopathy.

V 20/30
20/60
Slit lamp examination
Cornea: Clear OU
Anterior chamber: Deep and quiet OU
Iris: No rubeosis OU

Lens: Trace nuclear sclerosis OU
Applanation tonometry = 20/20 mm Hg (9:00 AM)
Gonioscopy: No rubeosis in the angle for 360 degrees.

Dilated funduscopic examination:
Right eye: Clinically significant macular edema seen on slit lamp biomicroscopy, large dot blot hemorrhages, and cotton-wool spots seen.
Left eye: Clinically significant macular edema seen on slit lamp biomicroscopy, cotton-wool spots, and large dot blot hemorrhages.
Fluorescein angiography: Macular edema OU

Comment
In summary, the patient, DC, has poorly controlled diabetes and he needs endocrinological follow-up and ophthalmic follow-up. His diagnosis is severe NPDR.

MACULAR EDEMA

Macular edema is one of the insidious manifestations of diabetic retinopathy which can be as subtle as one or two hard exudates in the macula to full-fledged hard exudate ring encompassing part of the macula and the fovea centralis region. Or it can present as a diffuse elevation of the inner retina filled with small cysts seen on slit lamp biomicroscopy. These diagnoses are easily made with optical coherence tomography (OCT), where the architecture of the retina and macula is well delineated.

Macular edema, which can exist with NPDR or proliferative diabetic retinopathy, involves the macula with swelling within the 10 layers of the retina. Macular edema has been defined by the landmark study, the Early Treatment Diabetic Retinopathy Study.[29] This study has defined for the retina-vitreous community the standard of care for the treatment of macular edema and diabetic retinopathy. For the past 20 years, early treatment of diabetic retinopathy denotes early laser when the clinician discovered macular edema seen on slit lamp biomicroscopy; now it has evolved to include macular edema as diagnosed by fluorescein angiography and or by ocular coherence tomography. Fast Fourier transform analysis of OCT, or spectral domain OCT, has changed the way that many retinal specialists have viewed macular edema. Thus, these new diagnostic tools have made it easier for clinicians to diagnose macular edema and initiate early treatment and maintain good vision for the patients.

CLINICAL CORRELATIONS

Patient complaints: Decrease in vision is noted on physical examination. Usually, 20/25 to 20/40 visual acuity or worse vision. The patient is symptomatic at near: reading books, doing close work, and decreased vision at the computer are the most common complaints. The patient may see a crooked line where the newspaper print may be distorted.

Caveats: Poor internal medicine or endocrinologic follow-up. Alcohol intake can add to the patient's daily calorie intake. The patient is a physician and he may be in denial of his disease.

Case Study (Fig. 1-3)

6–5–2005: Dr. AP is a 66-year-old Filipino male, practicing anesthesiologist, who presents with poor vision and a history of poor glycemic control. He denies hypertension. He has had insulin-dependent diabetes for the past 8 years. According to the patient, his HbA1c = 9%.

V 20/40
20/100
Slit lamp examination
Cornea: Clear OU
Anterior chamber: Deep and quiet
Iris: No rubeosis OU
Lens: 2 + nuclear sclerosis OU
Applanation tonometry = 18/18 mm Hg (3 PM)
Gonioscopy: No rubeosis 360 OU
Pigmented trabecular meshwork OU but open to ciliary body OU

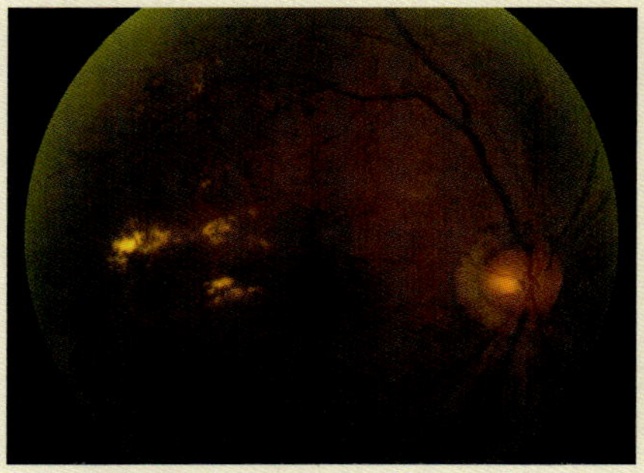

FIGURE 1-3. Macular edema and severe nonproliferative diabetic retinopathy.

Dilated fundus examination:

Right eye: Clinically significant macular edema, dot blot hemorrhages
Left eye: Clinically significant macular edema, dot blot hemorrhages

Comment:

Of note, this patient is noncompliant, is a physician and colleague. His management hinges on better glycemic control, laser for his clinically significant macular edema, and long-term ophthalmologic follow-up. The patient and his family need to be part of this sensitive discussion that glycemic control is important. The nurse in the office should provide American Diabetes Association pamphlets to the family. These noncompliant patients who need precise vision to maintain their livelihood are difficult to manage over the long term. It is best to involve an endocrinologist in addition to the internist who will reinforce the need for glycemic control.

PROLIFERATIVE DIABETIC RETINOPATHY

Approximately 700,000 Americans have proliferative diabetic retinopathy and 500,000 have macular edema. Approximately 65,000 new cases of proliferative diabetic retinopathy occur each year.

Proliferative diabetic retinopathy is the most severe form of diabetic eye disease affecting the retina. There is growth of new vessels from areas of the retina that are hypoxic from damage from hyperglycemia and cell death. The growth of new vessels lends itself to the name of "proliferation" of vascular growth. These new abnormal vessels bleed easily. With the bleeding, there is associated loss of vision, which may be abrupt or gradual. Treatment is laser, called panretinal photocoagulation or in severe cases, vitrectomy. In addition, in this severe form of diabetic retinopathy, traction retinal detachment can occur and in these instances, vitrectomy is done very quickly after diagnosis.

Testing involves ultrasound if there is no view of the retina landmarks, such as optic nerve or the retinal vessels. In addition, ERG and VER testing can be performed to evaluate test function and for prognosis for vision postoperatively. For proliferative diabetic retinopathy where there are new fronds of vessels but the vision is still preserved since there is no frank vitreous hemorrhage, laser photocoagulation is performed.

CLINICAL CORRELATIONS

Patient complaints: Gradual loss of vision in one eye, sudden loss of vision.

Caveats: Previous history of uncontrolled diabetes, elevated lipid profiles, history of recent infections of feet, feet ulcers, pneumonia, and hospitalizations that can cause sudden loss of glycemic control.

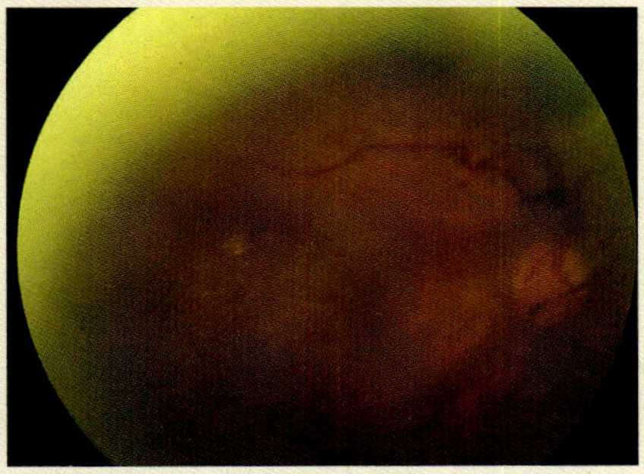

FIGURE 1-4. Proliferative diabetic retinopathy.

Case Study (Fig. 1-4)

10–29–2007: A 52-year-old Caucasian male, banker, who noted loss of vision. He has had an 8-year history of using insulin but his total duration of diabetes is 15 years. He has a sedentary lifestyle.

V Hand motion
20/80 NIPH
Slit lamp examination
Cornea: Clear OU
Anterior chamber: Deep and quiet OU
Iris: Normal OU, no rubeosis OU
Lens: 1 + nuclear sclerosis OU
Applanation tonometry = 14/14 mm Hg (10:00 AM)
Gonioscopy: Open 360 degrees OU, no rubeosis OU

Dilated funduscopic examination:

Right eye: Vitreous hemorrhage is seen, the optic nerve can be identified. Superiorly, there is a fibrovascular stalk OD. The blood is thickest at this area, superior optic disc. This is proliferative diabetic retinopathy.
Left eye: Vitreous hemorrhage is seen and the superior and inferior arcades can be identified. There is no retinal detachment.

Comment:

Proliferative diabetic retinopathy in a 52-year-old male who has a 15-year duration of diabetes and used insulin for the past 8 years. He needs to see an endocrinologist for better glycemic control. For every 1% decline of HbA1c, there is a 35% decline in diabetic retinopathy according to the United Kingdom Prospective Diabetes Study study. Pan retinal laser photocoagulation is recommended for both eyes. However, treatment may not be completed due to poor visualization. He may ultimately need vitrectomy.

DIABETES IN CHILDREN

Children are increasingly affected with diabetes. Twenty percent of the people <20 years of age are affected with diabetes. Thus, 1 in 500 children has diabetes or 200,000 children are affected. With the advent of fast foods and decreased school time for physical education, teen obesity has increased with an associated increase in the incidence of Type 2 diabetes in children and teens. This epidemic, which occurred in the last decade, has made diabetes a more common diagnosis in the practices of pediatrics and family medicine.

DURATION OF DIABETES AND TYPE 1 DIABETES

The duration of diabetes is a factor in the development of diabetic retinopathy. After 7 years of insulin-dependent diabetes mellitus (Type 1 or IDDM), approximately 50% of these patients have diabetic retinopathy. After 20-year duration of Type 1 diabetes, 90% of these patients have diabetic retinopathy. In the first few years of Type 1 diabetes, diabetic retinopathy rarely occurs (Table 1-8).

TABLE 1.8 Duration of Diabetes Mellitus

Duration (y)	Type I	Type II	Presence (%)
>7	x		50
≥20	x		90
≥15		x	25

CLINICAL CORRELATIONS

Patient complaints: When newly diagnosed, the patients are asymptomatic for retinal disease usually. Documentation of their retinal exam is useful with fundus photography.

They may complain of decreased vision with initiation of diabetic therapy.

Caveats: New insulin pump use, initiation of oral contraceptive use, and alcohol ingestion among teenagers.

Case Study (Fig. 1-5)

10–3–2007: CM is a 16-year-old white female, with a new insulin pump and transient visual changes after the fitting of the new insulin pump. She has had Type 1 diabetes in the past year.
Laboratory evaluation: HbA1c = 8.3 mg/dL.
Family history is significant for paternal grandmother and maternal grandfather with Type 2 diabetes

V 20/20
20/20
Pupils react to light and accommodation
Slit lamp examination
Cornea: Clear OU
Anterior chamber: Deep and quiet OU
Iris: Normal OU, no rubeosis
Lens: Clear OU, no abnormalities at the Y sutures OU
Applanation tonometry = 12/12 mm Hg (12:30 PM)
Gonioscopy: No rubeosis OU 360 degrees

Dilated funduscopic examination:
Right eye: No diabetic retinopathy seen
Left eye: No diabetic retinopathy seen

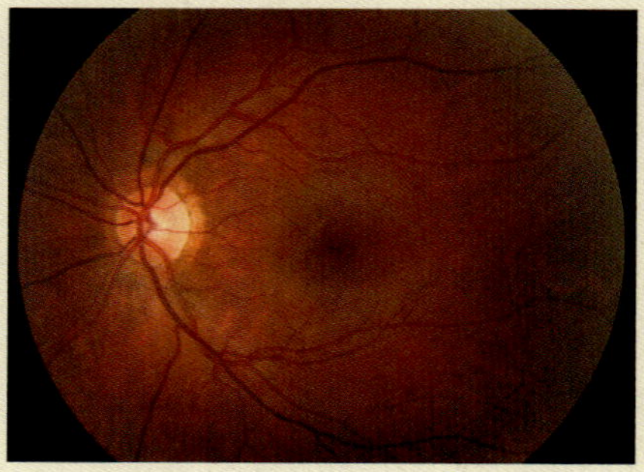

FIGURE 1-5. Photo OS, no diabetic retinopathy.

DIABETES AND THE RETINA

The changes in the retina that occur in diabetic retinopathy arise from an indolent course: from nonproliferative to proliferative diabetic retinopathy. In the early stages, there is capillary occlusion and in the later stages by fibrovascular proliferation and scar formation. In tissue culture, high concentrations of glucose can cause in vitro endothelial cell death. Clinically, anoxia in the diabetic retina occurs with the selective death of mural pericytes. The capillaries appear with a proliferation of endothelial cells and areas which lacked cells and became acellular, thus the term "ghost vessels." Pericyte loss and thickening of the residual basement membrane are early changes in the pathology of diabetic retinopathy. The occlusion of the capillary bed and consequent cell death can be seen with the fundus and fluorescein angiograph in the form of capillary nonperfusion.

These areas of nonperfusion are the areas of deficient blood flow. Ultimately, the loss of perfusion causes cell death at the retinal level, which in turn causes loss of vision.

The capillaries are found between the nerve fiber layer and the outer plexiform layer.

MICROANEURYSMS

One of the first signs of mild NPDR is microaneurysms. The appearance of the microaneurysm indicates capillary closure. They are usually found in the areas of occluded capillaries. Microaneurysms can occur at retinal layers between the superficial and deeper retinal layers.

The Airlie House classification defined a microaneurysm to be less than 125 μm. Larger areas would be classified as hemorrhages. Microaneurysms represent weakening of the capillary wall and loss of pericytes, causing outpouchings from the capillary wall.

More microaneurysms are seen by fluorescein angiography than can be seen clinically. Thus, the smallest microaneurysm can be seen with fluorescein dye. Generally, microaneurysms fill during the early venous phase and vary in size and shape as the study progresses.

THE FOVEAL AVASCULAR ZONE

This is the area that has no vascular structure but is purely populated by cone cells. The "avascular" nature of this area can be seen on a fluorescein angiography as an area without any fluorescence of the dye.

PROLIFERATIVE DIABETIC RETINOPATHY

When there is hypoxia or lack of oxygen delivered to the tissues of the retina, the consequent response of the retina is to create abnormal blood vessels, called neovascularization. It is now thought that there is a proliferation of vascular endothelial growth factors that cause the inflammation, which in turn causes abnormal bleeding in the retina. It is not clear whether it is indeed the release of vascular endothelial growth factors, ischemia, or the abnormalities in the alternative complement pathway that causes the formation of neovascular and abnormal blood vessels, but it is apparent that clinically these vessels exist and are a major cause of severe visual loss in severe proliferative diabetic retinopathy.

REFERENCES

1. http://www.diabetes.org/diabetes-statistics/cost-of-diabetes-in-us.jsp. Accessed 6 November 2008.
2. Wexler DJ, Nathan DM, Grant RW, et al. Prevalence of elevated hemoglobin A1c among patients admitted to the hospital without a diagnosis of diabetes. *J Clin Endocrinol Metab.* 2008;93:4238–4244.
3. www.diabetes.org/diabetesnewsarticle.jsp?storyID = 15351710&filename = 20070623/ADA200706231182625856641EDIT.xml. Accessed 16 November 2008.
4. Sinha R, Fisch G, Teague B, et al. There is a prevalence of impaired glucose tolerance among children and adolescents with marked obesity. *N Eng J Med.* 2002;346:802–810.
5. American Diabetes Association. Economic costs of diabetes in the US in 2007. *Diabetes Care.* 2008;31:596–615.
6. Narayan KMV, Boyle JP, Thompson TJ, et al. *JAMA.* 2003;290:1884–1890.
7. Harris MI. Medical care for patients with diabetes: Epidemiologic aspects. *Ann Int Med.* 1996;124:117–122.
8. Beckman JA, Creager MA, Libby P. Diabetes and atherosclerosis: Epidemiology, pathophysiology and management. *JAMA.* 2002;287:2570–2581.
9. http://www.diabetes.org/diabetes-statistics/prevalence.jsp. Accessed 16 November 2008.
10. Acton KJ, Burrows NR, Moore K, et al. Trends in diabetes prevalence among american indian and alaska native children, adolescents and young adults. *Am J Pub Health.* 2002;92(9):1485–1490.
11. http://www.cdc.gov/omhd/AMH/factsheets/diabetes.htm. Accessed 15 November 2008.
12. http://www.diabetes.org/diabetes-statistics/afrian-americans.jsp. Accessed 15 November 2008.
13. NHIS data 1993, http://www.blackhealthcare.com/BHC/Diabetes/Description.asp. Accessed November 16, 2008.
14. Roberts WL, Safar-Pour S, De BK, Rohlfing CL, Weykamp CW, Little RR. Effects of hemoglobin C and S traits on glycohemoglobin measurements by eleven methods. *Clin Chem.* 2005;51:776–778.
15. Hanis CL, Hewett-Emmett D, Bertin TK, et al. Origins of US Hispanics. implications for diabetes. *Diabetes Care.* 1991;14:618–627.
16. http://www.asiandiabetes.org/category/asian-diabetes-statistics/. Accessed 28 November 2008.
17. LaFrachi S. Diabetes during Pregnancy-United States, 1993–1995. *MMWR.* 1998; 47:408–414.

18. http://www.niddk.nih.gov/health/diabetes/pubs/dmstats/dmstats.htm#10. Accessed 16 November 2008.
19. Fuhimoto WY. *Diabetes in America: Diabetes in Asian and Pacific Islander Americans.* Bethesda, MD: National Diabetes Data Group; 1995.
20. http://www.cdc/omhd/AMH/factsheets/diabetes.htm.
21. Ogden CL, Carroll MD, Flegan KM. High body mass index for age among US children and adolescents, 2003–2006. *JAMA.* 2008;299(20):2401–2405.
22. www.cdc.gov/nccdphp/dnpa/bmi/index.htm. Accessed 12 December 2008.
23. Zimmet P, Alberti KGMM, Shaw J. Global and societal implications of the diabetes epidemic. *Nature.* 2001;414: 782–787.
24. Early Treatment Diabetic Retinopathy Study Research Group. Early photocoagulation for diabetic retinopathy. ETDRS report number 9. *Ophthalmology.* 1991;98:767–785.
25. Moss S, Klein R, Klein B. Factors associated with having eye examinations in persons with diabetes. *Arch Fam Med.* 1995;4:529–534.
26. Sprafka J, Fritsc T, Baker R, et al. Prevalence of undiagnosed eye disease in high-risk diabetic individuals. *Arch Int Med.* 1990;150:857–861.
27. Will JC, German RR, Schuman E, et al. Patient adherence to guidelines for diabetes eye care. *Am J Pub Health.* 1994;84:169–1671.
28. Harris MI, Klein R, Cowie CC, et al. Is the risk of diabetic retinopathy greater in non-Hispanic blacks and Mexican Americans than in non-Hispanic whites with Type 2 Diabetes? A US population study. *Diabetes Care.* 1998;21: 1230–1235.
29. Early Treatment Diabetic Retinopathy Study Research Group. Photocoagulation for diabetic macular edema. ETDRS report number 1. *Arch Ophthalmol.* 1985;103:1796–1806.

SUGGESTED READINGS

1. American Association of Clinical Endocrinology. Diabetes mellitus guidelines. *Endocr Pract.* 2007;13(suppl).
2. Early Treatment Diabetic Retinopathy Study Research Group. ETDRS report no. 12. Fundus photographic risk factors for progression of diabetic retinopathy. *Ophthalmology.* 1991;98:823–833.
3. Klein R, Klein BEK, Moss SE, et al. The Wisconsin epidemiologic study of diabetic retinopathy. VI. Retinal photocoagulation. *Ophthalmology.* 1987;94:747–753.
4. Klein R, Klein BEK, Moss SE, et al. The Wisconsin epidemiologic study of diabetic retinopathy. VIII. The incidence of retinal photocoagulation. Diabetic complications. *J Diabet Complications.* 1988;2:79–87.
5. National Society to Prevent Blindness. Operational Research Department. *Vision Problems in the U.S.: A Statistical Analysis.* New York, NY: National Society to Prevent Blindness; 1980:1–46.
6. Patz A, Smith RE. The ETDRS and Diabetes 2000 [Editorial]. *Ophthalmology.* 191;98:739–740.

CHAPTER 2

Pathophysiology of Diabetes

SYSTEMIC DISEASE AND DIABETES

Type 1 diabetes, also known as juvenile onset diabetes or insulin-dependent diabetes mellitus (IDDM), is a chronic condition of the pancreas in which there is little or no insulin, a hormone needed to convert sugar into energy. Although Type 1 diabetes can occur at any age, it appears during childhood or adolescence.

Currently, the American Diabetes Association recommends using the nomenclature that Type 1A diabetes is used for immune-mediated diabetes with its destruction of the islet beta cells of the pancreas,[1,2] whereas non–immune-mediated diabetes with severe insulin deficiency is termed Type 1B diabetes.[3]

Recent epidemiological studies show that the incidence of diabetes in children is now comparable in adults.[4] The international variation in incidence is now recognized. A child in Finland is almost 40 times more likely to develop Type 1 diabetes than a child in Japan, and the same child in Finland is 100 times more likely to get the disease than a child in the Zunyi region of China.[5] The EuroDiab collaborative study, registry involving 44 countries in Europe, indicates an annual rate of increase in the incidence of Type 1 diabetes of 3.4%, with a larger increase in some central and eastern European countries.[6] The largest rate of increase is seen in children aged 0 to 4. Type 1 diabetes is associated with other autoimmune conditions, the most common association is with thyroid disease.[7] The Belgian Diabetes Registry indicates that the prevalence of thyroid peroxidase autoantibodies is 22% in patients with Type 1 diabetes. Approximately 1 in 10 patients with Type 1 diabetes express transglutaminase IgA autoantibodies and more than half of these patients have celiac disease on intestinal biopsy. Approximately 1 in 50 people with Type 1 diabetes have 21-hydroxylase autoantibodies and approximately 25% of these patients progress to Addison disease.[8]

GENETICS

Genetic susceptibility and environmental factors are thought to provide the fundamental element for disease and potential targets for both prediction and prevention of disease.[9] More than 90% of patients who develop Type 1 diabetes have DR3, DQ2 or DR4, or DQ8 haplotypes, whereas fewer than 40% of normal controls have these haplotypes.[9] The DAISY (Diabetes Autoimmunity Study in the Young) in Denver, Colorado, found that bovine milk ingestion, enteroviral infection, or vaccination does not contribute to risk of diabetes. It is unclear that early ingestion of cereal or gluten increases Type 1 risk and needs further studies. This may involve aberrant immune response to cereal antigens in an immature gut system in susceptible individuals.

Alpha interferon has been implicated as an important cytokine linking viruses to the initiation of Type 1 diabetes. There are case reports of patients developing anti-islet autoantibodies, who then later manifest Type 1 diabetes, autoimmune endocrine disorders. Thus, neutralizing this cytokine, alpha interferon may potentially prevent the disease.

Compounds such as poly IC (a viral RNA mimicker) can induce alpha interferon which then can generate insulitis (selective beta cell destruction) and diabetes in animal models. Thus, there is a link between induction of diabetes and alpha interferon.[10]

PATHOGENESIS OF TYPE 1 DIABETES

Role of autoantibodies in the actual pathogenesis of Type 1 diabetes has not been established in humans. In general, Type 1 diabetes is considered a T-cell mediated disease. Examination of islet tissue obtained from pancreatic biopsy from patients with recent onset of Type 1 diabetes confirms insulitis, with the presence of an infiltrate composed of CD4 and CD8 T lymphocytes, B lymphocytes, and macrophages, suggesting that these cells have a role in the destruction of the beta cells.[11] Therapies directed against T cells have been shown to halt the disease process and prevent recurrent beta cell destruction after islet cell transplantation. Less is known about the nature and function of these T cells. The cause of the loss of tolerance to islet autoantigens is unknown. We understand neither why the immune system fails to suppress autoreactivity nor which autoantigens are critically involved in the initiation or progression of the disease. Some T cells are pathogenic, but others can regulate the disease process and thus form new targets for immunointervention.[12]

Examination of islet tissue obtained from pancreatic biopsy from patients with recent onset of Type 1 diabetes shows insulitis, with the presence of infiltrate composed of CD4 and CD8 T lymphocytes, B lymphocytes, and macrophages, suggesting that these cells have a role in the destruction of beta cells.[11]

Studies in mice show that anti-CD3 treatment prevented diabetes, thus subsequently spawning a new trial using humanized anti-CD3 antibody in patients with new onset Type 1 diabetes.[13]

To date, no treatment has been shown to prevent Type 1 diabetes in humans. More than 100 different treatments prevent Type 1 diabetes in the Nonobese diabetic (NOD) mouse model.[14] In the United States, the Diabetes Prevention Trial began in 1994 with the goal of determining whether antigen-based treatment with insulin (oral and parenteral insulin in relatives of high to moderate risk) would prevent or delay diabetes. The European Nicotinamide Diabetes Intervention Trial found no difference in the protection from diabetes when participants were assigned to either oral nicotinamide or placebo treatment.[1]

Thus, insulin is the main treatment of Type 1 Diabetes. The Diabetes Control and Complications Trial (DCCT) demonstrates the importance of strict metabolic control in delaying and preventing complications.[15]

The introduction of rapidly absorbed insulin analogs has reduced variability of insulin absorption and allows insulin administration in young children after meals. The insulin, glargine, functions as a very long acting insulin (peakless basal insulin).[16] Combinations of engineered very long acting insulin and rapid acting insulin can provide control and convenience similar to that obtained with insulin pumps.

The use of metformin alongside insulin has increased in patients with Type 1 diabetes. Recent studies have suggested that metformin might benefit Type 1 diabetes patients who are overweight, are receiving large doses of insulin, or have an HbA1c >8%.[17] The coexistence of insulin resistance in patients with Type 1 diabetes is a new area of interest. Islet cell transplantation is a consideration for the limited but important subset of patients with recurrent severe hypoglycemia not responsive to medical management.[18] However, inability to control autoimmunity and a lack of donor organs limit the application of islet transplantation.[19]

PATHOGENESIS OF TYPE 2 DIABETES MELLITUS

Type 2 diabetes is a result of insulin resistance, impaired beta cell insulin secretion. Excessive visceral adipose tissue in obesity contributes to these metabolic abnormalities. Coronary artery disease (CAD), a life threatening consequence of atherosclerosis, is the most common vascular consequence of insulin resistance.[19] The prevalence of CAD in Americans with Type 2 diabetes is two to four times greater than that in a nondiabetic patient population. The manifestations of CAD such as angina pectoris, myocardial infarction, and sudden death are twice as common in patients with Type 2 diabetes as in nondiabetic patients. The incidence of these manifestations is six times more common in diabetics versus nondiabetics.[20]

Type 2 Diabetes, Insulin Resistance and Obesity

Normal glucose metabolism requires the coordination of glucose production and glucose uptake. Hepatic glycogenolysis and gluconeogenesis become balanced with glucose uptake into skeletal muscle and adipose tissue in the fasting and postprandial states under the direction of neural influences and circulating hormones, insulin, glucagons, and incretins. There is a close association between obesity and insulin resistance. Intra-abdominal fat or adipose tissue is an active secretory organ. They secrete adipokines such as leptin and adiponectin. Leptin causes decrease insulin-mediated glucose uptake. Adiponectin increases insulin release and plays a role in anti-inflammatory effects in the vasculature. In obesity, leptin is increased and adiponectin is decreased.[21]

Adipose tissue releases free fatty acids (FFAs), cytokines, such as tumor necrosis factor–alpha (TNF-alpha), signaling proteins (angiotensin II), hormones, complement factors, and regulators of atherothrombosis (e.g., plasminogen activator inhibitor-1). Changes in the circulating levels of these substances play a role in the insulin resistant state of Type 2 diabetic patients who are overweight. In addition, these metabolites exert adverse effects in vascular endothelial and smooth muscle cells. TNF-alpha is elevated in adipose tissue in experimental models of obesity, suggesting that TNF-alpha plays a role in the systemic insulin resistance of Type 2 diabetes.[22] Both obesity and endothelial dysfunction are linked to Type 2 diabetes in the early inflammatory stages of atherogenesis. It is the endothelial cell dysfunction that mediates the two major long-term complications, cardiovascular disease and diabetic retinopathy.[22]

The increase in FFA in obesity leads to higher levels of fatty acid molecules within skeletal muscle and liver cells, which in turn cause insulin resistance. This is mediated by the activation of the signaling kinase, protein kinase C. Some of protein kinase C isoforms oppose the insulin action cascade.[23]

In response to insulin resistance associated with visceral obesity, pancreatic beta cell insulin secretion is augmented to maintain normal glucose level. Consequently, most obese patients are insulin resistant and hyperinsulinemic at the same time. These overweight Type 2 diabetics have impaired fasting glucose and impaired glucose tolerance.

LIFESTYLE MODIFICATIONS OF TYPE 1 DIABETES

Type 1 diabetic patients can be educated on estimating the carbohydrate content in their diets so that they can accurately match insulin administration during meals to carbohydrate intake by using insulin to carbohydrate ratios. Methods available for estimating carbohydrate intake are experience-based estimation, the exchange system, and carbohydrate counting. For those patients who use fixed daily doses of insulin, carbohydrate intake should be consistent in terms of the time of day and amount of food consumed each day.[24,25]

For planned exercise, patients should reduce their premeal bolus based on their level of anticipated activity to prevent hypoglycemia. Moderately intense exercise has been shown to increase glucose use by 2 to 3 mg/kg/min above usual requirements. Thus, a 70-kg person would need an additional 10 to 15 g of carbohydrate during moderate physical activity. More intense exercise would require the intake of more carbohydrates. As a result, unplanned physical activity usually requires supplemental carbohydrate intake to prevent hypoglycemia.[24]

LIFESTYLE MODIFICATION FOR TYPE 2 DIABETES

For patients with Type 2 diabetes, lifestyle modifications would be aimed at improving glycemia and dyslipidemia and reducing blood pressure and overall cardiovascular risk. The goal would be reduction of the intake of saturated and trans-fatty acids, cholesterol, and sodium and increase in physical activity.

A diet rich in fruits, vegetables, whole grains, nuts, and fiber would improve dyslipidemia and lower blood pressure and decrease cardiovascular risk. Patients should be encouraged to limit carbohydrate consumption by calculating the carbohydrate content of each meal based on grams of carbohydrate consumed or switching servings of food based on carbohydrate equivalents from exchange lists.[26]

For Type 2 diabetic patients using fixed doses of insulin, their carbohydrate intake should be consistent with the time of day and amount consumed on a daily basis.

Gestational Diabetes

Medical nutrition therapy, at the time of diagnosis, is aimed at food choices that allow for adequate energy intake to provide appropriate weight gain, normoglycemia, and absence of ketones. Weight loss during pregnancy is not recommended. However, obese or overweight women may benefit from modest exercise and carbohydrate restriction.

There are stringent glycemic targets during pregnancy; thus, frequent glucose monitoring and the maintenance of a dietary log will provide valuable information for possible meal plan adjustments.

Benefits of Exercise

The ADA recommends at least 150 min/week of moderate aerobic exercise (50% to 70% of maximal heart rate) and resistance exercise that targets all major muscle groups three times per week.[27] One exercise session can cause an acute decrease of plasma glucose levels in Type 2 diabetes patients. Postexercise enhancement of glucose metabolism, possibility for increased insulin sensitivity in muscle tissue may last for hours, even days. It is thought that more effective glycemic control may result from the additive effect of the exercise sessions and not from increased fitness.[28]

RISK FACTORS FOR DEVELOPMENT OF DIABETIC RETINOPATHY

Duration of Diabetes Mellitus

The Wisconsin Epidemiology Study of Diabetic Retinopathy (WESDR) found that 3.6% of patients with Type 1 diabetes whose disease occurred prior to age 30 are legally blind compared with 1.6% of patients with Type 2 diabetes whose disease occurred after age 30.[29]

Glycemic Control

Two studies, DCCT[15] for Type 1 diabetes and the United Kingdom Prospective Diabetes Study (UKPDS)[30] for Type 2 diabetes, demonstrate the efficacy of good glycemic control in preventing diabetic retinopathy. In the DCCT, the Type 1 diabetic patients, after a mean follow-up of 6.5 years, the groups of patients treated with intensive insulin therapy (multiple insulin injections during each day) have a mean glycosylated hemoglobin of 7.2% and have a reduction of progression of diabetic retinopathy or delayed development of diabetic retinopathy by 27% versus patients treated in a conventional manner (nonintensive insulin therapy). In the Type 2 diabetic patients in the UKPDS, intensive glycemic control reduces microvascular complications including diabetic retinopathy by 25% as compared to conventional therapy. Every percentage point of decrease of the HbA1c is associated with 35% risk reduction. Thus, the effort to achieve good glycemic control at the time of diagnosis is important.

Elevated Blood Pressure

In the WESDR, higher diastolic blood pressure is associated with increased progression of diabetic retinopathy and macular edema.[29] In the UKPDS, Type 2 diabetics with blood pressure of <150/85 have a 34% reduction in progression of diabetic retinopathy and a 47% decreased risk of deterioration in visual acuity compared with patients with blood pressure >185/105.[30]

Hypertension impairs autoregulation of retinal blood flow in diabetics compared with nondiabetics. It enhances endothelial damage and expression of vascular endothelial growth factor (VEGF) and its receptors in poorly controlled diabetes.

Hyperlipidemia

The WESDR shows that retinal hard exudates development is 50% more likely in patients with elevated total cholesterol or triglycerides and a significant risk factor for moderate visual loss.[31] The Early Treatment Diabetic Retinopathy Study shows an association between elevated baseline LDL and retinal hard exudates.[32]

Diabetic Nephropathy and Diabetic Retinopathy

Microalbuminuria is associated with diabetic retinopathy. In patients with known renal disease, their risk of diabetic retinopathy is increased and their diabetic retinopathy is accelerated as compared to those diabetic patients without renal disease.[33]

TREATMENT OF TYPE 2 DIABETES

The therapeutic goal of diabetes management is to achieve a HbA1c close to the normal range (4% to 6%), at least <6.5%. This requires the fasting blood glucose level of <110 mg/ dL and 2 hour postprandial glucose of <140 mg/dL. These biochemical targets confer benefits in the reduction of diabetic complications, for example, nephropathy, neuropathy, retinopathy, and cardiovascular morbidity and mortality. Unfortunately, Type 2 diabetes is a chronic and progressive disease which requires lifelong pharmacotherapy in addition to diet and exercise.

Oral Antiglycemics

Biguanides, Sulfonylureas, Thiazolidinediones (TZDs)[34]

Biguanides

Biguanides (Metformin, Glucophage, Glucophage XR, Glumetza) work by increasing insulin sensitivity in the liver by inhibiting hepatic gluconeogenesis, thereby reducing hepatic glucose production.[34]

Sulfonylureas

Sulfonylureas are the most widely prescribed drugs for Type 2 diabetes.[34] They are chlorpropamide (Diabinase), glipizide (Glucotrol, Glucotrol XL), glyburide (DiaBeta,

Micronase). The mechanism of action of sulfonylureas involves the augmentation of insulin release from pancreatic beta cells and the potentiation of action on its target cells.

Nonsulfonylurea Secretagogues

Repaglinide (Pradin), a benzoic acid derivative, and nateglinide (Starlix) are distinguished from the sulfonylureas because the former has short half-lives and does not contain the sulfonic acid moiety.[36] Thus, these are useful in patients with sulfa allergies.

Thiazolidinediones

TZDs are selective agonists for the nuclear receptor peroxisome proliferator-activated receptor–gamma (PPAR).[34] The role of PPARs in humans involves the regulation of gene transcription by two mechanisms: (a) transactivation and (b) transrepression. Transactivation is where activation occurs in the cytoplasm: PPARs bind to a retinoid X receptor/ retinoic acid receptor. The formation of this complex allows PPARs to be transported into the nucleus of an atom and bind to the promoter region of the regulated gene. The second mechanism is transrepression which is a DNA-independent pathway. This pathway interferes with other transcription pathways and may be responsible for the anti-inflammatory actions of TZDs.[35]

These mechanisms of action of TZDs create an increased insulin-stimulated glucose uptake by skeletal muscle cells, decreased hepatic glucose production, decreased lipolysis, and enhanced adipocyte differentiation.

Alpha-glucosidase Inhibitors

Alpha-glucosidase inhibitors delay the absorption of complex carbohydrates and inhibit postprandial glucose peaks and consequently lower postprandial insulin levels. In the United States, there are two alpha-glucosidase inhibitors: acarbose (Precose) and miglitol (Glyset).[34]

Dipeptidyl Peptidase IV Inhibitors

Dipeptidyl peptidase IV (DPP-IV) inhibitors are exenatide (Byetta) and sitagliptin (Januvia). As a background, glucagon-like peptide-1 (GLP-1) is an insulinotropic hormone secreted by L cells of the small intestine.[34] GLP-1 has several important biologic actions including the stimulation of insulin secretion in a glucose-dependent manner, inhibition of gastric emptying, and suppression of glucagon secretion and central anorexic activity. Patients with Type 2 diabetes exhibit reduced levels of active GLP-1 along with an impaired GLP-1 response to a glucose load. Endogenous GLP-1 is inactivated by the enzyme DPP-IV. DPP-IV inhibitors block this enzyme and thereby increase GLP-1.

ANATOMY OF THE RETINA

The retina is the innermost of the external layer of the eye, the sclera. The retina and choroid are the inner lining of the sclera. The retina is 350 μm thick in the equatorial part and 190 to 220 μm thick in the fovea and macula regions. This section concentrates on the retina, as this part of the anatomy is affected by diabetic retinopathy.

The central retina is cone-dominated and the peripheral retina is rod-dominated. There are 7 million cones and 120 million rods. At the center of the macula, there is a foveal pit where the cones are arranged in a hexagonal mosaic, which can be evaluated with fluorescein angiography as the foveal avascular zone or in electroretinography as the cone response in the 30 Hz flicker.

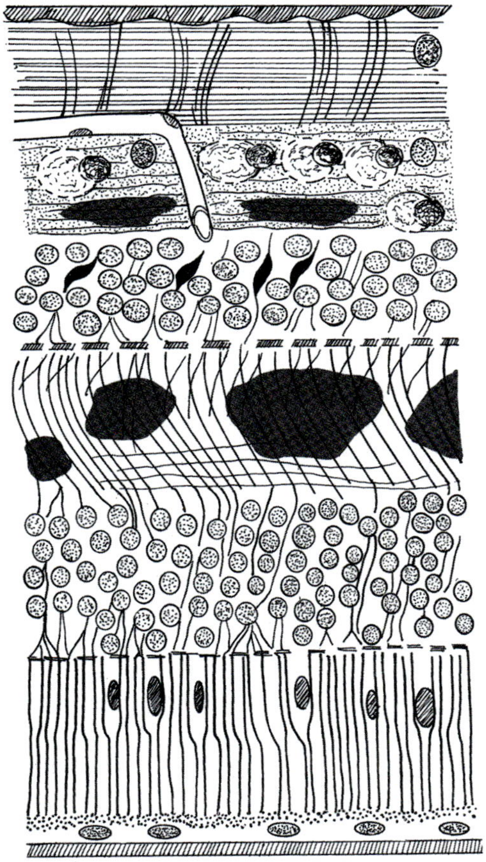

FIGURE 2-1. Diagram of the retina.

The Ten Layers of the Retina (Fig. 2-1)

1. Internal limiting membrane (ILM)
2. Nerve fiber layer
3. Ganglion cell layer
4. Inner plexiform layer
5. Inner nuclear layer
6. Outer plexiform layer (OPL)
7. Outer nuclear layer
8. External limiting membrane
9. Layer of rods and cones
10. Retinal Pigment Epithelium (RPE)

Layer 1—Internal Limiting Membrane

Muller cell footplates adhere to the vitreous interface from the ILM. These Muller cell footplates form the ILM. Clinically, these can be seen as small glistening dots in the vitreous interface in young people.

Layer 2—Nerve Fiber Layer

These are the axons of the ganglion cell layer and can be seen on clinical examination with fundus photography. Splinter-shaped hemorrhages can be seen in this layer. This is the site of cotton-wool spots or cytoid bodies.

Layer 3—Ganglion Cell Layer (Retinal Ganglion Cells)

The nuclei of the ganglion give rise to the optic nerve fibers. Axons are not myelinated until they get to the optic disc.

Midget retinal ganglion cells (RGCs) project to the parvocellular layers of the lateral geniculate nucleus. These cells are known as midget RGCs, based on the small sizes of their dendritic trees and cell bodies. Eighty percent of the RGCs are midget cells in the parvocellular pathway. They receive inputs from relatively few rods and cones. In many cases, they are connected to midget bipolars, which are linked to one cone each. They have slow conduction velocity and respond to changes in color, but respond only weakly to changes in contrast unless the change is great.[36]

Parasol retinal ganglion cells project to the magnocellular layers of the lateral geniculate nucleus. These cells are based on the large sizes of their dendritic trees and cell bodies. These cells make up 10% of RGCs. These cells, in contrast to the midget RGCs, receive inputs from many rods and cones. They have fast conduction velocity and can respond to low contrast stimuli. These cells are not sensitive to color.[36]

Bistratified RGCs project to the koniocellular layers of the lateral geniculate nucleus. These make up another 10% of RGCs and are in the koniocellular pathway. They receive inputs from intermediate numbers of rods and cones. They have moderate spatial resolution, moderate conduction velocity and can respond to moderate-contrast stimuli. They may be involved in color vision. They have large receptive fields that have only centers without surrounds. Their centers are always switched "ON" to the blue cone and "OFF" to both to the red and green cones.[37]

Photosensitive ganglion cells contain their own photopigment, melanopsin, which makes them respond directly to light even in the absence of rods and cones. They project to the suprachiasmatic nucleus via the retinohypothalamic tract for setting and maintaining circadian rhythms.

Layer 4—Inner Plexiform Layer

The inner plexiform layer is the synaptic layer where bipolar cells synapse with ganglion cells; amacrine cells modulate the synapses. This is where the action potential originates. All previous layers involve hyperpolarization or depolarization. The inner plexiform layer is thicker than the OPL.

Layer 5—Inner Nuclear Layer

The inner nuclear layer is where the bipolar nuclei are seen by light microscopy. The bipolar cells are the site of convergence of rods and cones. The nuclei of the horizontal cells are present in this layer.

Layer 6—Outer Plexiform Layer

In macular region, the layer of Henle is the synaptic layer where photoreceptors synapse with bipolar cells. Horizontal cells modulate the synapses. Cones and rods are synaptic upon bipolar and horizontal cells. Cones converge significantly less onto the bipolar cells than rods in this layer.

Layer 7—Outer Nuclear Layer

In light microscopy, this is the layer of the nuclei of the rods and cones.

Layer 8—External Limiting Membrane

On light microscopy, this is the rod and cone fibrils that form a network at the bases of the nuclei of the rods and cones.

Layer 9—Photoreceptors: Rods And Cones

This is the layer of the inner segment and outer segment of the rods and cones. The photoreceptor layer is also known as the neurosensory retina. There are two types of cells: the rods (one type) have high sensitivity, that is, they work best in lower light conditions, at darkness. They have the capacity for high amplification. They are saturated in low level of illumination. Rods have low temporal resolution and more convergence in that there are 100 million rods to 7 million cones.

Cones (three types) are divided into red, green, and blue cones. These have low sensitivity meaning that cones need the photopic response and work best in sunlight and low amplification saturated only in intense light. High temporal resolution means that they are densely crowded in the macula.

Layer 10—Retinal Pigment Epithelium

The RPE is one cell layer thick. The RPE contains melanin and it is derived embryologically from the outer portion of the optic cup. Of importance, this layer plays a role in various retinal diseases such as age-related macular degeneration, retinitis pigmentosa, and retinal detachment. In diabetes, this cell layer can seem slightly less pigmented than normal when seen on fluorescein angiography.

Experimental evidence shows that when diabetes is induced in animals by streptozotocin, the RPE shows a marked increase of membrane folding at its basal surface. Also, the RPE becomes "leaky" to small molecules such as found in fluorescein but not to larger molecules such as horseradish peroxidase.[38]

Recently, this cell layer is of interest for researchers, since this is where VEGF is produced.[39] The RPE has a dual role: light absorption and photoreceptor phagocytosis. While the majority of the light is absorbed by the rods and cones, the role of the RPE and its melanin pigment is to prevent backscattering of light, thereby producing more precise vision. The other role of the RPE is photoreceptor maintenance. The RPE participates in the cyclic phagocytosis of photoreceptors outer segments and sloughing off of membrane discs containing visual pigments.

CLINICOPATHOLOGIC CORRELATIONS

Vitreous and internal limiting membrane interface abnormalities: In early diabetic retinopathy, one can see the thickening in the ILM and the vitreous interface in diabetics. The ILM can be adherent to the vitreous in severe diabetic macular edema. The thickened premacular cortical vitreous can be present in diabetic macular edema. Native vitreous collagen with single cells is interspersed within the collagenous layer or a cellular monolayer which are seen in the ultrastructural features in autopsied diabetic eyes. Fibroblasts, fibrous astrocytes, myofibroblasts, and macrophages can be found in diseased ILM and the vitreous in diabetic macular edema[40] (Fig. 2-2).

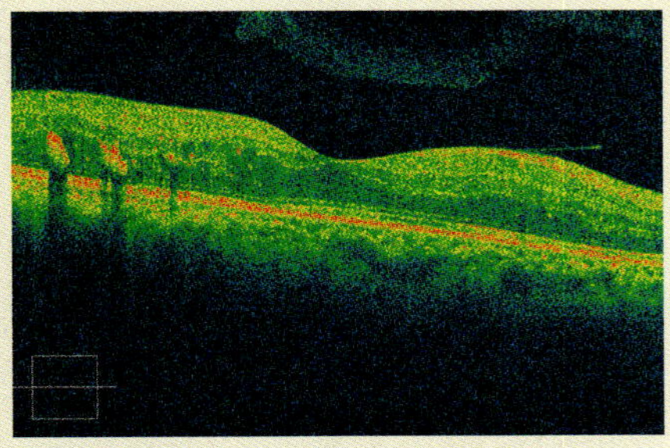

FIGURE 2-2. OCT scan of the ILM and vitreous interface.

Cotton-wool Spots

Cotton-wool spots occur in the nerve fiber layer and under the ILM. Cotton-wool spots are indicative of backup of axoplasmic flow. Histopathologically, the cotton-wool spots are cytoid bodies and are the swollen ends of ruptured axons in the nerve fiber layer in the infarcted area, just under the ILM (Fig. 2-3).

Diabetic Macular Edema

Diabetic macular edema occurs in the layer called Henle layer, which is the OPL. Pathologic examination of the retina for macular edema shows liquefaction necrosis of retinal capillary or venular endothelial cells.

The lumen of the blood vessels shows fibrin and proteinaceous material. The basement membrane of the capillary wall is thickened[41] (Fig. 2-4).

Pericyte degeneration plays a role. Mild to moderate amounts of fluid collections of Muller cells may result in macular edema. Excessive swelling and rupture or death of Muller cells produce pockets of fluid and cell debris. Adjacent neurons undergo similar changes secondarily.[42]

In the OPL, microcystoid degeneration of the macula or diabetic macular edema can occur. In diabetic macular edema, the presence of hard exudates causes pressure atrophy on the retina or enlargement of the intercellular spaces, thus resulting in microcystoid degeneration. These microcystoid retinal degenerative processes can lead to macular retinoschisis and even partial inner layer of schisis or complete macular hole formation (Fig. 2-5).

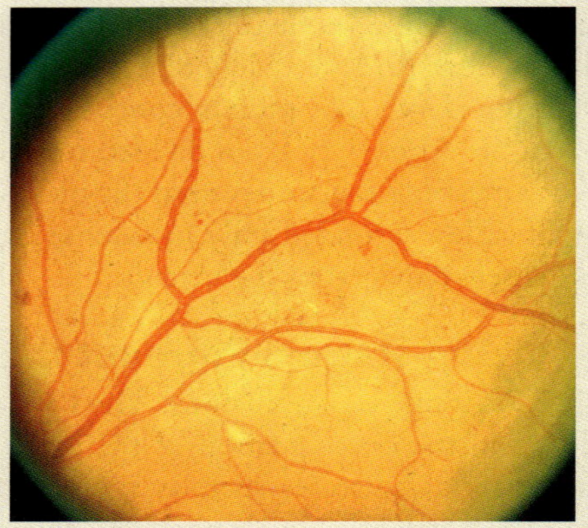

FIGURE 2-3. Cotton-wool spot.

Hard Exudates

In the OPL or Henle fiber layer, the exudates are seen pathologically as fat-filled (lipoidal) histiocytes. Massive exudation contains foamy histiocytes in the OPL. The concentration of exudates around diseased vessels causes circular pattern called circinate retinopathy[43] (Fig. 2-6).

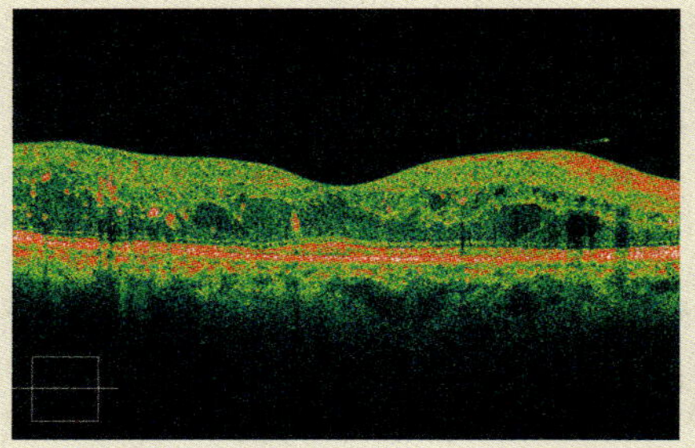

FIGURE 2-4. OCT scan of macular edema affecting OPL.

Vascular Changes

Vascular changes of the diabetic retina can occur anywhere between the nerve fiber layer and the OPL where venules and capillaries are found. On light microscopy, there is loss of capillary pericytes.

In the normal retinal capillary, the pericyte to endothelial cell ratio is 1:1. In the diabetic retinal capillary, the ratio of pericyte to endothelial cell is less than the 1:1 ratio due to the loss of pericytes[43] (Figs. 2-7 and 2-8).

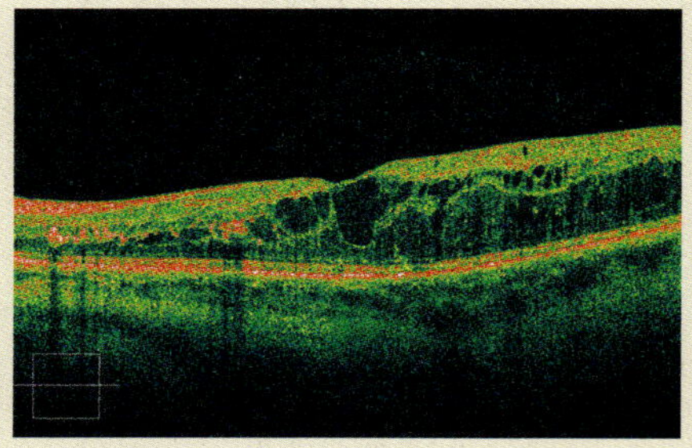

FIGURE 2-5. Cystic changes in macular edema.

Venous Dilatation and Venous Beading

Venous dilatations are irregularities in the venular walls. Arteriolar venular connections and thickened capillary basement membranes are found as well. Venous beading occurs when the dilated venular walls have the presence of saccular microaneurysms and appear clinically as "beading" on the veins (Fig. 2-9).

Intraretinal Microvascular Abnormalities

Arteriolar-venular connections are collaterals. The dilated cellular capillary arises from an arteriole and goes directly to a venule, bypassing the capillary bed. The dilated capillaries are "anuclear" capillaries which are nonfunctioning conduits for blood flow.[42,48] With the loss of pericytes, there is an associated increase in the number of retinal capillary microaneurysms. Microaneurysms are found on the arteriolar and venular sides of the capillary network. The formation of microaneurysms is thought to occur in the background of retinal ischemia.

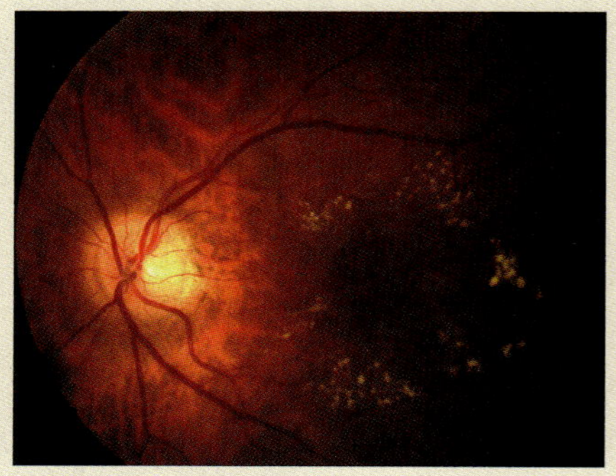

FIGURE 2-6. Hard exudates in circinate ring in diabetic retinopathy.

Microaneurysms are thin outpouchings from the wall of the capillary. As the endothelial cells proliferate and lay down increasing amount of basement membrane materials, the endothelial cells may disappear. Then, the

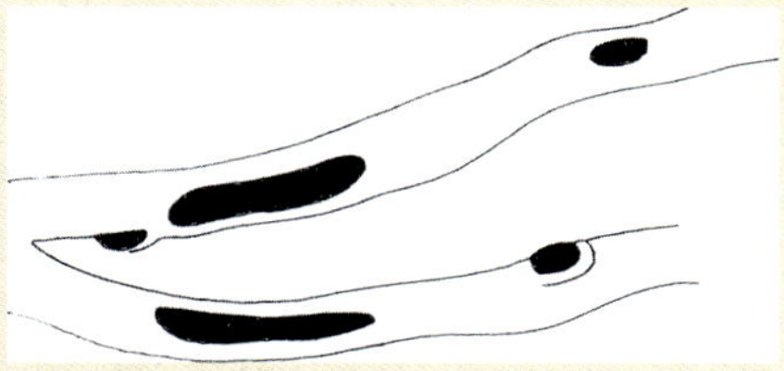

FIGURE 2-7. Diagram of pericyte and endothelial cell.

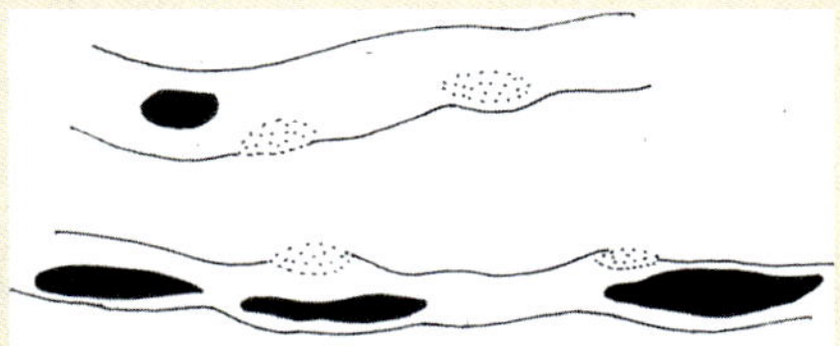

FIGURE 2-8. Diagram of pericyte loss.

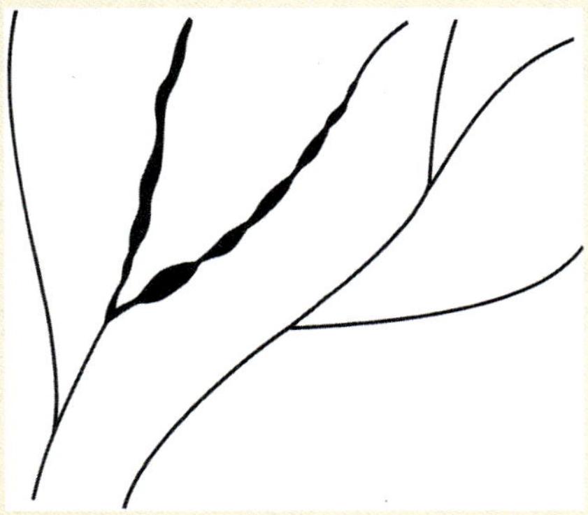

FIGURE 2-9. Venous beading.

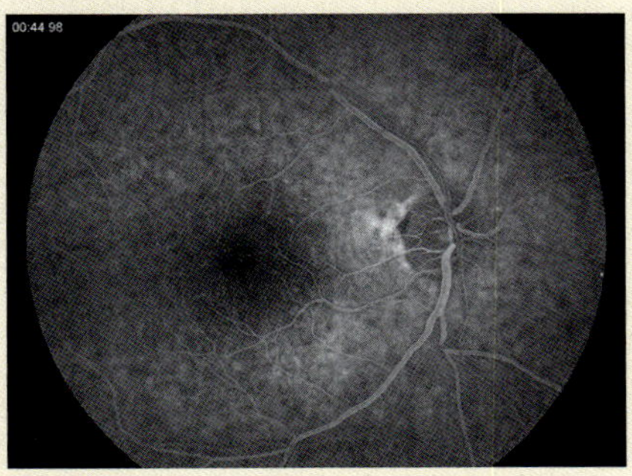

FIGURE 2-10. Fluorescein angiogram of microaneurysms.

next step is that the lumen of the microaneurysm may become occluded with the excess basement membrane material. More microaneurysms can be identified by fluorescein angiography or pathological specimen examination than with the clinical eye exam (Fig. 2-10).

Arteriovenular Shunts

Arteriolar-venular shunts or intraretinal microvascular abnormalities (IRMA) are secondary to hypoxic stimulus. These arteriolar-venular shunts demonstrate decreased blood flow.

Exudative Diabetic Retinopathy

Hard exudates are found in the macula in the OPL or Henle layer in the macula. In hyperlipidemic diabetic patients, with hard exudates, treatment of their hyperlipidemia leads to regression of hard exudates. Thus, the lipid content of the hard exudates may be manipulated by antilipid therapy.[44] Hard exudates can be removed by macrophage activity in 4 to 6 months.

Microcystoid Degeneration of the Macula

When hard exudates occur, the hard exudates cause pressure changes on the retinal surface such as atrophy on the retina or enlargement of the intercellular spaces. The resultant picture is microcystoid retinal degeneration. Severe cystic degeneration due to the hard exudates can lead to macular retinoschisis, partial inner layer of schisis, or complete macular hole formation.[42]

Vascular Endothelial Growth Factor

VEGF is found in the endothelial cells of the capillaries and the RPE. Blood retinal barrier breakdown in experimental diabetes is VEGF-dependent in the capillaries and venules of the superficial, inner retinal vasculature.[45]

Hemorrhages in Diabetic Retinopathy

Dot blot hemorrhages are located in the inner nuclear and can spread to OPL. Splinter-shaped hemorrhages are in the nerve fiber layer. Confluent hemorrhages are large and involve all the retinal layers.

Massive hemorrhages can break through the ILM into vitreous cavity and can extend into the subretinal space.[46]

PREPROLIFERATIVE DIABETIC RETINOPATHY

Pathologically, preproliferative diabetic retinopathy means increased retinal hemorrhages, cotton-wool spots, venous dilatation, and venous beading. The severity of preproliferative diabetic retinopathy increases with the increasing presence of the vascular abnormality.

PROLIFERATIVE DIABETIC RETINOPATHY

The proliferative phase of diabetic retinopathy is a vascular response to hypoxic retina. Many theories exist about the cause of the retina hypoxia in diabetes. The causes include retinal arteriolar and capillary closure, retinal capillary basement membrane alterations, immunogenic mechanism related to insulin, altered plasma proteins that cause platelet and red blood cell aggregation, increased blood viscosity, altered ability of the blood to transport oxygen, virus induction of diabetes mellitus, abnormal metabolic pathways in the retinal capillaries, and production of VEGFs.

Once the retina is hypoxic, presumably, the retinal blood vessels and the RPE are thought to elaborate the growth factors. Currently, it is thought that VEGFs play a role in the proliferation of neovascularization. Anti-VEGF therapy is beginning to be used for diabetic retinopathy.

The new blood vessels arise from retinal venules rather than from retinal capillaries, usually at the edge of an area of capillary nonperfusion. The new blood vessels or neovascularization may arise from retinal arterioles. These new abnormal blood vessels contain both endothelial cells and pericytes. These neovascular membranes can lie flat on the internal surface of the retina and are called epiretinal neovascular membranes. If the neovascular membranes become elevated, they are called preretinal neovascular membranes.

The neovascularization, which is initially intraretinal, breaks through the ILM and lies between it and the vitreous. Normal vitreous dynamics may cause a rupture of the new vessels leading to a vitreous hemorrhage.

With neovascularization, a fibrous component develops. This fibrous component leads to a retinal detachment. The majority of these are nonrhegmatogenous (without a hole) but have a tractional component. The fibrous tissue contracts as the neovascularization increases, and the neurosensory retina becomes elevated and pulled away from the RPE and a traction retinal detachment occurs.

Neovascularization

In streptozotocin-induced diabetes in the rat model, there is capillary embolization, noncellular capillaries, swelling, and distortion in endothelial cells. Thus, hyperglycemia in itself is toxic to the vascular tissue.[47]

Recently, VEGF is a potent selective mitogenic cytokine for endothelial cells and its expression can be induced by hypoxia. VEGFs have been isolated in the vitreous of diabetic patients undergoing vitrectomy.[48–51]

In fact, VEGF administered through gene therapy or protein injection has been proposed to enhance collateral vessel growth and prevent tissue necrosis under ischemic condition in cardiology. Thus, in ophthalmology, anti-VEGF therapy has been used for diabetic retinopathy in the form of bevacizumab (Avastin) since 2006.

REFERENCES

1. Devendra D, Liu E, Eisenbarth GS. Type 1 diabetes recent developments. *Brit Med J.* 2004;328:750–754.
2. American Diabetes Association. Report of the expert committee on the diagnosis and classification of diabetes mellitus. *Diabetes Care.* 1997;20:1183–1197.
3. Peterson JS, Hejnaes KR, Moody A, et al. Detection of GAD65 antibodies in diabetes and other autoimmune diseases using a simple radioligand assay. *Diabetes.* 1994;43:459–467.
4. Molbak AG, Christau B, Marner B, et al. Incidence of insulin-dependent diabetes mellitus in age groups over 30 years in Denmark. *Diabetes Med.* 1994;11:650–655.
5. Onkamo P, Vaananen S, Karvonen M, et al. Worldwide increase in increase of Type I diabetes—the analysis of the data on published incidence trends. *Diabetologia.* 1999;42:1395–1403.
6. EURODIAB ACE Study Group. Variation and trends in incidence of childhood diabetes in Europe. *Lancet.* 2000;355:873–876.
7. Devendra D, Eisenbarth GS. Immunologic endocrine disorders. *J Allergy Clin Immunol.* 2003;111:624–636.
8. De Block CEM, De Leeuw IH, Rooman RPA, et al. Belgian Diabetes Registry. Gastric parietal cell antibodies are associated with glutamic acid decarboxylase-65 antibodies and the HLA DQA1*0501-DQB1*0301 haplotype in Type 1 diabetes mellitus. *Diabetic Medicine.* 2001;17:618–622.

9. Atkinson MA, Eisenbarth GS. Type 1A diabetes: New perspectives on case pathogenesis and treatment. *Lancet.* 2001;358:221–229.
10. Moriyama H, Wen L, Abiru N, et al. Induction and acceleration of insulitis/diabetes in mice with a viral mimic (polyinosinic-polycytidylic acid) and an insulin self-peptide. *Proc Natl Acad Sci USA.* 2002;99:5539–5544.
11. Imagawa A, Hanafusa T, Itoh N, et al. Immunological abnormalities in islets at diagnosis paralleled further deterioration of glycemic control in patients with recent-onset Type I (insulin-dependent) diabetes mellitus. *Diabetologia.* 1999;42:574–578.
12. Roep BO. The Role of T Cells in the pathogenesis of Type 1 Diabetes: From cause to cure. *Diabetologia.* 2003;46: 305–321.
13. Herold KC, Hagopian W, Auger JA, et al. Anti-CD3 monoclonal antibody in new-onset Type 1A diabetes mellitus. *N Engl J Med.* 2002;346:1962–1968.
14. Atkinson MA, Leiter EH. The NOD mouse model of diabetes: As good as it gets? *Nat Med.* 1999;5:601–604.
15. Diabetes Control and Complications Trial Research Group. The effect of intensive treatment of diabetes on the development and progression of long-term complications in insulin-depending diabetes mellitus. *N Engl J Med.* 1993;329:977–986.
16. Bolli GB, Owens DR. Insulin glargine. *Lancet.* 2000;356:443–445.
17. Meyer L, Guerci B. Metformin and insulin in diabetes Type 1A: The first step. *Diabetes Care.* 2003;26:1655–1656.
18. Shapiro AM, Lakey JR, Ryan EA, et al. Islet transplantation in seven patients with Type 1A diabetes mellitus using glucocorticoid-free immunosuppressive regimen. *N Engl J Med.* 2000;343:230–238.
19. Resnick HE, Howard BV. Diabetes and cardiovascular disease. *Ann Rev Med.* 2002;52:245–267.
20. Laakso M. Cardiovascular disease in Type 2 diabetes: Challenge for treatment and preventation. *J Intern Med.* 2001;249:225–235.
21. Seufert J, Kieffer TJ, Leech CA, et al. Leptin supression of insulin secretion and gene expression in human pancreatic islets: Implications for the development of adipogenic diabetes mellitus. *J Clin Endocrinology Metab.* 1999;84: 670–676.
22. Hotamisligil GS, Spiegelman BM. Tumor necrosis factor alpha: A key component of the obesity-diabetes link. *Diabetes.* 1994;43:1271–1278.
23. Griffin ME, Marcucci M, Cline GW, et al. Free fatty acid-induced insulin resistance is associated with activation of protein kinase C theta and alterations in the insulin signaling cascade. *Diabetes.* 1999;48:1270–1274.
24. American Association of Clinical Endocrinologists medical guidelines for clinical practice for the management of diabetes mellitus. AACE Diabetes Mellitus Clinical Practice Guidelines Task Force. *Endocr Pract.* 2007;3(suppl 1): S1–S68.
25. Pan XR, Li GW, Hu YH, et al. Effects of diet and exercise in preventing NIDDM in people with impaired glucose tolerance. The Da Qing IGT and Diabetes Study. *Diabetes Care.* 1997;20:537–544.
26. Sacks FM, Svetkey LP, Vollmer WM, et al. The Dash-Sodium Collaborative Research Group. Effects on Blood Pressure of Reduced Dietary Sodium and Dietary approaches to Stop Hypertension (DASH) Diet. *N Engl J Med.* 2001;344:3–10.
27. American Diabetes Association. Diabetes mellitus and exercise (Position statement) *Diabetes Care.* 2001:24(suppl 1): S51–S55.
28. Schneider SH, Ruderman NB. Exercise and NIDDM. *Diabetes Care.* 1990;13:785–789.
29. Klein R, Klein BEK, Moss SE, et al. The Wisconisin epidemiology study of diabetic retinopathy II. Prevalence and risk of diabetic retinopathy when age of diagnosis is less than 30 years. *Arch Ophthalmol.* 1984;102:520–526.
30. Stratton IM, Adler AI, Neil HAW, et al. United Kingdom Prospective Diabetes Study Group. Association of glycaemia with macrovascular and microvascular complications of type 2 diabetes (UKPDS 35): Prospective observational study. *Brit Med J.* 2000;321:405–412.
31. Klein BE, Moss SE, Klein R, et al. WESDR XIII. Relationship of serum cholesterol to retinopathy and hard exudates. *Ophthalmology.* 1991;98:1261–1265.
32. Fong D, Segal PP, Myers F, et al. Subretinal fibrosis in diabetic macular edema: ETDRS Report no. 23. *Arch Ophthalmol.* 1997;115:873–877.
33. Olivarius, N deF, Andreasen AH, Keiding N, et al. Epidemiology of renal involvement in newly diagnosed middle aged and elderly diabetic patients. Cross sectional data from the population based study "Diabetes care in General Practice" Denmark. *Diabetologia.* 1993;36(10):1007–1016.
34. Goldstein BJ, Miller JL. *Contemporary Diagnosis and Management of The Patient with Type 2 Diabetes.* Newtown: Handbooks in Healthcare Co.; 2007:49.
35. Goldstein BJ, Miller JL. *Contemporary Diagnosis and Management of The Patient with Type 2 Diabetes.* Newtown: Handbooks in Healthcare Co.; 2007:61.
36. Field GD, Chichilnisky EJ. Information processing in the primate retina: Circuitry and coding. *Ann Rev Neurosci.* 2007;30:1–30.
37. Szmajda BA, Grunert U, Martin PR. Retinal Ganglion cell inputs to the koniocellular pathway. *J Comp Neurol.* 2008;510:251–268.
38. Grimes PA, Laties AM. Early morphological alteration of the pigment epithelium in streptozotocin–induced diabetes: Increased surface area of the basal cell membrane. *Exp Eye Res.* 1980;30:631–636.
39. Ming L, Amano S, Miyamoto K, et al. Insulin induced vascular endothelial growth factor expression in the retina. *Invest Ophthalmol Vis Sci.* 1999;40:3281–3286.
40. Gandorfer A, Rohleder M, Kampik A. Epiretinal pathology of vitreomacular traction syndrome. *Br J Ophthalmol.* 2002;86:902–909.
41. Yanoff M, Fine BS. *Ocular Pathology: A Text and Atlas.* Philadelphia, PA: Harper and Row; 1982:724.
42. Gandorfer A, Rohleder M, Grosselfinger S, et al. Epiretinal pathology of diffuse diabetic macular edema associated with vitreomacular traction. *Am J Ophthalmol.* 2003;139:638–652.
43. Yanoff M, Fine BS. *Ocular Pathology: A Text and Atlas.* Philadelphia, PA: Harper and Row; 1982:727.
44. Cusick M, Chew Y. Histopathology and regression of retinal hard exudates in diabetic retinopathy after reduction of elevated serum lipids. *Ophthalmology.* 2003;110:2126–2133.
45. Quam T, Qingwen X, Joussen AM, et al. VEGF-initiated blood-retinal barrier breakdown in early diabetes. *Invest Ophthalmol Vis Sci.* 2001;42:2408–2413.

46. Yanoff M, Fine *BS. Ocular Pathology: A Text and Atlas*. Philadelphia, PA: Harper and Row Publishers; 1982:731.
47. Cogan DG, Toussaint D, Kuwabara T. Retinal vascular patterns IV. Diabetic retinopathy. *Arch Ophthalmol.* 1961;66:366–378.
48. Aiello LP, Gardner TW, King GL, et al. Vascular endothelial growth factor in ocular fluid of patients with diabetic retinopathy and other retinal disorders. *N Engl J Med.* 1994;331:1480–1487.
49. Duh E, Aiello LP. Vascular endothelial growth factors and diabetes: The agonist and antagonist paradox. *Diabetes.*1999;48:1899–1906.
50. Veves A, King GL. Can VEGF reverse diabetic neuropathy in human subjects? *J Clin Invest.* 2001;107:1215–1218.
51. Shweiki D, Itin A, Soffer D, et al. Vascular endothelial growth factor induced by hypoxia may mediate hypoxia-initiated angiogenesis. *Nature.* 1992;359:843–845.

SUGGESTED READINGS

1. Abrams GW, Williams GA. "En bloc" excision of diabetic membranes. *Am J Ophthalmol.* 1987;103:302–308.
2. Ashton N. Injection of the retinal vascular system in the enucleated eye in diabetic retinopathy. *Br J Ophthalmol.* 1950;34:38–41.
3. Ashton N. The pathology of retinal microaneurysms. *Acta XVI Concilium Ophthalmol.* 1950;1:411–421.
4. Benson WE, Brown GC, Tasman W. *Diabetes and Its Ocular Complications.* Philadelphia, PA: WB Saunders Co; 1988.
5. Bloodworth JMB. Diabetic retinopathy. *Diabetes.* 1962;11:1–22.
6. Bohlen HG, Hankins KD. Early arteriolar and capillary changes in streptozotocin-induced diabetic rats and intraperitoneal hyperglycemic rats. *Diabetologia.* 1982;22:344–348.
7. Bresnick GH. Diabetic maculopathy: A crucial review highlighting diffuse macular edema. *Ophthalmology.* 1983;90:1301–1317.
8. Bresnick GH. Diabetic macular edema: A review. *Ophthalmology.* 1986;93:989–997.
9. Bresnick GH. Background diabetic retinopathy. In: Ryan S, ed. *Retina*, vol 2. St. Louis: CV Mosby Co; 1990: 327–366.
10. Bresnick GH, Condit R, Syrjala S, et al. Abnormalities of the foveal avascular zone in diabetic retinopathy. *Arch Ophthalmol.* 1984;102:1286–1293.
11. Bresnick GH, Davis MD, Myers FL, et al. Clinicopathologic correlations in diabetic retinopathy. II. Clinical and histologic appearances of retinal capillary microaneurysms. *Arch Ophthalmol.* 1977;95:1215–1220.
12. Bresnick GH, Engerman R, Davis MD, et al. Patterns of ischemia in diabetic retinopathy. *Trans Am Acad Ophthalmol Otolaryngol.* 1976;81:694.
13. Bresnick GH, Haight B, DeVenecia G. Retinal wrinkling and macular heterotopia in diabetic retinopathy. *Arch Ophthalmol.* 1979;97:1890–1895.
14. Catalano RA, Tanenbaum HL, Majerovics A, et al. White-centered hemorrhages in diabetic retinopathy. *Ophthalmology.* 1987;94:388–392.
15. Charles S, Flinn CE. The natural history of diabetic extramacular traction retinal detachment. *Arch Ophthalmol.* 1981;99:66–68.
16. Cunha-Vaz JG. Diabetic retinopathy. Human and experimental studies. *Trans Ophthalmol Soc UK.* 1972;92: 111–124.
17. Cunha-Vaz JG, Fonseca JR, de Abreau JRF, et al. Studies on retinal blood flow. II. Diabetic retinopathy. *Arch Ophthalmol.* 1978;96:809–811.
18. Dahl-Jorgensen K, Brinchmann-Hansen O, Hanssen KF, et al. Rapid tightening of blood glucose control leads to transient deterioration of retinopathy in insulin-dependent diabetes mellitus: The Oslo study. *Br Med J.* 1985;290: 811–815.
19. Davis MD. Vitreous contraction in proliferative diabetic retinopathy. *Arch Ophthalmol.* 1965;74:741–751.
20. Davis MD. Proliferative diabetic retinopathy. In: Ryan SJ, ed. *Retina*, vol 2. St. Louis: CV Mosby Co.; 1989: 367–402.
21. Davis MD, Norton EWD, Myers FL. The Airlie classification of diabetic retinopathy. In: Goldberg MF, Fine SL, eds. *Symposium on the Treatment of Diabetic Retinopathy.* Washington, DC: Public Health Service Publication No. 1840, US Government Printing Office; 1969.
22. Diabetic Retinopathy Study Research Group. A modification on the Airlie House classification of diabetic retinopathy. Report No 7. *Invest Ophthalmol Vis Sci.* 1981;21(part 2):210–226.
23. Dobree JH. Proliferative diabetic retinopathy: Evolution of the retinal lesions. *Br J Ophthalmol.* 1964;48:637–649.
24. Dobree JH. Simple diabetic retinopathy. Evolution of the lesions and therapeutic considerations. *Br J Ophthalmol.* 1970;54:1–10.
25. Early Treatment Diabetic Retinopathy Study Group. ETDRS Report No 1: Photocoagulation for diabetic macular edema. *Arch Ophthalmol.* 1985;103:1796–1806.
26. Early Treatment Diabetic Retinopathy Study Group. ETDRS Report No 7: Early treatment diabetic retinopathy study design and baseline patient characteristics. *Ophthalmology.* 1991;98:741–756.
27. Early Treatment Diabetic Retinopathy Study Group. ETDRS Report No 9: Early photocoagulation for diabetic retinopathy. *Ophthalmology.* 1991;98:766–785.
28. Early Treatment Diabetic Retinopathy Study Group. ETDRS Report No 10: Grading diabetic retinopathy from stereoscopic color fundus photographs – An extension of the modified Airlie House classification. *Ophthalmology.* 1991;98:786–806.
29. Early Treatment Diabetic Retinopathy Study Group. ETDRS Report No 11: Classification of diabetic retinopathy from fluorescein angiograms. *Ophthalmology.* 1991;98:807–822.
30. Early Treatment Diabetic Retinopathy Study Group. ETDRS Report No 12: Fundus photographic risk factors for progression of diabetic retinopathy. *Ophthalmology.* 1991;98:823–833.
31. Frank RN. On the pathogenesis of diabetic retinopathy. *Ophthalmology.* 1991; 98:586–592.
32. Goldbaum MH. Retinal depression sign indicating a small retinal infarct. *Am J Ophthalmol.* 1978;86:45–55.

33. Grunwald JE, Riva CE, Sinclair SH, et al. Laser doppler velocimetry study of retinal circulation in diabetes mellitus. *Arch Ophthalmol.* 1986;104:991–996.
34. Klein BEK, Davis MD, Segal P, et al. Diabetic retinopathy. Assessment of severity and progression. *Ophthalmology.* 1984;91:10–17.
35. Kohner EM, Dollery CT, Bulpitt CJ. Cotton-wool spots in diabetic retinopathy. *Diabetes.* 1969;18:691–704.
36. Kohner EM, Dollery CT, Paterson JW, et al. Arterial fluorescein studies in diabetic retinopathy. *Diabetes.* 1967;16:1–10.
37. Kohner EM, Hamilton AM, Saunders SJ. The retinal blood flow in diabetes. *Diabetologia.* 1975;11:27–33.
38. Kohner E, Henkind P. Correlation of fluorescein angiogram and retinal digest in diabetic retinopathy. *Am J Ophthalmol.* 1970;69:403–410.
39. Kohner EM, Sleightholm M, Kroc. Collaborative Study Group. Does microaneurysm count reflect severity of early diabetic retinopathy? *Ophthalmology.* 1986;93:586–589.
40. Kroc Collaborative Study Group. Blood glucose control and the evolution of diabetic retinopathy and albuminuria: A preliminary multicenter trial. *N Engl J Med.* 1984;311:365–372.
41. Lauritzen T, Frost-Larsen K, Larsen HW, et al. Two-year experience with continuous subcutaneous insulin infusion in relation to retinopathy and neuropathy. *Diabetes.* 1985;34:74–79.
42. Michels RG. Proliferative diabetic retinopathy. Pathophysiology of extraretinal complications and principles of vitreous surgery. *Retina.* 1981;1:1–17.
43. Muraoka K, Shimizu K. Intraretinal neovascularization in diabetic retinopathy. *Ophthalmology.* 1984;93:1440–1446.
44. Niki T, Muraoka K, Shimizu K. Distribution of capillary nonperfusion in early-stage diabetic retinopathy. *Ophthalmology.* 1984;91:1431–1439.
45. Patz A, Schatz H, Berkow JE, et al. Macular edema: An overlooked complication of diabetic retinopathy. *Trans Am Acad Ophthalmol Otolaryngol.* 1973; 77:34.
46. Ramsay WJ, Ramsay RC, Purple RL, Knobloch WH. Involutional diabetic retinopathy. *Am J Ophthalmol.* 1977;84: 851–858.
47. Shimizu K, Kobayaski Y, Muraoka K. Midperipheral fundus involvement in diabetic retinopathy. *Ophthalmology.* 1981;88:601–612.
48. Sigurdsson R, Begg IS. Organized macular plaques in exudative diabetic maculopathy. *Br J Ophthalmol.* 1980;64: 392–397.
49. Sinclair SH. Macular retinal capillary hemodynamics in diabetic patients. *Ophthalmology.* 1991;98:1580–1586.
50. Sinclair SH, Grunwald JE, Riva CE, et al. Retinal vascular autoregulation in diabetes mellitus. *Ophthalmology.* 1982;89:748–750.
51. Sleightholm MA, Aldington SJ, Arnold J, et al. Diabetic retinopathy: II. Assessment of severity and progression from fluorescein angiograms. *J Diabetic Complications.* 1988;2:117–120.
52. Sleightholm MA, Arnold J, Kohner EM. Diabetic retinopathy: I. The measurement of intercapillary area in normal retinal angiograms. *J Diabetic Complications.* 1988;11:113–116.
53. Small KW, Stefansson E, Hatchell DL. Retinal blood flow in normal and diabetic dogs. *Invest Ophthamol Vis Sci.* 1987;28:672–675.
54. Stefansson E, Landers MB III, Wolbarsht ML. Oxygenation and vasodilatation in relation to diabetic and other proliferative retinopathies. *Ophthalmic Surg.* 1983;14:209–226.
55. Taylor E, Dobree JH. Proliferative diabetic retinopathy: Site and size of initial lesions. *Br J Ophthalmol.* 1970;54:11–18.
56. Tso MOM, Cunha-Vaz JGF, Shin CY, et al. A clinicopathologic study of blood-retinal barrier in experimental diabetes. *Invest Ophthalmol Vis Sci.* 1979;18(suppl):169.
57. Yanoff M. Diabetic retinopathy. *N Engl J Med.* 1966;274:1344–1349.
58. Yoshida A, Feke GT, Morales-Stoppello J, et al. Retinal blood flow alterations during progression of diabetic retinopathy. *Arch Ophthalmol.* 1983;101:225–227.
59. Zatz R, Brenner BM. Pathogenesis of diabetic microangiopathy. The hemodynamic view. *Am J Med.* 1986;80: 443–453.

CHAPTER 3

National Clinical Trials and Classification

Laser photocoagulation began in the early 1960s with Meyer-Schwickerath using the xenon arc laser.[1,2] At that time, when surface neovascularization was directly treated with laser, regression of the neovascularization followed. Later, laser treatment was performed with the ruby laser and argon laser.[3–5]

The efficacy of laser photocoagulation was tested in several clinical trials. The two large randomized clinical trials were the British Multicentre Trial[6] using xenon arc and an American study, the Diabetic Retinopathy Study (DRS).[7–10] The National Eye Institute's DRS used both xenon arc and argon blue-green lasers to show that photocoagulation was successful in the management of proliferative diabetic retinopathy (PDR).

DIABETIC RETINOPATHY STUDY

The DRS began in 1971 as a multicentered, national, and prospective clinical trial. Its goal was to answer the question whether photocoagulation would prevent the development of severe visual loss in eyes with PDR. Retinopathy was classified using the modified Airlie House classification.[11] The Airlie House classification referred to a symposium held in 1968 discussing the current knowledge about the natural history and management of diabetic retinopathy (DR).[12]

The Airlie House classification included the seven standard photographic fields for DR.[11] Field 1 was centered on the optic disc, Field 2 was centered on the macula, Field 3 was centered on the area just temporal to the macula, Field 4 was superotemporal, Field 5 was inferotemporal, Field 6 was superonasal, and Field 7 was inferonasal.

In the DRS, one eye was randomized to treatment with either xenon arc or argon laser photocoagulation. The other eye was randomized as a "control" eye, that is, without treatment.

The DRS asked three questions[13,14]:

Does photocoagulation prevent severe vision loss from DR? Severe visual loss was defined as visual acuity <5/200 at each of the two consecutive follow-up visits at 4-month intervals of the study.

Was there a difference in the efficacy and safety of extensive scatter and focal treatment to surface neovascularization elsewhere (NVE), elevated NVE, and neovascularization at the disc (NVD) with argon laser, extensive scatter, and focal treatment to surface NVE with xenon arc?

Which stages of retinopathy benefit most by treatment and for which stages might treatment be of no benefit or harmful? (Table 3-1)

The DRS identified four new vessel-vitreous hemorrhage risk factors or retinopathy risk factors:

1. Presence of new vessels.
2. Location of new vessels on or within 1 disc diameter (DD) of the optic disc or NVD.
3. Severity of new vessels defined for NVD as equal to or greater than standard photograph 10A[11] or greater than one-fourth to one-third disc area in extent, or for NVE, NVE equal to or greater than one-half disc area.
4. Vitreous or preretinal hemorrhage.

TABLE 3.1 Definitions

Mild to moderate nonproliferative retinopathy
Microaneurysms
Intraretinal hemorrhages: mild to moderate in fewer than four quadrants
Hard exudates
Macular edema
Foveal avascular zone abnormalities

Moderate to severe nonproliferative retinopathy
1. Cotton-wool spots
2. Intraretinal hemorrhages: mild to moderate in four quadrants
3. Venous beading
4. IRMA

Severe nonproliferative retinopathy (ETDRS)
Any one of the following:
1. Severe intraretinal hemorrhages in four quadrants
2. Venous beading in two quadrants
3. Moderately severe IRMA in one quadrant

Very severe nonproliferative retinopathy (ETDRS)
Any two of the following:
1. Severe intraretinal hemorrhages in four quadrants
2. Venous beading in two quadrants
3. Moderately severe IRMA in one quadrant

Proliferative diabetic retinopathy
1. Neovascularization of the disc
2. Neovascularization of the retina elsewhere
3. Preretinal hemorrhage
4. Vitreous hemorrhage
5. Tractional retinal detachment
6. Neovascularization of the iris or angle or both

Eyes with three or four retinopathy risk factors were considered to be at highest risk for the development of severe visual loss.

High-risk groups:

Eyes with NVD ≥ to ¼ to ⅓ DD (Fig. 3-1).
Milder NVD if associated with vitreous or preretinal hemorrhage (Fig. 3-2).
NVE ≥ to ½ disc area if associated with vitreous or preretinal hemorrhage (Fig. 3-3).

Thus, after 2 years of follow-up, photocoagulation was found to reduce the risk of severe visual loss by more than 50% in eyes with high-risk retinopathy.[15] At 2 years, 11%

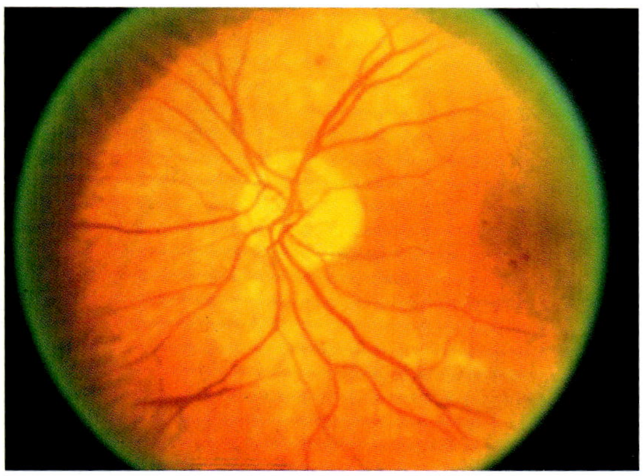

FIGURE 3-1. Disc neovascularization, standard photo 10A. (Courtesy of University of Wisconsin, Fundus Reading Center and Early Treatment Diabetic Retinopathy Study Research Group.)

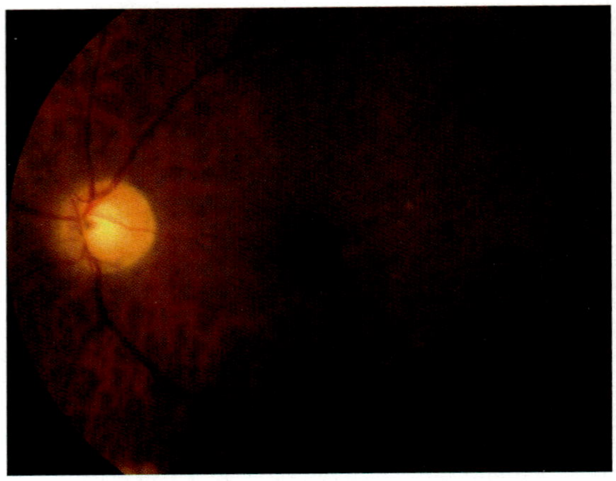

FIGURE 3-2. Retinal hemorrhages.

of the treated eyes and 26% of the control eyes with high-risk retinopathy developed severe visual loss.[15,16] At 4 years, 20% of the treated eyes and 44% of the control eyes developed severe visual loss. The clear treatment benefit was seen in longer follow-up.[14,15] In eyes with less than high-risk retinopathy, or severe nonproliferative diabetic retinopathy (NPDR), the same clear treatment benefit was not seen. Thus, at the time, the DRS did not recommend prompt treatment for these categories of eyes.[15,16]

In the DRS, the side effects of photocoagulation were noted: a decrease in visual acuity and constriction of the peripheral visual field. This constriction of the visual field occurred more frequently with xenon arc than argon laser photocoagulation. The constriction of the visual field was thought to be from the macular edema that occurred as a treatment effect in the xenon-treated eyes.[16,17]

EARLY TREATMENT DIABETIC RETINOPATHY STUDY

The Early Treatment Diabetic Retinopathy Study (ETDRS) was a multicentered, collaborative, prospective, and randomized clinical trial sponsored by the National Eye Institute. Between 1980 and 1985, the ETDRS recruited and enrolled over 3,700 patients.

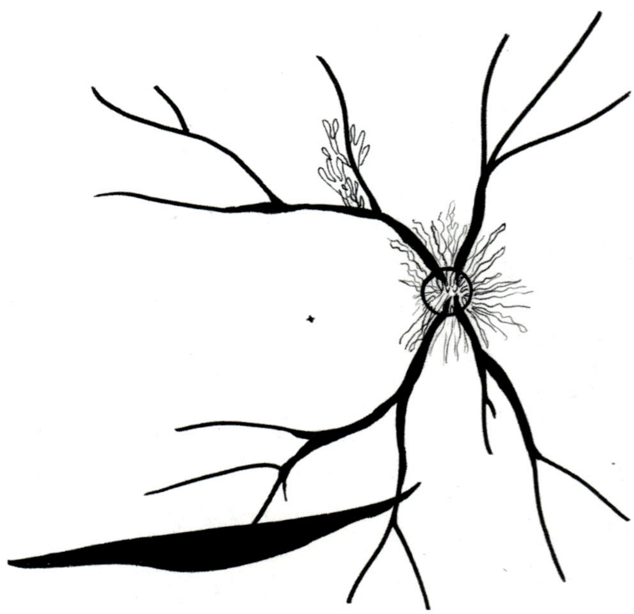

FIGURE 3-3. Neovascularization of the retina elsewhere and the optic disc neovascularization, meeting high-risk characteristics.

The ETDRS asked three questions:

1. Is photocoagulation effective in the treatment of diabetic macular edema (DME)?
2. Is aspirin effective in changing the course of DR?
3. When should panretinal photocoagulation be initiated so as to be the most effective in the management of DR?[18–24]

Clinically significant macular edema (CSME) has been defined by the ETDRS as (a) thickening of the retina at or within 500 μm of the center of the macula, (b) hard exudates at or within 500 μm of the center of the macula, if associated with thickening of the adjacent retina and not residual hard exudates remaining after the disappearance of retinal thickening, or (c) a zone or zones of retinal thickening of one disc area or larger, any part of which is within 1 DD of the center of the macula.[18,19]

The diagnosis of CSME was made by using slit lamp biomicroscopy and documented with stereoscopic fundus photography. Fluorescein angiography was required by the ETDRS only after the clinical diagnosis was made by slit lamp biomicroscopy.

Of note, the definition of macular edema was first made by slit lamp biomicroscopy. Thus, fluorescein angiography leakage without clinical thickening did not fulfill the definition of CSME according to the ETDRS criteria.

ETDRS asked three questions and provided answers:

1. Is photocoagulation effective in the treatment of macular edema?
   Focal photocoagulation reduced the risk of visual loss by approximately 50% in eyes with CSME. Visual loss was defined as the doubling of the visual angle or the loss of three lines or more using the ETDRS eye charts. Eyes with clinically significant edema with the central vision affected showed the greatest treatment benefit. Eyes with macular edema except without the characteristics meeting clinical significance did not demonstrate the same treatment benefit. Lastly, eyes with CSME except without involvement of the center of the macula showed a beneficial treatment effect midway between the two previously mentioned groups.[22]

   The greatest effect of this treatment was seen in eyes with visual acuity worse than 20/40. But all eyes demonstrated a favorable effect despite their visual acuity at entry. Although visual loss was significantly reduced, visual gain was minimal in those eyes with better than 20/40 vision at the onset of the study.

   The goal of treatment was to "maintain" visual acuity to prevent worsening of visual acuity caused by untreated macular edema, especially if clinical slit lamp, stereoscopic, biomicroscopic examination confirmed that the center of the macular was involved. In these cases, the ETDRS recommended prompt treatment, regardless of visual acuity, since it was statistically likely that visual loss will occur without laser.
2. Is aspirin beneficial to the treatment of DR?[24,25]
   The ETDRS found that daily ingestion of 650 mg of aspirin had no demonstrable effects on the progression of DR in 8 years of follow-up.[24] This aspirin study arm enrolled 3,711 patients with mild to severe nonproliferative or early PDR who were given 650 mg of aspirin or given placebo.
3. When to initiate photocoagulation for DR?
   In this part of the study, 3,711 patients with bilateral mild to severe nonproliferative or early proliferative retinopathy were enrolled. The eyes of these patients were classified into those with no macular edema, less severe retinopathy, and those with macular edema and more severe retinopathy (Table 3-2). One eye of each patient was randomized to early laser or deferral of treatment.[21–24]

The results of the study showed that the different types of laser treatment of full scatter or mild scatter photocoagulation were stated. Laser involving immediate full scatter reduced the threat of progression to high-risk retinopathy by 50%, whereas those strategies involving immediate mild scatter reduced the rate by 25%. However, the overall risk of visual loss was low for all eyes even with deferral of treatment. Eyes with more severe retinopathy and macular edema experienced only a 6.5% rate of visual loss at 5 years. No significant difference was noted in the rate of moderate or severe visual loss in eyes without macular edema between either treatment strategy or deferral of laser.

TABLE 3.2 Classification of DR

ETDRS levels of diabetic retinopathy

Nonproliferative diabetic retinopathy (NPDR)

Mild NPDR

At least one microaneurysm

Moderate NPDR

Hemorrhages or microaneurysms (H/Ma)

Soft exudates, venous beading (VB), and IRMAs definitely present.

Severe NPDR

H/Ma in all 4 quadrants

VB in 2 or more quadrants

IRMA in at least 1 quadrant

Very Severe NPDR

Any two or more of severe (NPDR) (above)

Proliferative diabetic retinopathy (PDR)

Early PDR

New vessels on the retina

Or new vessels on the optic nerve, less than standard photo 10A

High-Risk PDR

Eyes with three or four retinopathy risk factors are considered to be at highest risk for the development of severe visual loss.

1. Presence of new vessels.
2. Location of new vessels on or within 1 DD of the optic disc (NVD).
3. NVD and NVE: severity of new vessels defined for NVD as equal to or greater than standard photograph 10A or greater than one-fourth to one-third disc area in extent. For NVE, NVE equal to or greater than one-half disc area.
4. Vitreous or preretinal hemorrhage.

The results from this study showed that early laser reduced the risk of the need for vitrectomy and the risk of progression to high-risk retinopathy. The rate of progression from nonproliferative and early PDR to high-risk stages was discussed in the ETDRS.[26,27] Eyes with baseline, severe NPDR developed high-risk characteristics at a rate of 17% by the end of the first year, 44% by 3 years of follow-up, and 58% by 5 years of follow-up.

In summary, the acceleration of NPDR depended on severity of the retinal findings, such as intraretinal microvascular abnormalities (IRMAs) (Fig. 3-4), cotton-wool spots (Fig. 3-5), venous beading (Fig. 3-6), and venous loops, in two or more standardized photographic fields 4 to 7. The risk of attaining high-risk characteristics increased with time

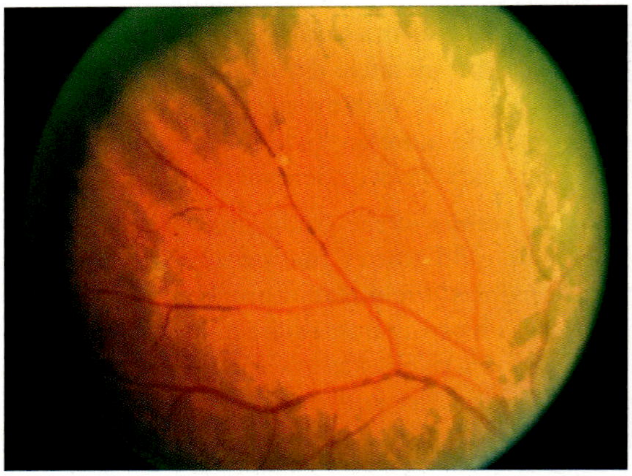

FIGURE 3-4. IRMA, standard photo 8A. (Courtesy of University of Wisconsin, Fundus Reading Center and Early Treatment Diabetic Retinopathy Study Research Group.)

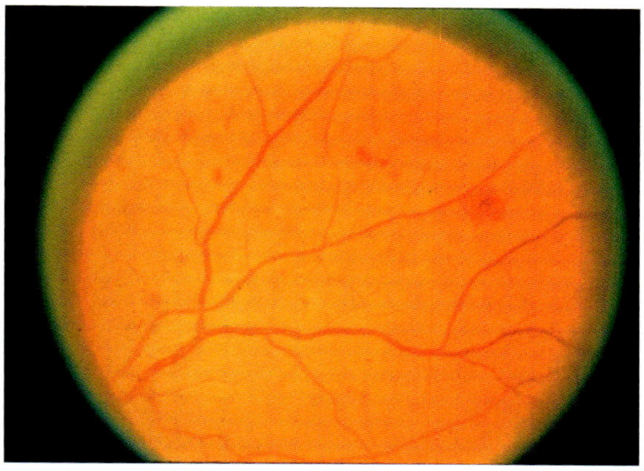

FIGURE 3-5. Cotton-wool spots, standard photo 2A. (Courtesy of university of Wisconsin, Fundus Reading Center and Early Treatment Diabetic Retinopathy Study Research Group.)

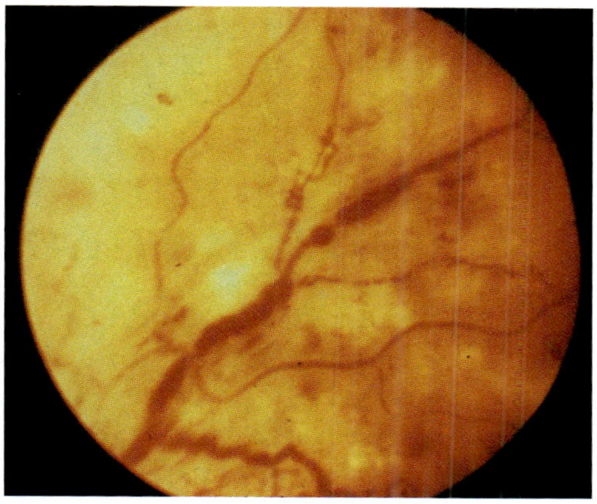

FIGURE 3-6. Venous beading.

and severity of disease seen on fundus examination.[26,27] In addition, reducing blood lipids and treating anemia slowed the progression of retinopathy. Improved glycemic control inhibited the progression of retinopathy as well.[28]

DIABETIC RETINOPATHY VITRECTOMY STUDY

The Diabetic Retinopathy Vitrectomy Study (DRVS) addressed the question of the timing of vitrectomy surgery for the management of PDR.[29] Between 1976 and 1980, the DRVS followed 744 eyes of 622 patients with severe PDR using conventional management such as laser photocoagulation. The eligibility criteria were that the patient had had a vitreous hemorrhage within 5 months and visual acuity of 5/200 or less. Patients eligible for the "very severe proliferative retinopathy with useful vision" group had extensive active fibrovascular proliferation and a visual acuity of 10/200 or better. Historically, DRVS was conducted at a time when most surgeons waited for the resolution of a vitreous hemorrhage for at least 1 year before performing vitrectomy.[30–35]

Of these eyes whose retina had four disc areas of new vessels, vision dropped from 10/30 to 10/50 at baseline to <5/200 at 2 years in 45% of the eyes. In eyes with baseline extramacular traction retinal detachments without active new vessels or vitreous hemorrhages, vision dropped to <5/200 in 14% of the eyes.[36]

Vitrectomy was needed in 25% of these eyes after 2 years of follow-up due to either new macular detachments or hemorrhage that did not clear after 1 year of follow-up.[37]

The DRVS defined Type 1 and Type 2 diabetes. Type 1 was defined as patients currently receiving insulin whose diabetes was diagnosed on or before age 20. Type 2 was defined as patients whose diabetes was diagnosed at 40 years or older, regardless of insulin use. An intermediate or mixed group was defined as patients whose diabetes was diagnosed between ages 21 and 39 years.

The DRVS found that there was a decisive advantage in early vitrectomy for Type 1 diabetes as compared with eyes in the control group at the 2-year follow-up visit.[37–39] The early treatment group maintained a higher proportion of eyes with 10/20 (36%) or better at the 2-year and 4-year follow-up periods, versus conventional treatment, in Type 1 diabetes.[40] By 4 years, it was 50% in the treated group versus 10% in the conventionally managed group that maintained 10/20 or better vision.

In Type 2 diabetes and the intermediate group, there was little difference between the two treatment groups at 2 years and 4 years of follow up.[40] Thus, the DRVS advocated early vitrectomy for eyes with severe visual loss from nonclearing vitreous hemorrhage of at least 5 months duration and they had vitrectomy performed in their sixth month of vitreous hemorrhage. The DRVS was a study performed when certain vitreoretinal techniques such as endophotocoagulation and micromanipulator instruments were not available.[36–40]

DIABETIC RETINOPATHY CLINICAL RESEARCH NETWORK

The Diabetic Retinopathy Clinical Research Network (DRCR.net), formed in 2002, was a multicentered, participatory group of academic medical centers and clinical practices with over 670 physicians throughout the United States focused on DME.[41] The study end points were visual acuity and OCT documented retinal thickness, and also included blood pressure and HbA1c measurements. The DRCR.net was funded by the National Eye Institute, part of the National Institutes of Health.[41]

There were four core centers within the DRCR.net that supported the operation and supplied the leadership of its ongoing studies. The core centers were Wilmer Ophthalmological Institute at Johns Hopkins in Baltimore, MD, the Coordinating Center at Jaeb Center for Health Research in Tampa, FL, the Fundus Photograph Reading Center at University of Wisconsin-Madison in Madison, WI, and the National Eye Institute in Washington, DC. These study groups were multicentered and randomized. However, they were on a smaller scale than that of the ETDRS or DRVS. These studies have been focusing on what will be of interest to retinal surgeons in the 21st century.[42]

Retinal Thickness on Stratus Optical Coherence Tomography in People with Diabetes and Minimal or No Diabetic Retinopathy

This 2008 study found that in minimal or no diabetic retinopathy (NDR), there was a difference between genders in the average central subfield thickness OCT 201 ± 22 μm: for males, average central subfield thickness was 209 ± 18 μm versus 194 ± 23 μm in females.[42] Thus, central subfield thickness in people with NDR or minimal DR was not statistically significantly different from that in controls (people without diabetes).[42]

A Pilot Study of Laser Photocoagulation for DME

Ongoing studies involve the use of macular or grid laser for the treatment of DME with the use of the OCT as a study end point. The study "A Pilot Study of Laser Photocoagulation for Diabetic Macular Edema" began its enrollment in September 2003 and was completed in August 2007.[43–45] The various results have been listed below.

A Pilot Study of Peribulbar Triamcinolone Acetonide for DME

Another small study of the DRCR.net is "A Pilot Study of Peribulbar Triamcinolone Acetonide for Diabetic Macular Edema."[46] This study planned to randomize 100 patients. A minimum of 40 eyes that have not received prior laser (or other treatment) for DME were randomized. Triamcinolone acteonide has been used since the 1990s, but no large clinical trial has been organized until now.

The objectives of this study were

1. To estimate the incidence of improvement of DME following a posterior peribulbar 40 mg injection of triamcinolone acetonide compared with laser.
2. To estimate the incidence of improvement of DME following an anterior peribulbar 20 mg triamcinolone acetonide injection compared with laser.

3. To estimate the incidence of intraocular pressure elevation and other complications with each type of injection.
4. To provide preliminary data comparing the incidence of improvement of DME with a peribulbar triamcininolone acetonide injection alone versus peribulbar triamcinolone acetonide injection followed by laser photocoagulation.

Visual acuity, OCT, and IOP were to be taken at the onset of the study and then at the first month. Afterward, visual acuity, OCT, and IOP were taken at months 2, 4, 8, 12, 24, and 36. Blood pressure was examined at onset, months 12, 24, and 36. HbA1c was taken at onset, months 4, 8, 12, 24, and 36.

Primary outcomes were measured by visual acuity on ETDRS eye charts. Secondary outcomes were measured by OCT: persistence or recurrence of DME either re-treated or meeting the criteria for re-treatment during the first 8 months; change in the area of retinal thickening and in the threat to or the involvement of the center of the macula which was estimated in color fundus photographs. The main safety outcomes were intraocular pressure elevation, glaucoma, cataractogenesis, ptosis, and complications of the injection procedure.

An Observational Study of the Development of DME Following Scatter Laser Photocoagulation[46]

The objectives of this study, utilizing a sample size of 150 study eyes, were the following:

1. To determine the incidence and extent of macular edema following scatter laser using OCT in eyes without macular edema prior to laser.
2. To explore whether the incidence and extent of macular edema variation according the number of sittings included in the treatment regimen.

The eyes under study received scatter laser according to two regimens:

1. One sitting with a minimum of 1,200 to a maximum of 1,600 burns, from peripheral arcades to beyond the equator.
2. Four sittings, each separated by 4 weeks, with 300 burns in each of the first two sittings and investigator judgment for the number of burns for the third and fourth sittings as long as the sum total of the four sittings was between 1,200 and 1,600 burns.

Primary outcome was the retinal thickening measured by OCT. Secondary outcome was measured by ETDRS visual acuity.

A Phase 2 Evaluation of Anti-VEGF Therapy for DME: Bevacizumab (Avastin)[46]

The objectives were

1. To assess the dose and the dose interval–related effects of intravitreally administered bevacizumab on central retinal thickness and visual acuity in subjects with DME.
2. To assess the effect of intravitreal bevacizumab combined with macular photocoagulation in DME.
3. To assess the safety of intravitreal bevacizumab in subjects with DME.

However, this study was not designed to study the efficacy of bevacizumab. This study was to determine if a phase 3 trial has merit in the future. The planned duration of follow-up was 70 weeks. Outcomes were to be measured by OCT and ETDRS visual acuity.

The major eligibility criteria included the following: age of the patient should be 18 years or greater and the study eye has a better corrected ETDRS score of 20/320 or better and ETDRS score of 20/32 or worse. The fellow eye has acuity of 20/400 or better and has not had anti-VEGF treatment within the past 3 months and there is no expectation of such treatment in the next 3 months.

The treatment was randomly assigned to the study eye:

1. Laser at baseline: If edema was present at 12 weeks, the eye can be treated with two intravitreal injections of 1.25 mg bevacizumab spaced 6 weeks apart.
2. 1.25 mg intravitreal injection of bevacizumab at baseline and 6 weeks.
3. 2.5 mg intravitreal injection of bevacizumab at baseline and 6 weeks.
4. 1.25 mg intravitreal injection of bevacizumab at baseline (sham injection at 6 weeks).
5. 1.25 mg intravitreal injection of bevacizumab at baseline, laser photocoagulation at 3 weeks, and intravitreal injection of 1.25 mg bevacizumab at 6 weeks.

Course of Response to Focal Photocoagulation for DME[46]

The eligibility criteria included age greater than or equal to 18 years, Type 1 or Type 2 diabetes, and DME involving the center of the macula (OCT central subfield thickness greater than or equal to 250 μm). The planned sample size was 110 eyes. The main outcome measurement was OCT.

OCT and visual acuity by ETDRS chart testing was done at onset, 8 weeks, 16 weeks, 24 weeks, 32 weeks, 40 weeks, and 48 weeks. The investigator intended to treat the DME with focal photocoagulation.

Comparison of Time-Domain OCT and Fundus Photographic Assessments of Retinal Thickening in Eyes with DME[47]

Two hundred fifty-nine participants enrolled in this trial. Type 2 diabetes was present in 93% of the participants. Mean duration of diabetes was 14 years and mean HbA1c was 8.1% (range = 4.6%–15%). Mean age of the study participants was 59 years. The study found that there was a moderate correlation between OCT and fundus photography of retinal thickening in patients with DME, slightly less correlation between OCT and vision and fundus photography and vision. Thus, OCT and fundus photography provide adjunctive, complementary information but neither can be a surrogate for visual acuity.

DME: What is Focal and What is Diffuse[48]

It is still unresolved as to what is diffuse and what is focal in the literature. Thus, further studies are needed.

PROTOCOL A—LASER PHOTOCOAGULATION OF DME

Comparison of the Modified ETDRS and Mild Macular Grip Laser Photocoagulation Strategies for DME[49]

Two hundred sixty-three subjects were evaluated with previously untreated DME. They were randomized to receive ETDRS laser treatment of direct/grid laser photocoagulation versus mild macular grid (MMG) laser. The MMG laser was potentially milder but more extensive. MMG grid meant mild burns occurred throughout the macula whether or not edema was present. About 162 eyes received the ETDRS technique of laser and 161 eyes received the MMG laser technique of laser. The main outcome measure was the change in OCT measurements at 12 months of follow-up. It was found that the MMG technique was less effective in reducing OCT measured retinal thickening than the ETDRS technique. However, the visual acuity after 12 months was not significantly different. Thus, modified ETDRS focal photocoagulation should continue to be the standard approach for DME.

PROTOCOL B—INTRAVITREAL TRIAMCINOLONE ACETONIDE VERSUS LASER STUDY

A Randomized Clinical Trial Comparing Intravitreal Triamcinolone Acetonide and Focal/Grid Photocoagulation for DME[50]

Eight hundred forty eyes of 693 patients with DME with visual acuity of 20/40 to 20/320 were included in the study. Of the 840 eyes, 330 eyes were randomized to focal/grid photocoagulation, 256 eyes were randomized to receive 1mg of preservative-free, intravitreal triamcinolone, and 254 eyes were randomized to receive 4 mg of preservative-free, intravitreal triamcinolone. Main outcome measures were visual acuity and OCT. Side effects were 10 mm Hg increased in 4% of the triamcinolone-treated eyes. Mean visual acuity was better than that of the laser group versus either triamcinolone-treated group.

Over a 2-year period, focal/grid photocoagulation was more effective and had fewer side effects than 1 mg or 4 mg doses of intravitreal triamcinolone for most patients with DME. The study supports that focal/grid photocoagulation was the standard with which other treatments were compared in clinical trials of DME.

PROTOCOL C—OCT DIURNAL VARIATION STUDY

Diurnal Variation in Retinal Thickening Measurement by OCT in Center-involved DME[51]

Using OCT, slight decreases were noted in retinal thickening in 156 eyes of 96 clinically diagnosed DME patients. Most eyes in this study showed little change of significance in the OCT central subfield thickening between 8 AM and 4 PM.

Reproducibility of Macular Thickness and Volume using Zeiss Optical Coherence Tomography in Patients with DME[52]

Central subfield thickness measurements were more reproducible than for other center point measurements. Retinal thickness expressed as a percent change was more reliable than absolute change. A change in central subfield thickness >11% was likely to be real. Scans with a standard deviation at the central point of ≥10% were less reproducible and thus may not be reliable as a method of documenting the change of retinal thickness between examinations. There was no effect in correlating central subfield thickness changes to the presence of cystoid macular edema, subretinal fluid, vitreomacular traction, or decreased visual acuity.

PROTOCOL E—PERIBULBAR TRIAMCINOLONE ACETONIDE STUDY

A Randomized Trial of Peribulbar Triamcinolone Acetonide with and without Focal Photocoagulation for Mild DME: A Pilot Study[53]

One hundred twenty-nine eyes of 109 patients were studied. They had mild DME and visual acuity of 20/40 or better. In cases of DME with good visual acuity, peribulbar triamcinolone with or without focal photocoagulation was not beneficial. A phase

3 clinical trial was warranted according to the authors of the Diabetic Retinopathy Clinical Research Network.

PROTOCOL F—PRP STUDY

Observational Study of the Development of DME Following Panretinal (Scatter) Photocoagulation Given in 1 or 4 Sittings[54]

Clinically meaningful differences were not found in OCT thickness or vision after prior photocoagulation (PRP) in one or four sessions.

PROTOCOL G—SUBCLINICAL DIABETIC MACULAR EDEMA STUDY

Retinal Thickness on Stratus Optical Coherence Tomography in People with Diabetes and Minimal or NDR[55]

Central subfield thickness on OCT scans in diabetic patients with minimal or NDR was similar to normal controls. There was a difference in central subfield thickness in men (209 ± 18 μm) versus women (194 ± 23 μm).

PROTOCOL H—BEVACIZUMAB (AVASTIN) PHASE 2 STUDY

A Phase 2 Randomized Clinical Trial of Intravitreal Bevacizumab for DME[56]

One hundred twenty-one eyes of 121 patients with DME with Snellen visual acuity of 20/32 to 20/320 were included in the study. Random assignment was made to five groups:

Group A: Focal laser at baseline (19 eyes)
Group B: Intravitreal injection of bevacizumab of 1.25 mg at baseline (22 eyes)
Group C: Intravitreal injection of bevacizumab of 2.5 mg at baseline and at 6 weeks (24 eyes)
Group D: Intravitreal injection of bevacizumab of 1.25 mg at baseline and sham injection at 6 weeks (22 eyes)
Group E: Intravitreal injection of bevacizumab of 1.25 mg at baseline and photocoagulation at 6 weeks (22 eyes)

Combining laser with intravitreal bevacizumab had no short-term benefits or untoward side effects. Compared with Group A, Groups B and C had a greater reduction in central subfield thickness reduction at 3 weeks and an average of one line improvement of visual acuity at 12 weeks. Groups B versus C had no significant OCT thickness or visual acuity improvements. Laser with intravitreal bevacizumab had no short-term benefits or untoward side effects. The study's conclusion was that intravitreal bevacizumab was helpful for some DME eyes in improving visual acuity but a phase 3 clinical trial was needed to ascertain whether treatment will be beneficial.

PROTOCOL H—BEVACIZUMAB (AVASTIN) PHASE 2 STUDY

Agreement Between Clinician and Reading Center Gradings of Diabetic Retinopathy Severity Level at Baseline in a Phase 2 Study of Intravitreal Bevacizumab for DME[57]

Clinicians grading scale used four levels: microaneurysms only, mild/moderate NPDR, severe NPDR, and PDR or PRP or both. The Reading Center used eight levels: microaneurysms only, mild NPDR, moderate NPDR, moderately severe NPDR, severe NPDR, mild PDR, moderate PDR, and high-risk PDR. The results showed that there was agreement in 89/118 (75%) eyes. In six eyes where there was a disagreement, five of the six eyes had subtle retinal neovascularization and one had a small preretinal hemorrhage found only in photographs. The study concluded that clinician grading placed eyes in broad baseline categories and that clinician grading had only moderate agreement with the Reading Center.

THE READ TRIAL

The study, Ranibizumab for the Edema of the Macula in Diabetes (READ) was sponsored by the Juvenile Diabetes Research Foundation to evaluate ranibizumab for the treatment of DME. The study rationale was based on the pathobiology of DME and the correlation between VEGF levels in aqueous and vitreous humor and neovascularization in diabetic patients with DR.[58,59]

The Phase I study, called READ-I, enrolled 20 patients with DME treated with repeated intravitreal injections of 0.5 mg of ranibizumab. The 0.5 mg dose of ranibizumab showed efficacy and safety for the 20 patients. The intravitreal injections of ranibizumab were given at months 1, 2, 4, and 6. By month 7, which was 1 month after the last intravitreal injection of ranibizumab, the median reduction of the excess foveal thickness as measured by OCT was 97%. There was a median improvement of 10 letters.

The READ-2 was the phase 2 randomized, multicentered, clinical trial sponsored by the Juvenile Diabetes Research Foundation. This part of the study enrolled 126 patients from 14 clinical centers throughout the United States.[60]

The primary end point would be the proportion of patients to have gained 15 letters or more and achieve a final vision of 50 letters (20/25) or better if baseline visual acuity is 40 letters (20/40) or better at 6 months. Eligibility criteria were (a) ETDRS visual acuity of 20/40 or worse, but better than or equal to 20/320 due to foveal thickening from DME; (b) baseline foveal thickness of 250 μm on OCT. The patients could have Type 1 or Type 2 diabetes.

Patients were randomized into three treatment groups: (a) ranibizumab only, (b) laser, and (c) ranibizumab and laser. In Group 1 (ranibizumab only), the patients were to receive injections of ranibizumab at baseline, months 1, 3, and 5 for a total of four injections. At the 6 month visit, the patients were reevaluated. If the patients met the re-treatment criterion, they received another injection of ranibizumab. After 18 months, the patients were reexamined every 8 weeks. If at any visit the patient met the re-treatment criterion, the patient received another injection. The re-treatment criterion was an absolute retinal thickness in OCT central subfield thickness of >250 μm at the time of study visit.

In Group 2 (laser), the patients received laser at baseline and were then reevaluated at month 3. If they met the re-treatment criterion, they were re-lasered. The patients returned at month 6, the primary time point. At month 6, if the patient needed re-treatment, he or she was given the option of having more laser or ranibizumab. Afterward, the patient returned every 2 months until month 24. If the patient met the re-treatment criterion, either laser or ranibizumab can be administered at the discretion of the investigator.

Laser can be administered at months 3, 6, 10, 14, 18, and 22. Ranibizumab can be administered at month 6, for every 2 months thereafter, if the re-treatment criteria was met. At months 8, 12, 16, 20, 24, ranibizumab or no treatment was the option for the patient. Laser was not an option at those visits. The re-treatment criterion was an absolute retinal thickness in OCT central subfield thickness of >250 μm at time of study visit.

Group 3 (ranibizumab and laser) patients received one injection of ranibizumab at baseline followed by laser on day 7. The patients were reexamined at month 3, where the investigator gave another injection of ranibizumab and performed laser on day 7. Then, the patients were reassessed at month 6, as in both Groups 1 and 2. If the Group 3 patients met the criterion for re-treatment, then the investigator gave another injection of ranibizumab and laser on day 7, unless the investigator felt that the laser was not appropriate and laser was omitted. The patients were followed every 12 weeks until month 24, the secondary time end point for all three study groups. At any study visit, if the re-treatment criterion was met, the investigator injected ranibizumab and performed laser at day 7. The Re-treatment criterion was an absolute retinal thickness in OCT central subfield thickness of >250 μm at time of study visit.

THE ACCORD STUDY

The Action to Control Cardiovascular Risk in Diabetes (ACCORD) Study was a randomized clinical trial to determine change in cardiovascular morbidity and mortality in participants with Type 2 diabetes by intensive blood glucose control, intensive blood pressure control, lowering serum triglycerides, and raising serum high density lipoprotein.[61] It recruited 10,251 patients. There was the intensive group of 5,128 patients and standard group of 5,123 patients.

The key inclusion criteria were (a) stable Type 2 diabetes; (b) glycosylated hemoglobin of 7.5% to 11%; (c) age 40 to 79 years with cardiovascular disease (CVD); (d) age 55 to 79 years with anatomic evidence of significant atherosclerosis, albuminuria, left ventricular hypertrophy or at least two additional risk factors for CVD; dyslipidemia, hypertension, currently smoking, and obesity.

The mean age of the recruited patients was 62.2 years with a median glycosylated hemoglobin of 8.1%. The intensive therapy group had a targeted HbA1c below 6.0%. The standard treatment group had a targeted HbA1c of 7.0% to 7.9%. Of these patients, 38% were women and 35% had a previous cardiovascular event. The primary outcome was a composite of nonfatal myocardial infarction, nonfatal stroke, or death from CVD. The finding of higher mortality in the intensive therapy group led to a discontinuation of intensive therapy after a mean of 3.5 years of follow-up. About 257 patients of the intensive therapy group versus 203 patients of the standard therapy group died ($p = 0.04$).

The conclusion of the ACCORD Study showed that the use of intensive therapy to target normal HbA1c levels for 3.5 years increased mortality and did not significantly decrease major cardiovascular events. The findings delineated the previously unrecognized harm of intensive glucose lowering in high-risk patients with Type 2 diabetes.

The ACCORD Eye Study: A Substudy of the ACCORD Study

The ACCORD Eye study evaluated the primary microvascular outcome of ACCORD.[62] The main outcome variable was the progression of DR of at least three steps on the ETDRS scale. The study enrolled 3,537 patients. The 4-year follow-up will be available in 2010.

REFERENCES

1. Meyer-Schwickerath G. *Light Coagulation.* St Louis: CV Mosby Co; 1960.
2. Meyer-Schwickerath G, Gerke E. Bjerrum Lecture: Treatment of diabetic retinopathy with photocoagulation. *Acta Ophthalmol.* 1983;61:756–768.
3. Aiello LM, Beethan WP, Balodimas MC. Ruby laser photocoagulation in treatment of diabetic proliferating retinopathy. In: Goldberg MF, Fine SL, eds. *Symposium on the Treatment of Diabetic Retinopathy.* Public Health Service Publication No. 1890, Washington, DC: US Government Printing Office; 1969.
4. Okum E. Summary of papers on treatment techniques in photocoagulation. In: Goldberg MF, Fine SL, eds. *Symposium on the Treatment of Diabetic Retinopathy.* Public Health Service Publication No. 1890, Washington, DC: US Government Printing Office; 1969.
5. Zweng HC. The treatment of diabetic retinopathy by laser photocoagulation. In: Goldberg MF, Fine SL, eds. *Symposium on the Treatment of Diabetic Retinopathy.* Public Health Service Publication No. 1890, Washington, DC: US Government Printing Office; 1969.
6. British Multicentre Study Group. Photocoagulation for PDR. A randomized trial using xenon arc. *Diabetologia.* 1984;26:109–115.
7. Diabetic Retinopathy Study Research Group. Preliminary report on effects of photocoagulation therapy. *Am J Ophthalmol.* 1976;81:383–396.
8. Diabetic Retinopathy Study Research Group. Photocoagulation treatment of proliferative diabetic retinopathy: The second report of diabetic retinopathy/vitrectomy study findings. *Am J Ophthalmol.* 1979;97:654–655.
9. Diabetic Retinopathy Study Research Group. DRS Report No. 3: Four risk factors for severe visual loss in diabetic retinopathy. *Arch Ophthalmol.* 1979;97:654–655.
10. Diabetic Retinopathy Study Research Group. DRS Report No. 6: Design, Methods and Baseline results. *Invest Ophthalmol Vis Sci.* 1981;21:149–209.
11. Diabetic Retinopathy Study Research Group. DRS Report No. 7: A modification on the Airlie House classification of diabetic retinopathy. *Invest Ophthalmol Vis Sci.* 1981;21(part 2):210–226.
12. Goldberg MF, Jampol LM. Knowledge of diabetic retinopathy before and 18 years after the Airlie House Symposium on treatment of diabetic retinopathy. *Ophthalmology.* 1987;94:741–746.
13. Diabetic Retinopathy Study Research Group. DRS Report No 8: Photocoagulation treatment of proliferative diabetic retinopathy; clinical applications of DRS findings. *Ophthalmology.* 1981;88:583–600.
14. Diabetic Retinopathy Study Research Group. DRS Report No 4: Diabetes 1979. International Congress Series No. 500. *Proceedings of the 10th Congress of the Internal Diabetes Federation*, Vienna, Austria, September 1979; 789–794.
15. Diabetic Retinopathy Study Research Group. DRS Report No 14: Indications for photocoagulation treatment of diabetic retinopathy. *Int Ophthalmol Clin.* 1987;274:239–252.
16. Diabetic Retinopathy Study Research Group. DRS Report No 5: Photocoagulation treatment of proliferative diabetic retinopathy: Relationship of adverse treatment effects to retinopathy severity. *Dev Ophthalmol.* 1981;2:248–261.
17. Ferric FL, Podgor MJ, Davis MD, Diabetic Retinopathy Study Research Group. DRS Report No 12: Macular edema in diabetic retinopathy study patients. *Ophthalmology.* 1987;94:754–760.
18. Early Treatment Diabetic Retinopathy Study Research Group. DRS Report No 1: Photocoagulation for diabetic macular edema. *Arch Ophthalmol.* 1985;103:1796–1806.
19. Ferris FL. Photocoagulation for diabetic macular edema: Results of the Early Treatment Diabetic Retinopathy Study. *Contemp Ophthalmic Forum.* 1986;4:25–31.
20. Early Treatment Diabetic Retinopathy Study Research Group. ETDRS Report No. 2: Treatment techniques diabetic macular edema. *Ophthalmology.* 1987;94:761–774.
21. Early Treatment Diabetic Retinopathy Study Research Group. ETDRS Report No. 3: Techniques for scatter and local photocoagulation treatment of diabetic retinopathy. *Int Ophthalmol Clin.* 1987;27:254–264.
22. Early Treatment Diabetic Retinopathy Study Research Group. ETDRS Report No. 4: Photocoagulation for diabetic macular edema. *Int Ophthalmol Clin.* 1987; 27:265–272.
23. Early Treatment Diabetic Retinopathy Study Research Group. ETDRS Report No. 7: Early treatment diabetic retinopathy study design and baseline patient characteristics. *Ophthalmology.* 1991;98:741–756.
24. Early Treatment Diabetic Retinopathy Study Research Group. ETDRS Report No. 8: Effects of aspirin treatment on diabetic retinopathy. *Ophthalmology.* 1991;98:757–765.
25. DAMAD Study Group. Effect of ASA alone and ASA plus dipyridamole in early diabetic retinopathy. *Diabetes.* 1989;38:491–498.
26. Early Treatment Diabetic Retinopathy Study Research Group. ETDRS Report No. 9: Early Photocoagulation for diabetic retinopathy. *Ophthalmology.* 1991;98:766–785.
27. Early Treatment Diabetic Retinopathy Study Research Group. ETDRS Report No. 12: Fundus photographic risk factors for progression of diabetic retinopathy. *Ophthalmology.* 1991;98:823–833.
28. Davis MD, Fisher MR, Gaugnon RE, et al. Risk factors for high risk proliferative diabetic retinopathy and severe visual loss: Early Treatment Diabetic Retinopathy Study No.18. *Invest Ophthalmol Vis Sci.* 1998;39:233–252.
29. Machemer R, Buettner H, Norton EWD, et al. Vitrectomy: A pars plana approach. *Trans Am Acad Ophthalmol Otolaryngol.* 1971;75:813–820.
30. Machmer R, Blankenship G. Vitrectomy for proliferative diabetic retinopathy associated with vitreous hemorrhage. *Ophthalmology.* 1981;88:643–646.
31. Shea M. Early vitrectomy in proliferative diabetic retinopathy. *Arch Ophthalmol.* 1983;101:1204–1205.
32. Michels RG, Rice TA, Rice EF. Vitrectomy for diabetic vitreous hemorrhage. *Ophthalmology.* 1983;95:12–21.
33. O' Hanley GP, Canny CLB. Diabetic dense premacular hemorrhage. *Am J Ophthalmol.* 1983;95:507–511.
34. Ramsay RC, Knoblock WH, Cantrill HL. Timing of vitrectomy for active proliferative diabetic retinopathy. *Ophthalmology.* 1986;93:283–289.
35. Aaberg TM, Abrams GW. Changing indications and techniques for vitrectomy in management of complications of diabetic retinopathy. *Ophthalmology.* 1987;94:775–779.
36. Diabetic Retinopathy Vitrectomy Study Group. DRVS Report No 1: Two-year Course of visual acuity in severe proliferative diabetic retinopathy with conventional management. *Ophthalmology.* 1985;92:492–502.

37. Diabetic Retinopathy Vitrectomy Study Group. DRVS Report No 2: Early vitrectomy for severe vitreous hemorrhage in diabetic retinopathy. Two-year results of a randomized trial. *Arch Ophthalmol.* 1985;103:1644–1652.
38. Diabetic Retinopathy Vitrectomy Study Group. DRVS Report No 3: Early vitrectomy for severe proliferative diabetic retinopathy in eyes with useful vision. Results of a randomized trial. *Ophthalmology.* 1988;95:1307–1320.
39. Diabetic Retinopathy Vitrectomy Study Group. DRVS Report No 4: Early vitrectomy for severe proliferative diabetic retinopathy in eyes with useful vision. Clinical application of results of a randomized trial. *Ophthalmology.* 1988;95: 1321–1334.
40. Diabetic Retinopathy Vitrectomy Study Group. DRVS Report No 5: Early vitrectomy for severe vitreous hemorrhage in diabetic retinopathy. Four-year results of a randomized trial. *Arch Ophthalmol.* 1990;108:958–964.
41. www.drcr.net. Accessed 12 February 2009.
42. Bressler NM, Edwards AR, Antoszyk AN, et al. Retinal thickness on stratus optical coherence tomography in people with diabetes and minimal or no diabetic retinopathy. *Am J Ophthalmol.* 2008;145:894–901.
43. Diabetic Retinopathy Clinical Research Network, Browning DJ, Glassman AR, Aiello LP, et al. Relationship between optical coherence tomography-measured central retinal thickness and visual acuity in diabetic macular edema. *Ophthalmology.* 2007;114:525–536.
44. Davis MD, Bressler SB, Aiello LP, et al. Diabetic Retinopathy Clinical Research Network Study Group. Comparison of time-domain OCT and fundus photographic assessments of retinal thickening in eyes with diabetic macular edema. *Invest Ophthalmol Vis Sci.* 2008;49:1745–1752.
45. Writing Committee for the Diabetic Retinopathy Clinical Research Network, Fong DS, Strauber SF, Aiello LP, et al. Comparison of the modified Early Treatment Diabetic Retinopathy Study and mild macular grid laser photocoagulation strategies for diabetic macular edema. *Arch Ophthalmol.* 2007;125:469–480.
46. http://public.drcr.net/publications/PublicationList.php. Accessed 8 March 2009.
47. Davis MD, Bressler SB, Aiello LP, et al. Comparison of time-domain OCT and fundus photographic assessments of retinal thickening in eyes with diabetic macular edema. *Invest Ophthalmol Vis Sci.* 2008;49:1745–1752.
48. Browning DJ, Altawel MM, Bressler NM, et al. Diabetic Macular Edema: What is focal and what is diffuse. *Am J Ophthalmol.* 2008;146:649–655.
49. Writing committee of DRCRnet. Comparison of the modified early treatment diabetic retinopathy study and mild macular grip laser photocoagulation strategies for diabetic macular edema. *Arch Ophthalmol.* 2007;125:469–480.
50. DRCR network. A randomized clinical trial comparing intravitreal triamcinolone acetonide and focal/grid photocoagulation for diabetic macular edema. *Ophthalmology.* 2008;115:1447–1459.
51. DRCR network. Diurnal variation in retinal thickening measurement by oct in center-involved diabetic macular edema. *Arch Ophthalmol.* 2006;124:1701–1707.
52. DRCR Network. Reproducibility of macular thickness and volume using zeiss optical coherence tomography in patients with diabetic macular edema. *Ophthalmology.* 2007;114:1520–1525.
53. DRCT Network. A randomized trial of peribulbar triamcinolone acetonide with and without focal photocoagulation for mild diabetic macular edema: A pilot study. *Ophthalmology.* 2007;114:1190–1196.
54. DRCR Network. Observational study of the development of diabetic macular edema following panretinal (scatter) photocoagulation given in 1 or 4 sittings. *Arch Ophthalmol.* 2009;127:132–140.
55. Bressler NM, Edwards AR, Antonszyk AN, et al. Retinal thickness on stratus optical coherence tomography in people with diabetes and minimal or no diabetic retinopathy. *Am J Ophthalmol.* 2008;145:894–901.
56. DRCR Network. A phase 2 randomized clinical trial of intravitreal bevacizumab for diabetic macular edema. *Ophthalmology.* 2007;114:1860–1867.
57. Scott IU, Bressler NM, Bressler SB, et al. Agreement between clinician and reading center gradings of diabetic retinopathy severity level at baseline in a phase 2 study of intravitreal bevacizumab for diabetic macular edema. *Retina.* 2008;28:36–40.
58. Aiello L, Avery R, Arrigg P, et al. Vascular endothelial growth factor in ocular fluid of patients with diabetic retinopathy and other retinal disorders. *N Engl J Med.* 1994;331:1480–1487.
59. Nguyen QD, Shah M, Tatlipinar S, et al. Vascular endothelial growth factor is a critical stimulus for diabetic macular edema. *Am J Ophthalmol.* 2006;142:961–969.
60. Do DV, READ-2 Research Group. The READ trial: Ranibizumab in the treatment of diabetic macular edema. *Presented at the Annual Retina Subspecialty Day 2008.* Atlanta, 8 November 2008.
61. The ACCORD Study Group. Effects of intensive glucose lowering in type 2 diabetes. *N Engl J Med.* 2008;358: 2545–2559.
62. Chew EY, Ambrosius WT, Howard LT, et al. for the ACCORD Study Group. Rationale, design, and methods of the action to control cardiovascular risk in Diabetes Eye Study (ACCORD-EYE). *Am J Cardiol.* 2007;99:103i–111i.

CHAPTER 4

Diagnostic Testing

FUNDUS PHOTOGRAPHY

Standard fundus photography at the ophthalmologist's office now includes a basic digital funduscopic camera or a wide-field nonmydriatic camera. In fact, many optometric offices have nonmydriatic cameras. Operating nonmydriatic cameras requires no training, and hence no need for skilled ophthalmic photographers. The ophthalmologist has instant documentation to show to the patient. The nonmydriatic camera requires a pupil size of at least 3.7 mm in order to obtain a good quality retinal image.

The regular, digital fundus camera is a specialized low-power microscope with an attached camera designed to photograph the interior of the eye, the retina, optic disc, and macula. The optical design of the camera is based on the principle of the monocular indirect ophthalmoscope. The fundus camera provides an upright magnified view of the fundus. A typical camera has views of 30, 35, or 50 degrees of the retinal area. The camera's 2.5× magnification allows some variation of the magnification through auxiliary lenses from 15 degrees, which provides 5× magnification, to 140 degrees with a wide angle lens, which minifies the image by half.

The observation and illumination systems follow dissimilar paths. The observation light is focused via a series of lenses through a donut-shaped aperture. It then passes through a central aperture to form an annulus before passing through the camera objective lens and through the cornea onto the retina.

The light reflected from the retina is passed through the unilluminated hole in the donut, all formed by the camera's internal illumination system. Because the light paths of the two systems are independent, reflections of the light source captured in the formed image are minimal.

The image forming rays continue toward the low-powered telescopic eyepiece. When the button is pressed to take a picture, a mirror interrupts the path of the illumination system slowing the light from the flash bulb to pass into the eye. Simultaneously, a mirror falls in front of the observation telescope and redirects the light onto the capturing medium, typically a film or digital charge-coupled device. Because of the eye's tendency to accommodate while looking through a telescope, it is imperative that the exiting vergence is parallel in order for a focused image to be formed on the capturing medium.

Because of this accommodation, nonmydriatic cameras are not as successful as the regular fundus cameras in recording the details of the retina. However, if the patient's eye is dilated, the nonmydriatic camera can be effective.

In color fundus photography, the retina is illuminated by white light and examined in full color. Color fundus photography is the standard photograph in ophthalmology (Fig. 4-1).

In red-free photography, the imaging light is filtered to remove red colors, improving contrast of vessels and other structures. Red-free photographs show small hemorrhages, microaneurysms, and hard exudates with more clarity than color fundus photos (Fig. 4-2).

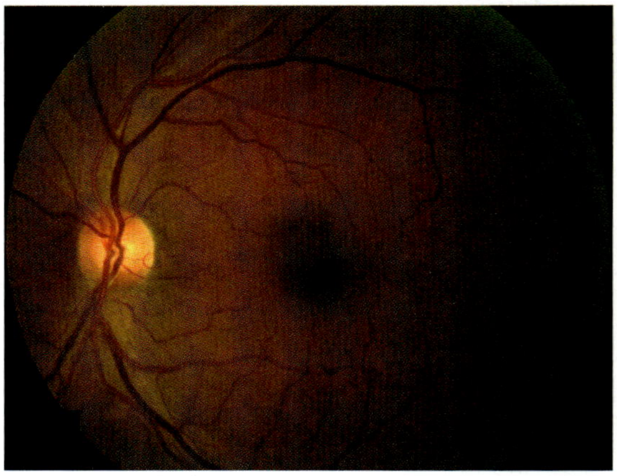

FIGURE 4-1. Color fundus photograph of microaneurysms.

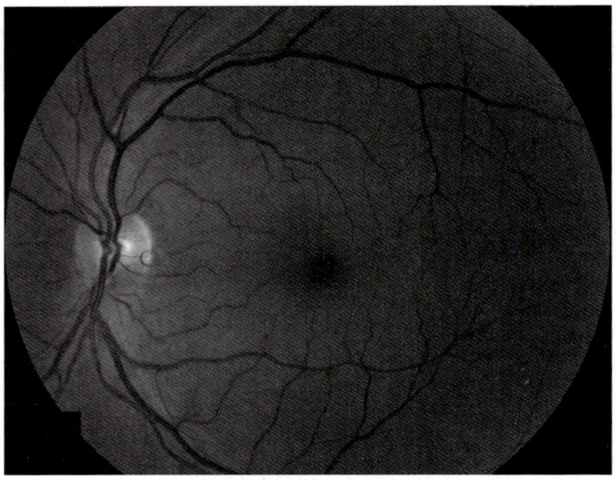

FIGURE 4-2. Red-free photograph of Figure 4-1, microaneurysms are shown clearly.

FLUORESCEIN ANGIOGRAPHY AND INDOCYANINE GREEN ANGIOGRAPHY

In fluorescein angiography, the vessels are brought into high contrast by the intravenous injection of a fluorescent dye. The retina is illuminated with an excitation color which fluoresces the light of another color where the dye is present. By using a filter to exclude the excitation color and passing the fluorescent color, a very high contrast image of the vessels is produced. A timed sequence of photos showing the progression of the dye into the vessels reveals the flow dynamic and the different layers of the retina. Thus, different areas of the retinal architecture are delineated (Fig. 4-3).

Indocyanine green dye angiography (ICG) is another method to capture the flow of the dye in the deeper tissue, the choroid. In approximately 15% of patients with nonproliferative diabetic retinopathy, ICG can reveal additional microvascular complications in diabetes not seen with conventional fluorescein angiography[1] (Fig. 4-4).

Seven Standard Diabetic Photographic Fields

This is a technique of taking a series of photos, using the stereoscopic setting on the digital fundus camera. All of these fields utilize a 35-degree field of view. Field 1 is centered

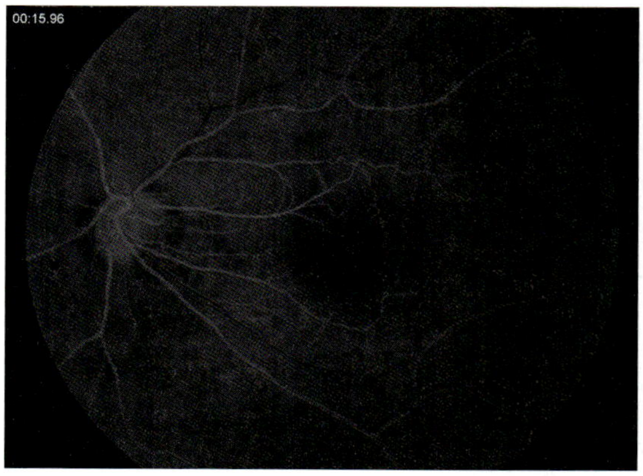

FIGURE 4-3. Fluorescein angiogram sequence, beginning with AV phase and progressing to midtransit.

FIGURE 4-4. Indocyanine green dye photograph.

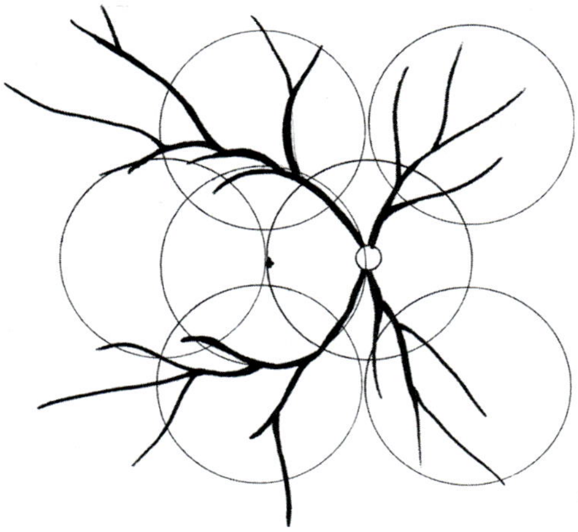

FIGURE 4-5. Diagram of seven standard photographic fields.

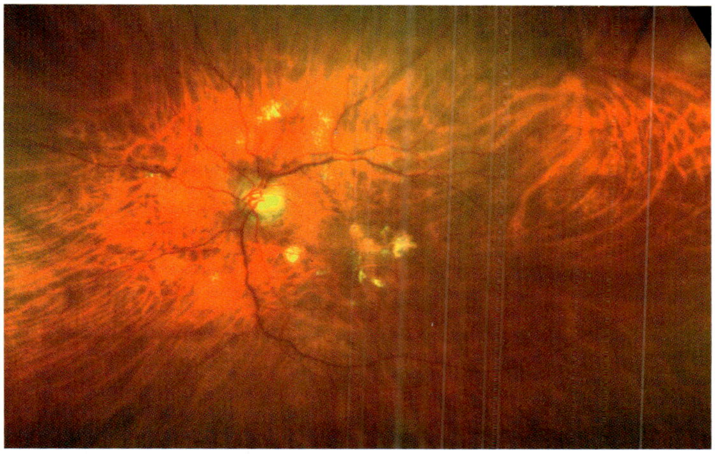

FIGURE 4-6. Optomap scan of diabetic retinopathy. (Courtesy of Optos PLC, Queensferry House, Carnegie Business Campus, Dunfermline, Fife, Scotland KYII 8GR, UK.)

on the optic nerve. Field 2 is centered on the macula; Field 3 temporal to the macula; Field 4 superotemporally, excluding the optic disc; Field 5 inferotemporally, excluding the optic disc; Field 6 superonasally along the arcades, excluding the optic disc; and Field 7 inferonasally, excluding the optic disc (Fig. 4-5).

There is the ultrawide field fundus camera (Optomap), which uses red and green laser lights to scan the retina. A spinning polygon at 30,000 rpm produces a scanning laser ophthalmoscope.[2] There is a 200-degree field of view of the retina. The red and green light wavelengths scatter less than that of white light. Therefore, they can penetrate cataracts, corneal opacities, and vitreous hemorrhage better than white light. Optomap photographs the retina up to the ora serrata. This type of camera is available and has provided clinicians with the capability of documenting widespread diabetic ischemia previously not recordable (Figs. 4-6 and 4-7). The Optomap is useful in the documentation of intraocular tumors.

Optical Coherence Tomography

Optical Coherence Tomography (OCT) is based on white light interferometry for in vivo ocular eye measurements and imaging of biological tissues, especially the human eye.[3]

The optical set up is white light or low-coherence interferometry. The light source is of low coherence and broad bandwidth. This type of light is created by superluminescent

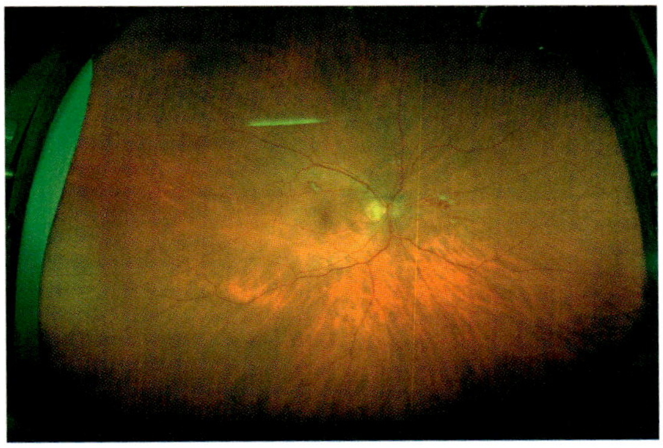

FIGURE 4-7. Optomap scan of the retina.

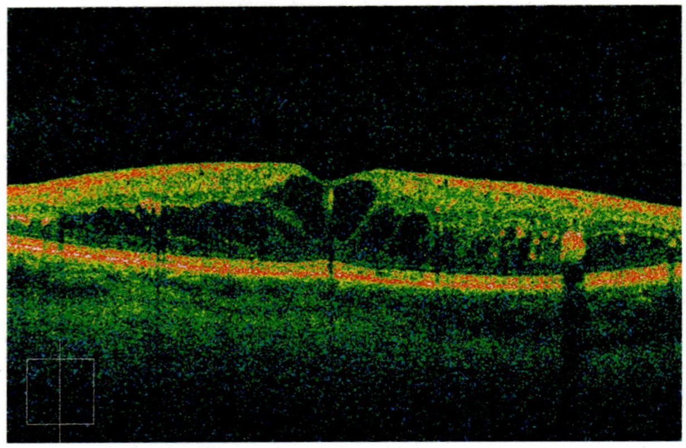

FIGURE 4-8. OCT scan of macular edema.

diode (SLD) laser such as the femtosecond laser. The light is split into and recombined from reference and sample arm respectively.[4,5]

This ophthalmic imaging technique is similar to ultrasound. But instead of measuring sound echoes, low-coherence interferometry measures the echo time delay of light. The Stratus OCT (Carl Zeiss, Meditech, Dublin, CA) is based on time domain detection technology where all time delays are measured sequentially. Thus, 400 axial scans are acquired in 1 second. Stratus OCT uses a SLD light source with a wavelength of 820 nm and a bandwidth of 25 nm to achieve a resolution of 10 to 12 μm. The slow acquisition speed leads to sparse scan patterns. Motion artifacts are common but are resolved with digital smoothing.

Light in an OCT system is divided into two arms: a sample arm aimed at the item of interest and a reference arm, a mirror. The combination of reflected light from the sample arm and reference light from the reference arm gives rise to an interference pattern. Only the reflected nonscattered light is coherent, that is, this coherent light retains the optical phase that causes light rays to propagate in one or another direction.

In the OCT instrument, an optical interferometer is used to detect only coherent light. The interferometer strips off scattered light from the reflected light needed to generate an image. In the process, depth and intensity of light reflected from the subsurface feature is obtained. A three-dimensional image can be built up by scanning, as in sonar or a radar system.

This technique is limited to imaging 1 to 2 mm below the surface of the biological tissue because at greater depths, the proportion of light that escapes without scattering is too small to be detected (Fig. 4-8).

Spectral Domain or Fourier Domain OCT

The broadband interference is acquired with spectrally separated detectors. The depth scan can be immediately calculated by a Fourier transform from the acquired spectra, called spectroscopic signal analysis, thus the name Spectral Domain OCT or Frequency Domain OCT. The signal analysis is done without the movement of the reference arm. The depth analysis is done by inverse Fourier transformation of a backscattered light spectrum to produce axial scans. This feature improves imaging speed dramatically, which reduces losses during a single scan to improve the signal-to-noise ratio of the detection elements.

Thus, the acquisition time is improved by 20 to 100 times of the conventional OCT. The faster acquisition time leads to the reduction of motion artifact, preserves true retinal topography, and allows "3D data sets."[6–9]

OCT, first popular in the mid-1990s, has now become the standard of care for retina-vitreous specialists. It is useful in describing diabetic macular edema versus macular gliosis or macular hole formation (Fig. 4-7).

The optical coherence scans number 20,000 to 40,000 A-scans per second providing information of the retina architecture. Specifically, the clinician can view the vitreous interface with the internal limiting membrane for macular gliosis, macular hole, and macular pseudohole formation. The inner layers of the retina can be seen in pathological states in diabetic retinopathy, for example, macular cysts in diabetic macular edema. The size of the cysts can be measured and seen using this technique. The retinal pigment epithelium can be seen if the area is separated from the retina in a retinal pigment epithelial detachment or bleeding under the retinal pigment epithelium in disease entities such as age-related macular degeneration. The current iteration of the software has now allowed 25,000 to 27,000 A-scans per second. The resulting axial resolution is approximately 5 μm.[10–14]

Heidelberg Retinal Angiography and OCT

Heidelberg retinal angiography (HRA) with OCT has an acquisition speed of 40,000 A-scans per second. It has a digital axial resolution of 3.8 μm. It uses a scanning laser ophthalmoscope, along with an eye tracking device, to scan the retina and its blood vessels while obtaining an OCT, in real time. This method allows for precise tracking of the retinal lesion from examination to examination. Images are acquired point-by-point and reconstructed with a computer, allowing three-dimensional reconstructions of topologically complex objects.

The confocal laser scanning microscope, part of the Spectralis system, contains a laser beam which passes through a light source aperture, and then the laser beam is focused by an objective lens into a small, diffraction-limited, focal volume within a fluorescent specimen. A mixture of emitted fluorescent light as well as reflected laser light from the illuminated spot is recollected by the objective lens. A beam splitter separates the light mixture by allowing only the laser light to pass through and reflecting the fluorescent light in the detection apparatus. After passing the pinhole, the fluorescent light is detected by a photodetection device, photomultiplier tube or avalanche photodiode. Thus, the light signal is transformed into an electrical signal that is recorded by the computer.

The detected light originating from an illuminated volume element within the specimen represents one pixel in the resulting image. As the laser scans over the plane of the specimen, a whole image is obtained pixel-by-pixel and line-by-line.

The computer can generate a three-dimensional picture of a specimen by assembling a stack of these two dimensional images from successive focal planes[15] (Figs. 4-9 and 4-10).

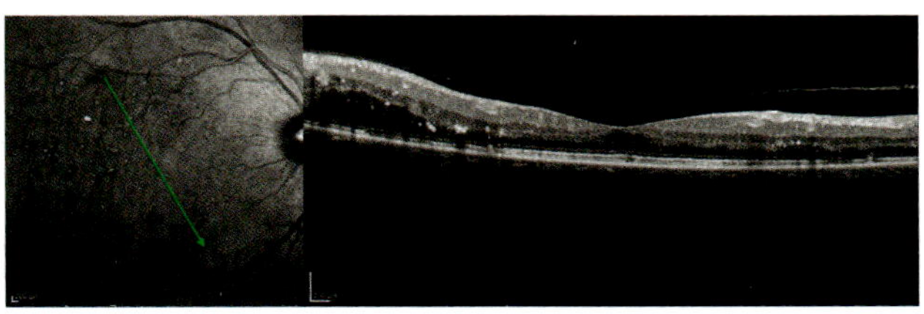

FIGURE 4-9. Spectralis scan of diabetic retinopathy. (Courtesy of Heidelberg Engineering, 1499 Poinsettia Ave., Suite 160, Vista, CA 92081.)

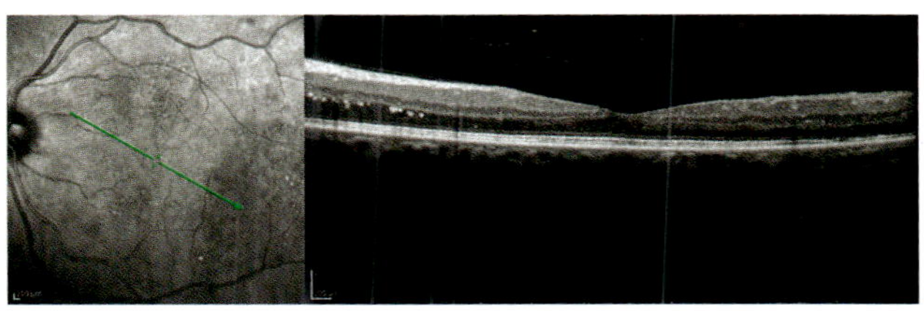

FIGURE 4-10. Spectralis scan of diabetic retinopathy. (Courtesy of Heidelberg Engineering, 1499 Poinsettia Ave., Suite 160, Vista, CA 92081.)

Fundus Autofluoresence

The camera has a filter that shines light onto the retina, and the response shows the activity of the rod/cone interface with the retinal pigment epithelium. Fundus autofluorescence (FAF) uses a fundus spectrophotometer[5] and an excitation light of a short wavelength. FAF is derived mainly from retinal pigment epithelium's lipofuscin granules with a broad emission spectrum from 500 to 750 nm and a peak at about 630 nm.[16–20] The Heidelberg Spectralis system uses three models for FAF imaging: Spectralis HRA, Spectralis FA + OCT, and Spectralis HRA + OCT.

The Spectralis HRA uses a confocal Scanning Laser Ophthalmoscope (cSLO) to show the spatial distribution of FAF over large retinal areas to be documented.[7–9] The use of a confocal system and a monochromatic light allows high spatial resolution imaging of a sharp image in a selected plane and avoids lens fluorescence. To study FAF, cSLO usually utilizes an argon blue laser of 488 nm, the same wavelength as that used for fluorescein angiography, and a barrier filter with a short wavelength cut off at 495 nm to separate the excitation from the emitted fluorescent light. To amplify the autofluorescence signal, single images are usually averaged after eye movement correction. In cases of nystagmus or poor fixation, this may be difficult. To date, this method has been used for age-related macular degeneration and geographic atrophy, inherited retinal dystrophies with its abnormal retinal pigment epithelium. However, this method may prove useful in other diseases such as diabetes where the retinal pigment epithelium is abnormal in patients with diabetic retinopathy.[21]

Clinical Applications of Fluorescein Angiography

Fluorescein angiography is important for the evaluation of blood flow indirectly and directly evaluating the anatomy of the different layers of the retina. The initial flow of the fluorescein dye goes into the venous system, into the capillaries, and then into the arterial system. This is still the most easily accessible method for clinicians to evaluate flow and the possible delay of flow in vasculopathic diseases such as diabetes (Fig. 4-3).

For example, if the first appearance of fluorescein dye occurs at 15 seconds in the arteriovenous phase after a standard 5-second injection time in one patient with background diabetic retinopathy and macular edema, this same injection sequence in another diabetic patient with severe proliferative diabetic retinopathy and macular edema may result in the fluorescein dye showing up in the arteriovenous phase at 20 seconds. This difference in flow may be an indicator of delay in flow in these two diabetic patients.

In the midtransit of the fluorescein angiogram, the ophthalmologist may identify areas of capillary nonperfusion or neovascularization (Fig. 4-9), which would lead to different treatment options than if no fluorescein angiography had been performed. Or, if in the late transit, there is profound macular edema as demonstrated by massive hyperfluorescence at the macula region. This picture may then convince the retinal specialist of the need for closer follow-up examinations. For example, a newly diagnosed Type 2 diabetic patient may need to be seen more frequently than every 6 months.

Sodium fluorescein is a well-tolerated dye in the majority of patients. If patients are concerned about fluorescein allergy, we suggest that they take the vial and see an allergist for testing.

In diabetic patients with macular edema and nonproliferative diabetic retinopathy, fluorescein angiography can be used to evaluate areas of capillary nonperfusion. Capillary nonperfusion would lead to the use of earlier scatter photocoagulation. Fluorescein angiography would identify areas of neovascularization of the retina elsewhere, a feared complication of diabetic retinopathy. Any areas of retinal neovascularization would lead to possible earlier treatment of scatter photocoagulation or closer monitoring of the patient to prepare for eventual need for panretinal photocoagulation (PRP), as we expect acceleration of diabetic retinopathy.

Fluorescein angiography is useful to monitor residual macular edema after previous laser. Comparison photographs and angiographic frames from previous examinations can be used to evaluate the resolution or progression of residual macular edema.

Clinical Applications of Indocyanine Green Angiography

ICG Angiography looks at the choroidal circulation. This type of angiography may be used to follow in patients with diabetes with an abnormal presentation of diabetic retinopathy or those patients who have choroidal lesions, unrelated to the underlying systemic disease of diabetes. For example, diabetic patients with choroidal tumors would have this procedure performed. This test utilizes an iodine-based dye, and thus, patients with iodine allergy would not be candidates for this test. More allergic reactions occur with ICG dye than with sodium fluorescein dye.

Patients who are candidates for the ICG dye test in a diabetic population would include new patients with loss of central vision, who are diabetic but whose fundus photo does not show typical diabetic microaneurysmal dilatation. If you suspect another form of retinal disease involving anastomoses with the choroidal circulation to the retinal circulation, the ICG angiography is useful.

Other Testing

Visual Field

Visual field tests can quantify the extent of visual loss in diabetic patients with diabetic retinopathy. Visual fields can also monitor the progression of diabetic retinopathy in follow-up examinations. The visual field evaluates the diabetic patients for comorbid risk factors such as glaucoma. In addition, visual field testing can evaluate those diabetic patients with unexplained visual loss. One should consider open-angle glaucoma in the differential diagnosis, since glaucoma has been one of the associated health risks with diabetes. It has been well known that diabetic retinopathy decreases blood flow to the retina, and as a corollary, it is not unexpected to see low-tension glaucoma in diabetic patients.

Visual fields can be offered in the following modes:

a. Confrontational Visual Field: At the bedside, the examiner's peripheral hand movements are brought from the far periphery to the near periphery in four quadrants, using counting fingers.
b. Amsler Grid: This small test evaluates macular vision in diabetic patients. This is useful as a screening test for diabetics who are newly diagnosed or for those diabetics who present to the internal medicine practice complaining of loss of near vision. In an ophthalmologist's office, the use of the Amsler Grid can be done with the testing of the visual acuity, as a way to determine more clearly the patient's chief complaint.
c. Static Perimetry (Humphrey Zeiss field analyzer—"24-2" or Octopus): These automated visual field machines use a fixed light source which is either a stationary, pinpoint light source or projected dots within a large Ganzfeld bowl.
d. Kinetic Perimetry (also known as the traditional Goldmann Perimeter): This test produces an island map of peripheral visual perception. Fixation monitoring as well as movement of light source is necessary to perform this test.
e. Frequency Doubling Perimetry (Humphrey Zeiss field analyzer—"30-2"): This test uses varying intensities of a shimmering grid of light in standardized sectors of the peripheral and central visual field. It is particularly useful in detecting early glaucoma field loss and can be 40% more sensitive than that of standard static or kinetic perimetry.

For diabetic patients, there may be visual field changes related to the loss of peripheral vision from their diabetic retinopathy, even if untreated. After laser photocoagulation such as PRP, there may be some additional visual field loss. It is important to document a baseline visual field in these diabetic patients before and after PRP as they are at risk for glaucoma in the future.

In diabetic macular edema patients, it is important to document their preexisting visual field loss before their initial macular laser.

In diabetic patients who later develop glaucoma, visual field changes may be gradual or abrupt. Thus, the clinician should monitor for optic disc changes for increased cup-to-disc ratios and follow gonioscopy for rubeosis in the diabetic patient. The patient's optic nerve changes can be sequentially examined with the Heidelberg Retinal Tomography or the OCT.

In diabetic patients who have had loss of vision not correlated with retinal findings, a visual field test may identify glaucoma. Normal-tension glaucoma can occur in diabetic patients. Diabetic patients who have not had laser may complain of loss of contrast sensitivity at night or difficulty ambulating in dark movie theaters or parking lots. These patients may have normal vision (20/20 to 20/40) but complain of loss of vision out of proportion with their retinal exam.

Electrodiagnostic Testing

The Electroretinogram

The oscillatory potential is the classical method of evaluating diabetic retinopathy, but newer methods of evaluating retinal function exist with the use of 30-Hz Flicker, implicit times and amplitudes.[22–24] Bresnick et al.[25–27] described oscillatory potentials in diabetic retinopathy. Oscillatory potentials are extracted from the ERG B wave by a computer-automated mechanism which increases the low-frequency band-pass filter to 60 Hz and leaves the high-frequency band-pass filter at the usual setting of about 300 Hz.

Much of visual function testing in diabetics has been used for prognosis in severe diabetics or for those diabetics with profound and severe visual loss in assessing their low vision status. Oscillatory potentials and its amplitude have been affected in patients with no diabetic retinopathy to background diabetic retinopathy.[25–27]

Thirty-Hertz flicker is useful in testing the loss of retinal function especially its implicit times. This is becoming more popular among clinicians because the ERG can provide prognostication of future visual function after laser or surgery.[23,26,28]

Modern electrodiagnostic testing now involves the use of the DTL electrode which is a noncontact electrode. No longer is the Burian-Allen or jet contact lens electrode the contact electrode of choice for a busy clinical practice. The DTL electrode uses a silver-coated filament, approximately 10-0 nylon suture to be placed in the cul-de-sac in the tear film of the tarsal conjunctiva.[29] There is still a ground electrode and a forehead electrode as previously described.[30]

The testing protocol is the standard ISCEV, International Society of Clinical Electrophysiology and Vision.[31] Dark adaptation of 20 minutes is performed in a blackened room, without any light entry. This can be accomplished by bilaterally patching a patient in a darkened room. The scotopic or dark-adapted ERG starts with a small, dim white light, a brighter white light flash, then a lit Ganzfeld bowl with a white flash, and then the 30-Hz Flicker to test the cone response. The oscillatory potentials are removed from the photopic part of the ERG by the computer which extracts the oscillatory potentials and analyzes them using the software programs in all of the commercially available ERG systems.

Patients who present for the first time with severe diabetic retinopathy are candidates for ERG testing. The ERG will quantify the degree of ischemia for the clinician. While photographic methods evaluate the retinal anatomy, the ERG evaluates the function. In nonproliferative or proliferative retinopathy: look for a baseline and repeat after onset of medical treatment to stabilize diabetes or as a method of following patients who are being treated with bevacizumab (Avastin) and who are not responding to treatment. The degree of ischemia seen in the B waves or oscillatory potentials or delayed implicit times of the 30-Hz Flicker may be useful information. This consistent delay of implicit times despite treatment may suggest earlier laser intervention is needed or that bevacizumab (Avastin) may be needed for adjunctive therapy (Fig. 4-11).

Visual Evoked Response

The visual evoked response (VER) can measure accurately the foveal function. The potentials recorded are "indirect" measures of the fovea. These potentials which are generated in the occipital cortex represent the end stages of the visual response with stimulation of

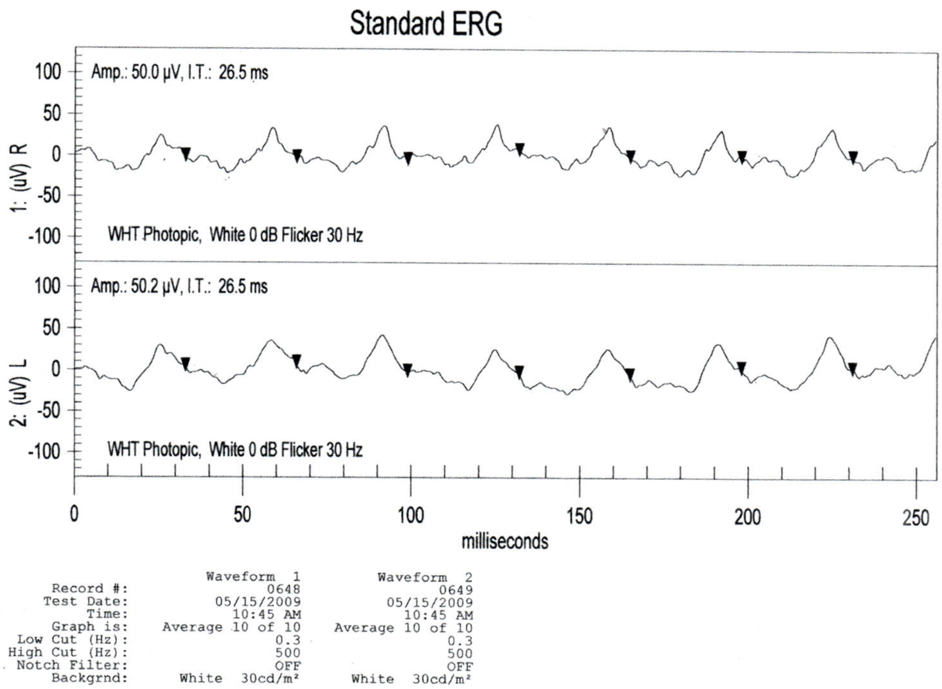

FIGURE 4-11. ERG: 73-year-old female with newly diagnosed diabetes. OD (**Top**), OS (**Bottom**). ERG normal (70–79 years old): amplitude = 103.06 ± 9.50, implicit time = 26.69 ± 0.93. The patient's amplitude is decreased when compared to normal, age-matched standards. (Courtesy of LKC Technologies, Gaithersburg, Maryland. www.KLC.com, Database: C:\EMRIN\EMDATA.mdb.)

the retina. To elicit maximal cortical activity, a computer-generated checkerboard pattern allows the fovea to detect the presence of the pattern, not a change in luminance. This type of stimulus ensures that areas remote from the fovea do not contribute to the resulting waveforms[32] (Fig. 4-12).

Changing the size of the squares in the checkerboard helps to determine visual acuity. Loss of contrast sensitivity for such large stimuli has been noted in macular degeneration, cataract, and optic neuritis.[32–36] Thus, optic nerve function in severe proliferative diabetic retinopathy, preoperative and postoperative evaluations of severe visual loss in proliferative diabetic retinopathy, can also be evaluated with the visual evoked reponse.[32]

Ultrasonography

Ultrasound is used for the examination of diabetic patients with opaque media. The anterior vitreous base in vitreous hemorrhages can be evaluated with ultrasound. Determining retinal detachment status or the retina integrity in a diabetic patient with a dense cataract or severe vitreous hemorrhage requires the use of ultrasound. Sometimes, the ultrasound can be deceiving in the case of a dense vitreous hemorrhage and blood on the hyaloid face. The resulting ultrasound may mimic a retinal detachment. Thus, it is important to change the decibel status by going higher on the decibel switch and having the patient look in the six cardinal positions to create a dynamic ultrasound picture of his posterior pole. Ultrasounds can be used to follow diabetic patients with a vitreous hemorrhage if there is a worsening of vision or new appearance of traction retinal detachment on successive B-scans[37] (Fig. 4-13).

While examining the vitreous in its fluid or gellike state in the eye, one can get an idea of the structure of the vitreous by asking the patient, whose eyes are closed, to move up, down, in all the cardinal positions, and the vitreous will then move. This will give the

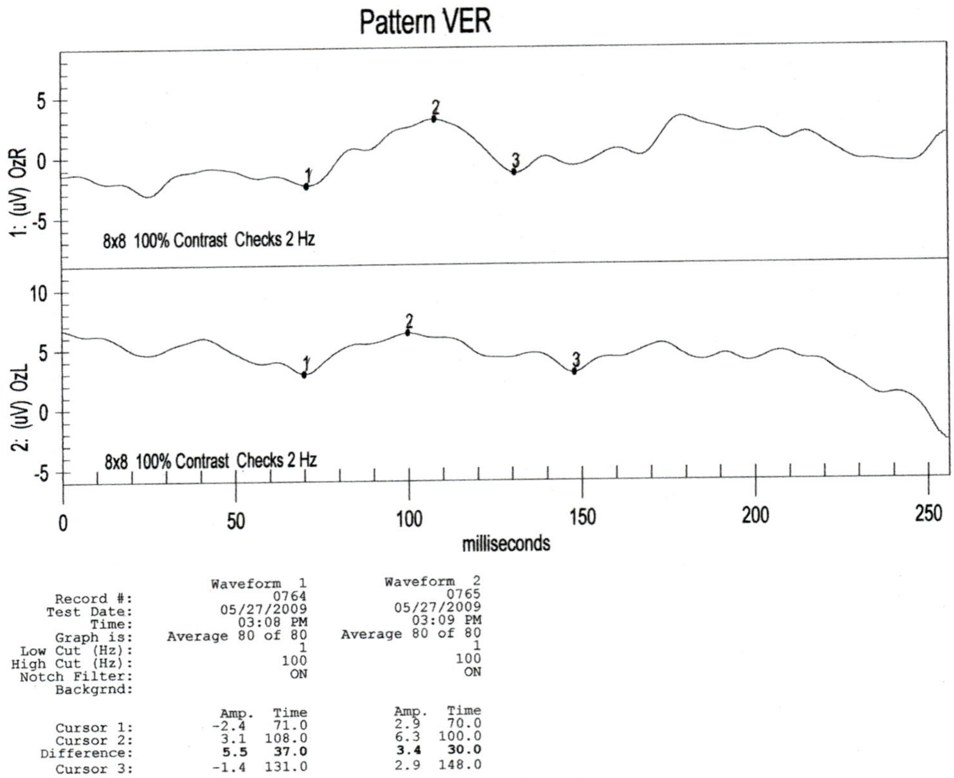

FIGURE 4-12. VER: 54-year-old male with 2 years of Type 2 diabetes. OD (**Top**), OS (**Bottom**). VER normal (50–59 years old): amplitude = 11.8 ± 2.8, implicit time = 98.2 ± 6.6. The patient's amplitude is decreased when compared to normal, age-matched standards. (Courtesy of LKC Technologies, Gaithersburg, Maryland. www.KLC.com, Database: C:\EMRIN\EMDATA.mdb.)

clinician a "dynamic vitreous examination." In gellike vitreous, there is minimal movement seen. With fluid vitreous and abnormal vitreous as in vitreous hemorrhage, these eye movements, with the ultrasound probe on the eye, will reveal whether the vitreous is freely moving and the retina is attached without any relation to the movement of the vitreous or if there is an underlying rhegmatogenous retinal detachment. In those cases of a bullous retinal detachment, one can see the operculum with the vitreous using this dynamic

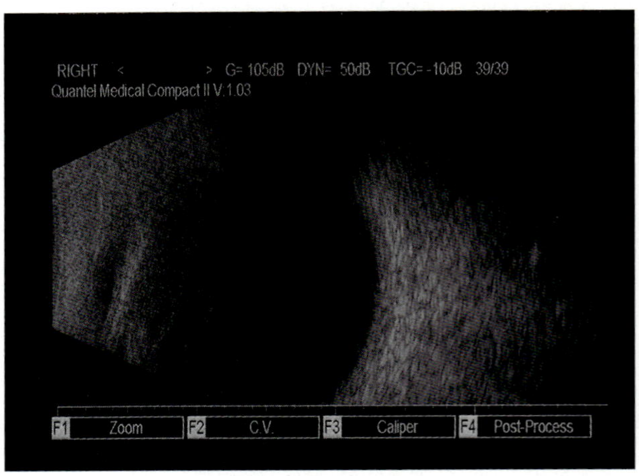

FIGURE 4-13. USG: mild vitreous hemorrhage at 12:00.

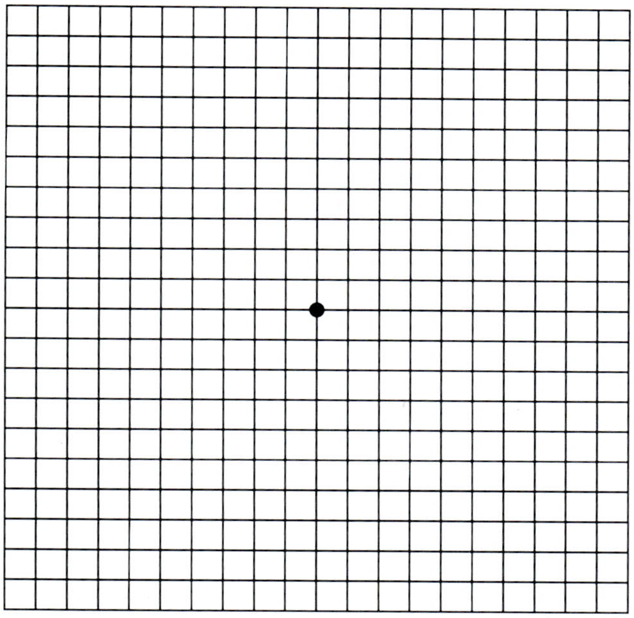

FIGURE 4-14. Amsler grid.

approach to vitreous examination.[37] In the cases of a vitreous hemorrhage and traction retinal detachment, the vitreous stands can be seen attached to the fibrotic membranes of the traction retinal detachment.

Preoperatively, prior to vitrectomy, ultrasound examination is important. A retinal detachment underneath a dense vitreous hemorrhage would necessitate immediate surgery, whereas a vitreous hemorrhage without a retinal detachment can be scheduled in a timely, less emergent manner. B-scan ultrasound can be used for the examination of the retina prior to cataract surgery as well.

For the cataract surgeon who has a diabetic patient with a dense cataract, it is important to evaluate the retina prior to surgery so as to provide some visual prognosis outcome for the patient and his family. In diabetic patients who have not been seen by any ophthalmologist or any eye care provider, an opaque media may mean an occult mass lesion such as a melanoma. In addition, vitreous hemorrhages or opaque media, the ultrasound is important to identify any hidden masses, melanomas, before cataract surgery.

Amsler Grid Testing

This is very useful in testing macular edema laser outcomes or in the evaluation of residual macular edema after laser. It is useful for testing the fellow eye, as well (Fig. 4-14).

Color Vision Testing

Patients, who have had previous PRP or macular laser, may exhibit an acquired blue-yellow loss of color vision. Color vision testing can help monitor the loss of visual function if no electrophysiology equipment is available. For more advanced color vision testing, these patients need the 100-hue color test. The Ishihara color plates are inadequate for color vision screening for red-green deficiency.

REFERENCES

1. Weinberger D, Kramer M, Priel E, Gaton D, Axer-Siegel R, Yassur Y. Indocyanine green angiographic findings in nonproliferative diabetic retinopathy. *Am J Ophthalmol.* 1998;126(2):238–247.
2. http://www.optos.com/us/Products-Services/About-optomap-products/optomap-Retinal-Exam. Accessed 16 February 2009.
3. Huang D, Swanson EA, Lin CP et al. Optical coherence tomography. *Science.* 1991;254:1178–1181.
4. Hee MR, Izatt JA, Swanson EA et al. Optical coherence tomography of the human retina. *Arch Ophthalmol.* 1995;115:325–332.

5. Fercher AF, Hitzenberger CK, Kamp G, Elzaiat SY. Measurements on intraocular distances by backscattering spectral interferometry. *Opt Commun.* 1195;117:43–48.
6. Cabrera Fernandez D, Salinas HM, Puliafito CA. Automated detection of retinal layer structures on optical coherence tomography images. *Optics Express.* 2005;13(25):10200–10216.
7. Jiao S, Wu C, Knighton RW, Gregori G, Puliafito CA. Registration of high-density cross sectional images to the fundus image in spectral-domain ophthalmic optical coherence tomography. *Optics Express.* 2006;14(8):3368–3376.
8. Wehbe H, Ruggeri M, jiao S, Gregori G, Puliafito CA, Zhao W. Automatic retinal blood flow calculation using spectral domain optical coherence tomography. *Optics Express.* 2007;15(23):15193–15206.
9. Jiao S, Knighton R, Huang X, Gregori G, Puliafito CA. Simultaneous acquisition of sectional and fundus ophthalmic images with spectral domain optical coherence tomography. *Optics Express.* 2005;13(2):444–452.
10. Wojtkowski M, Leitgeib R, Kowalczyk A, Bajraszewski T, Fercher AF. In vivo human retinal imaging by Fourier domain optical coherence tomography. *J Biomed Opt.* 2002;7:457–463.
11. Leitgeb RA, Drexler W, Unterhuber A, et al. Ultrahigh resolution Fourier Domain optical coherence tomography. *Optics Express.* 2004;12:2156–2165.
12. Wojtkowski M, Bajraszewski T, Gorczynska I, et al. Ophthalmic imaging by spectraloptical coherence tomography. *Am J Ophthalmol.* 2004;138:412–419.
13. Srinivasan VJ, Wojtkowski M, Witkin AJ, et al. High definition and 3-dimensional imaging of macular pathologies with high speed ultra-high –resolution of optical coherence tomography. *Ophthalmology.* 2006;113:2054–2056.
14. Wojtkowski M, Srinivasan VJ, Fujimoto J, et al. Three dimensional retinal imaging with high speed ultrahigh resolution optical coherence tomography. *Ophthalmology.* 2005;112:1734–1736.
15. http://en.wikipedia.org/wiki/confocal_laser_scanning_microscopy. Accessed 23 November 2008.
16. Delori FC. Spectrophotometer for noninvasive measurement of intrinsic fluorescence and reflectance of the ocular fundus. *Appl Optics.* 1994;33:7439–7452.
17. Delori FC, Dorey CK, Staurenghi G, Arend O, Goger DG, Weiter JJ. In vivo fluorescence of the ocular fundus exhibits retinal pigment epithelium lipofuscin characteristics. *Invest Ophthalmol Vis Sci.* 1995;36:718–729.
18. von Rückmann A, Fitzke FW, Bird AC. Distribution of fundus autofluorescence with a scanning laser ophthalmoscope. *Br J Ophthalmol.* 1995;79:407–412.
19. von Rückmann A, Fitzke FW, Bird AC. Fundus autofluorescence in age-related macular disease imaged with a laser scanning ophthalmoscope. *Invest Ophthalmol Vis Sci.* 1997;38:478–486.
20. von Rückmann A, Fitzke FW, Bird AC. Distribution of pigment epithelium autofluorescence in retinal disease state recorded in vivo and its change over time. *Graefes Arch Clin Exp Ophthalmol.* 1999;237:1–9.
21. http://www.revophth.com/index.asp?page=1_781.htm. Accessed 16 February 2009.
22. Satoh S, Iijima H, Imai M, Abe K, Shibuya T. Photopic electroretinogram implicit time in diabetic retinopathy. *Jpn J Ophthalmol.* 1994;38:178–184.
23. Tahara K, Matsura T, Otori T. Diagnostic evaluation of diabetic retinopathy by 30-Hz flicker electroretinography. *Jpn J Ophthalmol.* 1993;37:204–210.
24. Wu G, Severns M. Dyslipidemia and diabetic retinopathy. Retina Society. Fairmont Scottsdale Princess Hotel, Scottsdale. 28 September 2008.
25. Bresnick G, Palta M. Oscillatory Potential amplitudes: Relation to the severity of diabetic retinopathy. *Arch Ophthalmol.* 1987;105:929–933.
26. Bresnick G, Palta M. Temporal aspects of the electroretinogram in diabetic retinopathy. *Arch Ophthalmol.* 1987;105: 660–664.
27. Bresnick G, Palta M. Predicting the progression to diabetic retinopathy. *Arch Ophthalmol.* 1987;105:810–814.
28. Holopigian K, Greenstein VC, Seiple W, Hood DC, Carr RE. Evidence for photoreceptor changes in patients with diabetic retinopathy. *Invest Ophthalmol Vis Sci.* 1997;38:2355–2365.
29. Berezovsky A, Perera JM, Salomao SR, Rogerio dos Santos V, Schor P. Validation of a new fiber electrode prototype for clinical electroretinography. *Arq Bras Oftalmol.* 2008;71:316–320.
30. Carr RE, Noble KG, Siegel IM. *Visual Electrodiagnostic Testing: A Practical Guide for the Clinician.* Baltimore, MD: Williams and Wilkins; 1982:15–23.
31. Marmor MF, Holder GE, Seeliger MW, Yamamoto S. Standard for clinical electroretinography. *Doc Ophthalmol.* 2004;108:107–114.
32. Carr RE, Noble KG, Siegel IM. *Visual Electrodiagnostic Testing.* 38–40.
33. Sjöstrand J, Frisen L. Contrast sensitivity in macular disease. *Acta Ophthalmol.* 1977;55:507–514.
34. Hess R, Woo G. Vision through cataracts. *Invest Ophthalmol Visual Sci.* 1978;17:428–435.
35. Arden GB. The visual evoked response in ophthalmology. *Proc R Soc Med.* 1973;66:1037–1043.
36. Bass SJ, Sherman J, Bodis-Wollner I, Nath S. Visual evoked potentials in macular disease. *Invest Ophthalmol Vis Sci.* 1985;26:1071–1074.

SUGGESTED READINGS

1. Aiello LM, Rand LI, Briones JC, Wafai MZ, Sebestyen JG. Diabetic retinopathy in Joslin Clinic patients with adult-onset diabetes. *Ophthalmology.* 1981;88:619–623.
2. American Academy of Ophthalmology. *Preferred Practice Pattern: Diabetic Retinopathy.* San Francisco, CA: American Academy of Ophthalmology; 1989.
3. Barr CC. Estimation of the maximum number of argon laser burns possible in panretinal photocoagulation. *Am J Ophthalmol.* 1984;97:697–703.
4. Diabetes 2000 symposium at the annual meeting of the American Academy of Ophthalmology Anaheim, California, October, 1991.
5. Early Treatment Retinopathy Study Research Group. ETDRS Report No 3. Techniques for scatter and local photocoagulation treatment of diabetic retinopathy. *Int Ophthalmol Clin.* 1987;27:254–264.
6. Early Treatment Diabetic Retinopathy Study Research Group. ETDRS Report no. 7. Early treatment diabetic retinopathy study design and baseline patient characteristics. *Ophthalmology.* 1991;98:741–756.

7. Early Treatment Diabetes Retinopathy Study Research Group. ETDRS Report No. 9. Early photocoagulation for diabetic retinopathy. *Ophthalmology.* 1991;98:766–785.
8. Early Treatment Diabetic Retinopathy Study Research Group. ETDRS Report No. 10. Grading diabetic retinopathy from stereoscopic color fundus photographs- an extension of the modified Airlie House classification. *Ophthalmology.* 1991;98:786–806.
9. Early Treatment Diabetic Retinopathy Research Group. ETDRS Report No. 12. Fundus photographic risk factors for progression of diabetic retinopathy. *Ophthalmology.* 1991;98:823–833.
10. Early Treatment Retinopathy Study Research Group. ETDRS Report No. 13. Fluorescein angiographic risk factors for progresson of diabetic retinopathy. *Ophthalmology.* 1991;98:834–840.
11. Garcia JPS, Garcia P, Finger PT. Dynamic ultrasound movements of the Eye and orbit. *Br J Ophthalmol.* 2006;90: 395–520.
12. Javitt JC, Aiello LP, Bassi LJ, Chiang YP, Canner JK. Detecting and treating retinopathy in patients with type I diabetes mellitus. *Ophthalmology.* 1991;98:1565–1574.
13. Javitt JC, Canner JK, Frank RG, Steinwachs DM, Sommer A. Detecting and treating retinopathy in patients with type I diabetes mellitus. *Ophthalmology.* 1990;9:483–495.
14. Javitt JC, Canner JK, Sommer A. Cost effectiveness of current approaches to the control of retinopathy in type I diabetes. *Ophthalmology.* 1989;96:255–264.
15. Klein BEK, Davis MD, Segal P, et al. Diabetic retinopathy. Assessment of severity and progression. *Ophthalmology.* 1984;91:10–17.
16. Klein BEK, Moss SE, Klein R, et al. The Wisonsin Epidemiologic Study of Diabetic Retinopathy. XIII. Relationship of serum cholesterol to retinopathy and hard exudates. *Ophthalmology.* 1991;98:1261–1265.
17. Klein R. The epidemiology of diabetic retinopathy: Findings from the Wisconsin Epidemiologic Study of Diabetic Retinopathy. *Int Ophthalmol Clin.* 1987;27:230–238.
18. Klein R, Klein BEK, Moss SE, Davis MD, DeMets DL. The Wisconsin Epidemiologic Study of Diabetic Retinopathy II. Prevalence and risk of diabetic retinopathy when age at diagnosis is less than 30 years. *Arch Ophthalmol.*1984;102: 520–526.
19. Klein R, Klein BEK, Moss SE, Davis MD, DeMets DL. The Wisconsin Epidemiologic Study of Diabetic Retinopathy. III. Prevalence and risk of diabetic retinopathy when age at diagnosis is 30 or more years. *Arch Ophthalmol.* 1984;102: 527–532.
20. Klein R, Klein BEK, Moss SE, Davis MD, DeMets DL. The Wisconsin Epidemiologic Study of Diabetic Retinopathy. VII. Diabetic nonproliferative retinal lesions. *Ophthalmology.* 1987;94:1389–1400.
21. Klein R, Klein BEK, Moss SE, Davis MD, DeMets DL. The Wisconsin Epidemiologic Study of Diabetic Retinopathy. IX. Four year incidence and progressions of diabetic retinopathy when age at diagnosis is less than 30 years. *Arch Ophthalmol.* 1989;107:237–243.
22. Klein R, Klein BEK, Moss SE, Davis MD, DeMets DL. The Wisconsin Epidemiologic Study of Diabetic Retinopathy. X. Four-year incidence and progression of diabetic retinopathy when age at diagnosis is less than 30 years. *Arch Ophthalmol.* 1989;107:244–249.
23. Klein R, Klein BEK, Neider NW, et al. Diabetic retinopathy as detected using ophthalmoscopy, a non-mydriatic camera and standard fundus camera. *Ophthalmology.* 1985;92:485.
24. Klein R, Klein BEK, Syrjala SE, Davis MD, Meuer MM, Magli Y. Wisconsin Epidemiologic Study of Diabetic Retinopathy. I. Relationship of diabetic retinopathy to management of diabetes. Preliminary report. In: Friedman EA, L'Esperance FA, eds. *Diabetic Renal-retinal Syndrome* (Vol 2). New York, NY: Grune & Stratton; 1982; 2:21–40.
25. Moss SE, Kline R, Kessler SD, Richie, KA. Comparison between ophthalmology and fundus photography of diabetic retinopathy. *Ophthalmology.* 1985;92:62–67.
26. Palmberg P, Smith M, Waltman S, et al. The natural history of retinopathy in insulin-dependent juvenile-onset diabetes. *Ophthalmology.* 1981;88:613–618.
27. Reddy VM, Zamora R, Olk RJ. A comparison of the size of the burn produced by Rodenstock and Goldman contact lenses. *Am J Ophthalmol.* 1991;112:212–214.
28. Sussman EJ, Tsiaras WG, Soper KA. Diagnosis of diabetic eye disease. *JAMA.* 1982;247:3231–3234.
29. The Diabetes Retinopathy Study Research Group. Photocoagulation treatment of proliferative diabetic retinopathy. *Am J Ophthalmol.* 1978;85:82–106.
30. The Diabetes Retinopathy Study Research Group. DRS Report No. 3. Four risk factors for severe visual loss in diabetic retinopathy. *Arch Ophthalmol.* 1979;97:654–655.
31. The diabetes Retinopathy Study Research Group. DRS Report No. 6 Design, methods, and baseline results. *Invest Ophthalmol Vis Sci.* 1981;21:149–209.
32. The diabetes Retinopathy Study Research Group. Report No. 14. Indications for photocoagulation treatment of diabetic retinopathy. *Int Ophthalmol Clin.* 1987;27:239–252.

CHAPTER 5

Examination of the Diabetic Patient

HISTORY

When taking the history of the diabetic patient, be aware of other entities that can contribute to the severity of diabetic retinopathy, such as hypertension, kidney disease, hyperlipidemia, ischemic heart disease, or peripheral vascular disease.[1–3] Look for metabolic syndrome in patients who are overweight, obese, diabetic and have a history of dyslipidemia. Lastly, always inquire about their cholesterol and triglyceride levels in these diabetic patients. Smoking history is important as nicotine can cause acceleration of the diabetic retinopathy. Ask about the fasting blood sugar and glycosylated hemoglobin (HbA1c) as an assessment of the overall status of diabetes in the patient about to be evaluated for diabetic retinopathy. If the patient cannot remember his glucose level or HbA1c or any of his past blood sugar levels, the patient is probably not fully informed about the importance of such laboratory indices with respect to his diabetic retinopathy.

Duration of Diabetes

Duration of diabetes is an important question for the patient. The longer the duration of diabetes, the greater the risk of diabetic retinopathy. In Type 1 diabetes, the longer the duration of diabetes, the greater the risk for increasing severity of diabetic retinopathy. In Type 2 diabetes, after 15 years of diabetes, there will be increased risk of diabetic retinopathy. After diabetes has been present for 20 years, almost all persons in whom the onset of diabetes occurred before age 30 years have some evidence of diabetic retinopathy, and about 50% have proliferative diabetic retinopathy. In persons who are 30 years or older when diabetes is diagnosed, while they are at lower risk for retinopathy, retinopathy may be their first symptom of diabetes.[4]

Past Ocular History

Ask the patient about previous laser or eye surgery history. When did the diabetic patient first note eye problems or vision problems?

Review of Systems: These are some of the pertinent and related issues that have some influence on vision and diabetic retinopathy.

Glaucoma can be present in patients with longstanding diabetic retinopathy or in patients with rapid deterioration of vision due to proliferative diabetic retinopathy. There is neovascular glaucoma to consider in those diabetic patients whose vision is decreasing rapidly over a short period of time. Open-angle glaucoma can occur in Type 2 diabetic patients.

Thyroid disease does not affect the retina unless it is severe and causes optic disc edema. Thyroid disease can occur in diabetic patients and present as severe dry eye. If there is proptosis in the setting of thyroid disease and diabetes, send the patient for an endocrinology evaluation.

Other endocrine abnormalities can occur with diabetes. This one caveat should be considered when the diabetic patient sees an endocrinologist at the time of diagnosis.

TABLE 5.1 Examination of the Diabetic Eye Patient

Correlate vision loss to the retina findings
Eyelids and pupils:
III nerve palsy and eyelid abnormalities
Papillary abnormality
Slit lamp examination:
Rubeosis iridis, iris atrophy
Cataract

Fundus examination
Review of system checklist
Hypertension (silver wiring or copper wiring, poor flow seen on angiogram)
Hyperlipidemia (hard exudate rings)
Cardiovascular disease (transient ischemic attack by history with loss of vision suddenly, emboli)
Smoking (attenuated arterioles or capillary nonperfusion or ischemic retina)
Obesity and Metabolic Syndrome (expect poor glycemic control and retinopathy)

Diabetes history
Duration of Diabetes (the greater the duration, the worse the retinopathy)
Type 1 diabetes versus Type 2 diabetes
Gestational diabetes in the past (acceleration of diabetes over pregnancy)
Diabetes and pregnancy (acceleration of diabetes over pregnancy)
Poor glycemic control (expect diabetic retinopathy at first visit to ophthalmologist's office)

Obesity has been linked to the epidemic of diabetes in teens in America for the past decade. Adipocytes are now thought to play a role in insulin resistance in Type 2 diabetic patients. Thus, obesity is a risk factor in the development of diabetes.

Poor lipid metabolism with its associated hypercholesterolemia and hypertriglyceridemia plays a role in diabetic complications, such as heart disease, heart attacks and transient ischemic attacks. If there is loss of vision, the dilated funduscopic examination may show areas of ocular ischemia.

Family History

Do members of the family have diabetes, Type 1 or Type 2 diabetes? Do family members who are diabetic have eye disease that lead to blindness or amputation or kidney dialysis? Is there a history of stroke and/or cardiovascular disease in the family? Ask about glaucoma in family members. Open-angle glaucoma is common among Type 2 diabetic patients. Rubeotic glaucoma is common in Type 1 diabetics who have been in poor glycemic control (Table 5-1).

EXAMINATION

Visual Acuity

Visual acuity can tell you if the patient is seeing 20/40 or better **and therefore able to** perform the activities of daily living or continue to drive legally. Visual acuity at 20/40 to 20/60 range may signify macular edema. Visual acuity at the level of 20/200 or worse signifies legal blindness. Vision worse than 20/200 suggests that the patient might have proliferative diabetic retinopathy and requires close monitoring with an ophthalmologist.

Pupils

The pupillary examination will show brisk response to light and accommodation. Diabetic patients who have never had previous eye surgery but exhibit a sluggish but symmetrical

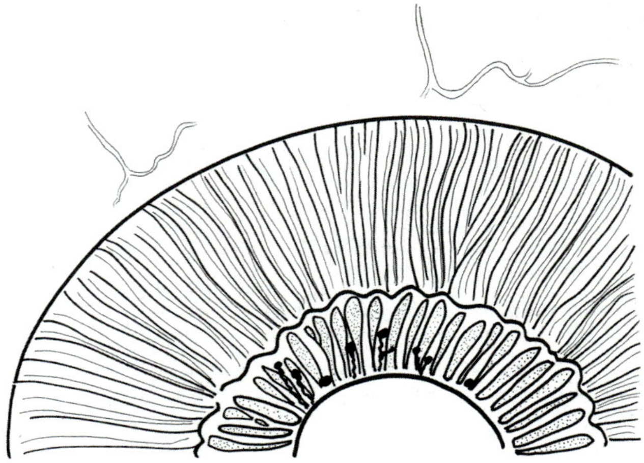

FIGURE 5-1. Iris neovascularization, diagram.

papillary response may have iris atrophy or an abnormality of the iris at the sphincter muscle. Thus, there is an inability of the iris to contract properly. In these patients with sluggish but equal papillary responses, it is important to look for rubeosis iridis on the slit lamp examination (Fig. 5-1). It is these same eyes that will have a poor ability to respond to dilating and diagnostic drops.

Extraocular Movements

The extraocular movements may reveal a III nerve palsy or VI nerve palsy from diabetes. Look for superior oblique palsy for IV nerve palsy. Is there a new onset of diplopia or head tilt in a diabetic patient?

Eyelids

Look for symmetric lid position of the eyelids. If there is ptosis of long-standing duration, the **ophthalmologist** will see creases of the ipsilateral frontalis muscle.

SLIT LAMP EXAMINATION

Cornea

Is the cornea clear? Are there signs of previous scars from old recurrent corneal abrasion? Is there corneal edema? Is there abnormal punctuate staining of the cornea from dry eye? Look at **Descemet** membrane for folds suggesting corneal dysfunction in diabetic patients with long-standing diabetic retinopathy. Is the patient at risk for corneal epithelial defect in the future? Are there areas of corneal thinning?

Anterior Chamber

Is there evidence of cell and flare which one would find in rubeosis iridis? Is there chronic flare which would mean long-standing inflammation in the diabetic eye? The long-standing inflammation could be due to rubeosis iridis or recent panretinal laser photocoagulation. Is the chamber deep or is there a risk of angle-closure glaucoma?

Iris

Look for rubeosis iridis under low-power and then under high-power magnification. Look in the crypts of the iris to find rubeosis iridis. Look at the iris margin to find early pinpoint rubeosis iridis. In brown-eyed patients, it is especially difficult to identify small tufts of neovascularization. Looking for iris neovascularization would entail a darkened room with an intense but narrowed slit beam at the pupillary margin.

Lens

Look for a diabetic cataract in noncompliant diabetics or diabetic patients who have been suddenly out of control of long-standing Type 1 diabetes. Type 1 diabetics usually exhibit early cataract formation. Look at the Y suture in the center of the lens. There may be isolated abnormalities near the Y suture suggesting a severe illness in childhood, especially common in Type 1 diabetic patients. The lens opacity may correlate to the first time the patient was diagnosed with diabetes in childhood.

Gonioscopy

Look at the angle by Goldmann three-mirror or the Zeiss four-mirror lens. Angle neovascularization is very common in diabetic patients with proliferative diabetic retinopathy. Press on the angle to view small fronds of neovascularization which might be hidden from **the view**.

EXAMINATION OF THE RETINA (SEE CHAPTER 3)

In examining the retina, the use of the direct ophthalmoscope, indirect ophthalmoscope, Goldmann contact lens, hand held 60-D lens, and 90-D lens are all useful. The 90-D lens is small, fits into a pocket, and can be used at all times. Direct ophthalmoscope has been less utilized in a retina practice since retinal specialists have myriad equipment and cameras to examine the retina and the optic nerve.

However, the direct ophthalmoscope is useful as a screening tool for evaluating the optic nerve before we examine the optic nerve using the 90-D lens. The direct ophthalmoscope is a useful teaching tool for medical students and general internal medicine colleagues who are not trained to use the indirect ophthalmoscope.

The retina is extremely important part of the diabetic eye examination since so much pathology can occur while the patient may be relatively asymptomatic. For example, optic nerve cupping, optic disc neovascularization, trace macular edema, cotton-wool spots in the periphery, and microaneurysms all can be existent while the patient sees 20/20.

Optic Nerve

Starting out with the optic nerve head, the examination can begin at the slit lamp. The 90-D lens or 60-D lens can do the job. The optic nerve can be examined for fine fronds of neovascularization (Fig. 5-2), flame-shaped hemorrhages as in glaucoma. Glaucoma can occur with diabetic patients. While the etiology is unclear about the association of glaucoma and diabetes, optic disc pathology and abnormalities can be seen in the examination of a diabetic patient.[5] A recent study involving 76,000 women in the Nurses Health Study shows there is a 70% increased risk of developing open-angle glaucoma in women with diabetes as compared to women without diabetes.[6–8] At the optic nerve, look for abnormalities of the caliber of the vessels or unusual circumferential vessels which would also indicate increased cupping and therefore increased glaucomatous risk.

Then, look at the nerve fiber layer emanating from the optic nerve. Is it abnormal? This is the baseline information. If this area changes sequentially over time, this would make the clinician think about glaucoma in the setting of diabetes.

The optic nerve can demonstrate atrophy from long-standing quiescent proliferative diabetic retinopathy. Optic nerve atrophy can be seen in patients with a history of heavy panretinal photocoagulation, overall retinal atrophy, and attenuation of the retinal

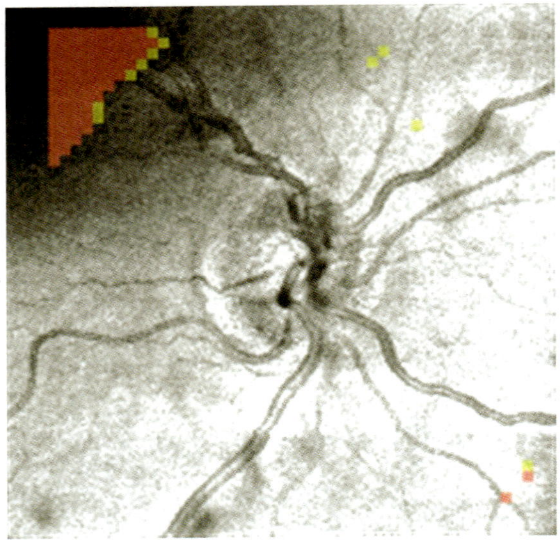

FIGURE 5-2. Optic nerve neovascularization, diagram.

arterioles in all four quadrants. These patients may have had 25 years or more of diabetes and may have 20/20 to 20/40 vision in the center, but there is a pale optic nerve. It is unclear whether the atrophy is from open-angle glaucoma or from low-tension glaucoma due to chronic poor blood flow to the optic nerve.

Optic disc edema can occur in diabetic patients. This is usually nonarteritic anterior ischemic optic neuropathy (NAION).[9] The systemic diseases associated with this entity include hypertension, diabetes, and prior history of cardiovascular disease such as a past history of a myocardial infarction. Arteritic AION is due to giant cell arteritis which has severe risk of visual loss. In NAION, the visual loss is less severe, but NAION is more common than the arteritic AION. The vision loss in NAION is painless. The patient may complain of loss of vision upon awakening.

In arteritic AION, the disc is chalky white, pale, and swollen. Ischemia in multiple vascular regions can occur as central retinal artery occlusion, choroidal infarction, anterior segment ischemia, and extraocular muscle ischemia causing diplopia. Arteritic AION is associated with pain, scalp tenderness, pain when brushing hair, jaw claudication, and pain while chewing. Temporal arteries may be prominent and tender. Sedimentation rate can be obtained to verify the diagnosis.

In NAION, atherosclerosis, arteriolar sclerosis is thought to affect the circulation of the optic nerve head. The posterior ciliary arteries feed the optic nerve head, and these are affected in hypertension and diabetes.

In arteritic AION, similar anatomy is affected. Giant cells affect the posterior ciliary arteries, the orbital vessels, and the central retinal artery (Table 5-2).

TABLE 5.2 Checklist for the Retinal Examination: Optic Disc

Field 1 optic disc
Disc edema (think nonarteritic AION)
Disc pallor (think arteritic AION, low-tension glaucoma)
Optic nerve neovascularization
Cup to disc ratio
Flame-shaped hemorrhage at the optic disc (think glaucoma)
Optociliary shunt vessels at the disc (think old branch vein occlusion)
Look for emboli in the lumen of vessels in TIA complaints

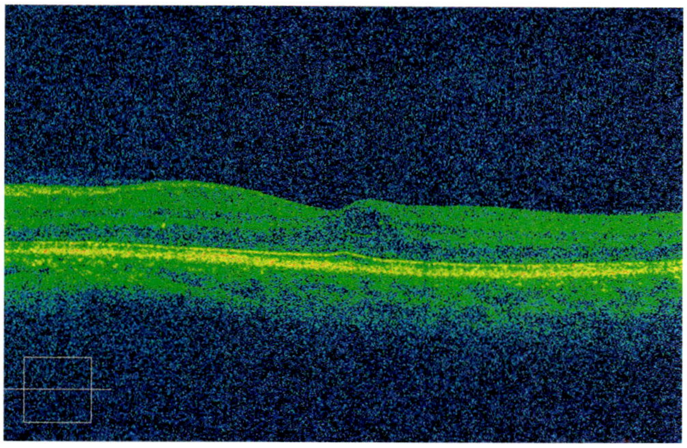

FIGURE 5-3. OCT scan: Mild macular edema, V 20/40.

The Macula at the Slit Lamp

The macula can be evaluated at the slit lamp using the 90-D lens. The interface of the vitreous and macula should be invisible. Once there is a demarcation, then you are seeing a posterior vitreous detachment, partial or total. In addition, the vitreous interface with the macula is important in the development of the macular cysts and macular edema in diabetic patients. In rare instances, the vitreous and internal limiting membrane interface warns us of the macular hole formation in Type 2 diabetic patients who have coexisting hypertension.[10–12]

Macular edema can be seen by looking at the area, using retroillumination techniques to scan the surface of the retina. The OCT scan serves as an adjunct enabling the clinician to view the irregularities on the surface of the vitreous and internal limiting membrane interface. The OCT can colorfully diagram the abnormalities. Any irregularity can be subtle, but it will be seen on the OCT scan. Or the OCT can demonstrate macular edema which is barely seen by slit lamp biomicroscopy (Fig. 5-3). Note that this irregularity in macular edema, cystic type, is less pronounced than that found in macular gliosis.

At the macula, you can also see large cysts and blebs of fluids that will be magnified by the optics of the 90-D lens or 60-D lens. The anterior-posterior distortion of the 90-D lens will be greater than that of the 60-D lens. Thus, the macular cysts will appear to be more elevated in the anterior-posterior direction (coming toward you in the vitreous plane)in the 90-D lens than in the 60-D lens.[13]

At the macula, look for radiating folds of fluid as well. These can also be seen with gliosis after long-standing macular laser (Tables 5-3 and 5-4).

After Macular Laser

There may be gliosis on the surface, there can be widening of the macular laser burns, and there can be scar formation at the macula from old laser burns. All of this occurs months

TABLE 5.3 Checklist for the Retinal Examination: Macula

Field 2 macula
Macular edema
Hard exudates
Dot blot hemorrhages
Cotton-wool spots
Ghost vessels
Microaneurysms

TABLE 5.4 Checklist for the Retinal Examination: Temporal to the Macula

Field 3 temporal to the macula
Hard exudates
Dot blot hemorrhages
Cotton-wool spots
Ghost vessels
Microaneurysms

and years after cellular repair mechanisms throughout the different layers of the macula. Recurrent and/or residual macular edema can occur as well.

Slit lamp biomicroscopy with the 60-D or 90-D lens allows the clinician to evaluate the macula and fovea. Look for macular edema with slit lamp biomicroscopy. Look at the vitreous with slit lamp biomicroscopy. During this examination, one could look for any abnormalities of the retina-vitreous interface with the 90-D lens. Subtle neovascularization can be seen in a darkened room with low illumination to medium illumination at the slit lamp.

At the slit lamp, one could also examine the retina within the arcades. Within the arcades, the posterior pole, there is usually a site where the pathology correlates with the visual acuity or Amsler grid findings. If you look carefully, you could correlate visual field abnormalties with cotton-wool spots or clusters of microaneurysms with macular edema and hence decreased vision. These areas of abnormal venous abnormalities such as IRMA (intraretinal microvascular abnormalities) or venous beading would signal severe nonproliferative diabetic retinopathy. The foveal capillary net would be part of the examination with a 90-D lens. The artery-to-vein ratio, if abnormal, would signal hypertensive changes in addition to diabetic retinopathy which could be further identified with fluorescein angiography.

ASSOCIATED SYSTEMIC DISEASES

Hypertension

As we all know, diabetic patients often have associated hypertension or cardiovascular disease. Slit lamp biomicroscopy and a 90-D lens would allow for the detection of hypertensive changes, such as silver wiring or copper wiring which denotes hyalinization of the arterioles (Fig. 5-4). In addition, the presence of more hard exudates than microaneurysms would lead the clinician to think of hyperlipidemia in the diabetic patient.

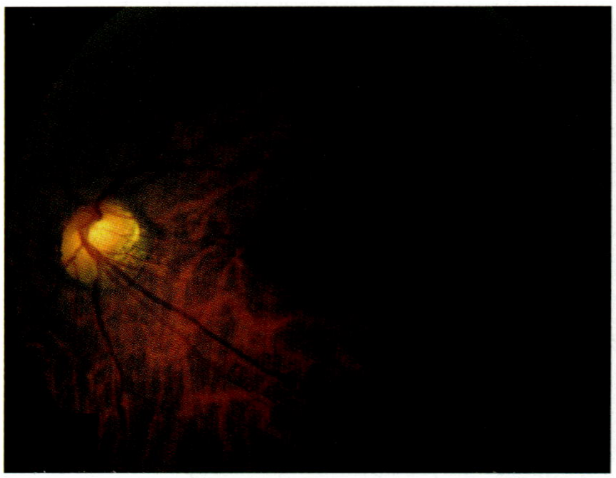

FIGURE 5-4. Hypertensive arteriolar narrowing, superotemporal to optic nerve.

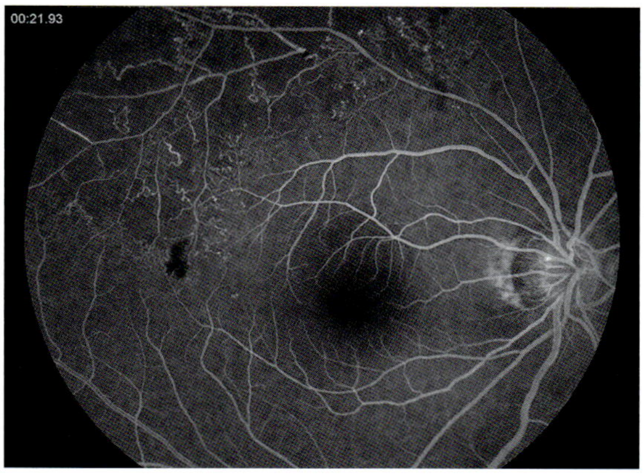

FIGURE 5-5. Featureless retina: Capillary nonperfusion on fluorescein angiogram.

The presence of "featureless" retina in between the arteries and veins would make the clinician consider the presence of capillary nonperfusion (Fig. 5-5). At this point, think of ordering a fluorescein angiogram to document the changes that you suspect.

The lack of capillary nonperfusion can be exacerbated by uncontrolled hypertension, smoking, and collagen vascular disease in the diabetic patient. Cardiovascular disease or carotid disease in a diabetic patient leads to greater risk of proliferative diabetic retinopathy at an accelerated rate.

Cardiovascular Disease

In diabetic patients with severe ischemic heart disease, one would expect to see a relatively quiet retina, with little macular edema but rather loss of capillaries and loss of retinal function. The arterioles will be narrowed; the color of the retina in one eye versus the other eye would be different in some cases, especially in the setting of asymmetric carotid disease.

Patients with ischemic heart disease who present with the loss of vision have retinal findings that appear "normal," that is, without cotton-wool spots, hard exudates. However, the retina is actually manifesting capillary nonperfusion. This is the time to do a fluorescein angiogram whereupon one could see areas of capillary nonperfusion in several quadrants of the retina.

Using indirect ophthalmoscopy, look for traction retinal detachments, abnormal neovascularization in the periphery, schisis cavities, and abnormalities of the vitreous interface at the areas of the retina, anterior to the equator (Table 5-5).

Traction Retinal Detachments

These can be emanating from the macula, extending to the arcades. These cases need to be scheduled for surgical intervention once the patient's blood sugar is evaluated and

TABLE 5.5 Checklist for the Retinal Examination: Equator

Field 4 (superotemporal), field 5 (inferotemporal), field 6 (superonasal), field 7 (inferonasal)
Hard exudates
Dot blot hemorrhages
Cotton-wool spots
Ghost vessels
Microaneurysms
Areas of capillary nonperfusion
Neovascularization elsewhere

stabilized. At this stage of proliferative diabetic retinopathy, the patient usually has some cardiovascular issues or EKG abnormalities. Thus, preoperative clearance with the internist or primary care physician is needed prior to having the surgery.

Abnormal neovascularization of the periphery is difficult to see with the indirect ophthalmoscope; however, with the ophthalmologist appropriately dark adapted, one can see fine fronds of neovascularization. They are seen usually in areas of the retina that seem paler in color or different in color than other quadrants of the retina in the same eye. These areas can be examined in the seven standard fields of fundus photography. Lastly, if you suspect neovascularization elsewhere (extramacular), you can order a fluorescein angiogram.

Schisis Cavities and Retinal Holes

Schisis cavities can exist outside the areas of the arcades and outside the areas of panretinal photocoagulation. Retinal holes can exist in high myopes who are diabetic. Look for peripheral pathology while you are examining the diabetic eye. Diabetic patients may have small atrophic holes in the periphery. It is important to examine the diabetic patient's ora serrata as well.

THE VITREOUS AND INDIRECT OPHTHALMOSCOPY

The vitreous can be abnormal in the diabetic patient. The vitreous interface at the macula can be adherent to the cystic changes in the macula in long-standing macular edema. The vitreous can be adherent and scarred to areas of the macula after macular laser if there was past inflammation. In areas of successfully treated and quiescent macular edema, the vitreous face will have been detached from the retina.

In patients with a light vitreous hemorrhage, there is a presence of red blood cells in the vitreous gel in the area of Cloquet canal (Fig. 5-6). This area is easily seen with a slit lamp biomicroscopy with a 90-D lens.

Vitreous Changes in High Myopia and Diabetes

The vitreous is abnormal and full of synergetic cavities in diabetic patients with >6 D of myopia. In myopic patients, their vitreous is liquefied earlier than age 40: there is increased vitreous liquefaction with increasing degrees of myopia. Because of the abnormal collagen

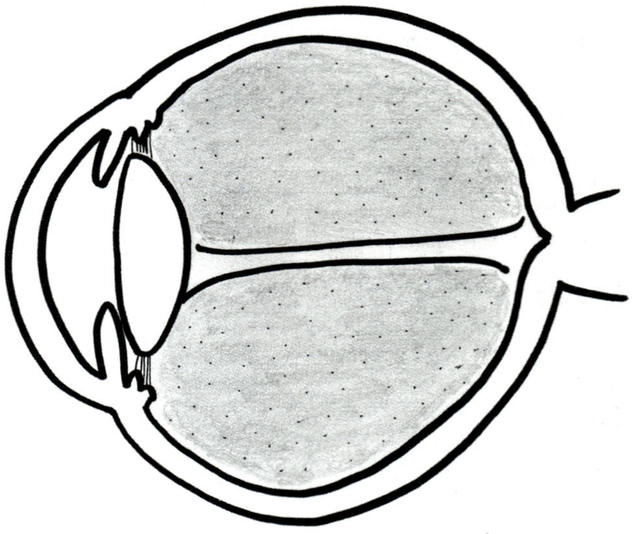

FIGURE 5-6. Schematic diagram of Cloquet Canal: Clear, central zone through the vitreous where the hyaloid artery originated in the embryonic eye.

in myopic eyes, these eyes have a tendency for retinal holes, abnormal vitreous collagen, and schisis cavities. When these same patients with high myopia develop diabetic retinopathy, their myopic retinal risk factors are added with diabetic retinopathy risks. Thus, for these patients, there is a need for more thorough retinal examinations—looking at their vasculature as well as their peripheral retina.[14–17]

Diabetic Myopes: Retinal Holes and Schisis

Because of the abnormal collagen in myopic eyes, these eyes have a tendency for retinal holes, abnormal vitreous collagen, and schisis cavities. When these same patients with high myopia develop diabetic retinopathy, their myopic retinal risk factors are added with diabetic retinopathy risks. Thus, for these patients, they have need for more thorough retinal examination looking at their vitreous and retinal interface in the macula as well as their peripheral retina.

REFERENCES

1. Chew EY, Ambrosius WT, Howard LT, et al. for the ACCORD Study Group. Rationale, design, and methods of the Action to Control Cardiovascular Risk in Diabetes Eye Study (ACCORD-EYE). *Am J Cardiol.* 2007;99:103i–111i.
2. The Action to Control Cardiovascular Risk in Diabetes Study Group. Effects of intensive glucose lowering in type 2 diabetes. *N Engl J Med.* 2008;358(24):2545–2559.
3. The ACCORD Study Group. Action to Control Cardiovascular Risk in Diabetes (ACCORD) Trial: Design and methods. *Am J Cardiol.* 2007;99:21i–33i.
4. Ferris FL, Davis MD, Aiello LM. Treatment of diabetic retinopathy. *N Engl J Med.* 1999;341:667–678.
5. Aiello LM, Wand M, Liang G. Neovascular glaucoma and vitreous hemorrhage following cataract surgery in patients with diabetes mellitus. *Ophthalmology.* 1983;90:814–820.
6. http://www.medicinenet.com/script/main/urt.asp?astidekey = 89226. Accessed 21 January 2009.
7. Pasquale L, Kang J, Manson J, et al. Prospective study of the Type 2 Diabetes Mellitus and Risk of Primary Open Angle Glaucoma in Women. *Ophthalmology.* 2006;113:1081–1086.
8. de Voogd S, Ikram M, Wolfs R, et al. Is Diabetes Mellitus a risk factor for open angle glaucoma? The Rotterdam Study. *Ophthalmology.* 2006;113:1827–1831.
9. Jacobson DM, Vierkant RA, Belongia EA. Nonarteritic anterior ischemic optic neuropathy: A case control study of potential risk factors. *Arch Ophthalmol.* 1997;115:1403–1407.
10. Takahashi M, Trempe CL, Schepens CL. Biomicroscopic evaluation and photography of posterior vitreous detachment. *Arch Ophthalmol.* 1980;98:665–669.
11. Keikehashi A, Kado M, Akiba J, et al. Variations of posterior vitreous detachment. *Br J Ophthalmol.* 1997;81:527–532.
12. Nasrallah FP, Van de Velde F, Jalkh AE, et al. Importance of the vitreous in young diabetics with macular edema. *Ophthalmology.* 1989;96:1511–1516.
13. Kakehashi A, Schepens CL, Trempe CL. Vitreomacular Observations I. Vitreomacular adhesion and hole in the premacular hyaloid. *Ophthalmology.* 1994;101:1515–1521.
14. Ozdek SC, Onol M, Gürelik G, et al. Scanning Laser polarimetry in normal subjects and patients with myopia. *Br J Ophthalmol.* 2000;84:264–267.
15. Richards AJ, Scott JD, Snead MP. Molecular genetics of rhegmatogenous retinal detachment. *Eye.* 2002;16:388–392.
16. Fledelius HC. Is myopia getting more frequent? Across sectional study of 1416 Danes age 16 years. *Acta Ophthalmol (Copenh).* 1983;61:545–559.
17. Bishop PN. Structural macromolecules and supramolecular organization of vitreous gel. *Prog Retin Eye Res.* 2000;19: 323–344.

SUGGESTED READINGS

1. Aiello LM, Rand LI, Briones JC, et al. Diabetic retinopathy in Joslin Clinic patients with adult-onset diabetes. *Ophthalmology.* 1981;88:619–623.
2. Ansell PL, Marshall J. Laser-induced phagocytosis in the pigment epithelium of the Hunter dystrophic rat. *Br J Ophthalmol.* 1976;60:819–828.
3. Blankenship GW. Diabetic macular edema and argon laser photocoagulation: A prospective randomized study. *Ophthalmology.* 1979;86:69–75.
4. Bresnick GH. Diabetic maculopathy: A critical review highlighting diffuse macular edema. *Ophthalmology.* 1983;90:1301–1317.
5. British Multicentre Study Group. Photocoagulation for diabetic maculopathy. A randomized controlled clinical trial using the xenon arc. *Diabetes.* 1983;32:1010–1016.
6. Casswell AG, Canning CR, Gregor ZJ. Treatment of diffuse diabetic macular edema: A comparison between argon and krypton lasers. *Eye.* 1990;4:668–672.
7. Clover GM. The effects of argon and krypton photocoagulation on the retina: Implications for the inner and outer blood retinal barriers. In: Gitter KA, Schatz H, Yannuzzi LA, et al., eds. *Laser Photocoagulation of Retinal Disease.* San Francisco, CA: Pacific Medical Press; 1988:11–18.

8. Crues AF, Williams JC, Willan AR. Argon green and krypton red laser treatment of diabetic macular edema. *Can J Ophthalmol.* 1988;23:262–266.
9. Early Treatment Diabetic Retinopathy Study Research Group. ETDRS Report No. 1. Photocoagulation for diabetic macular edema. *Arch Ophthalmol.*1985;103:1796–1806.
10. Early Treatment Diabetic Retinopathy Study Research Group. ETDRS Report No 2. Treatment techniques and clinical guidelines for photocoagulation of diabetic macular edema. *Ophthalmology.* 1987;94:761–774.
11. Early Treatment Diabetic Retinopathy Study Research Group. ETDRS Report No 4. Photocoagulation for diabetic macular edema. *Int Ophthalmol Clin.* 1987;27:265–272.
12. Early Treatment Diabetic Retinopathy Study Research Group. ETDRS Report No. 9. Early photocoagulation for diabetic retinopathy. *Ophthalmology.* 1991;98:766–785.
13. Early Treatment Diabetic Retinopathy Study Research Group. ETDRS Report No 10. Grading diabetic retinopathy from stereoscopic color fundus photographs – An extension of the modified Airlie House classification. *Ophthalmology.* 1991;98:786–806.
14. Ferris FL, Patz A. Macular edema. A complication of diabetic retinopathy. *Surv Ophthalmol.* 1984;28:452–461.
15. Ferris FL, Podgor MJ, Davis MD. The Diabetic Retinopathy Study Research Group, Report No. 12. Macular edema in diabetic retinopathy study patients. *Ophthalmology.* 1987;94:754–760.
16. Kayazawa F, DeJesus GT, Miyake K. Grid-pattern laser photocoagulation for diabetic diffuse macular edema (the Japanese experience). In: Gitter KA, Schatz H, Yannuzzi LA, et al., eds. *Laser Photocoagulation of Retinal Disease.* San Francisco, CA: Pacific Medical Press; 1988:65–68.
17. Kinyoun J, Barton F, Fisher, et al. Detection of diabetic macular edema: Ophthalmology versus photography. Early Treatment Diabetic Retinopathy Study Report No. 5. *Ophthalmology.* 1989;96:746–751.
18. Klein R, Klein BEK, Moss SE. Visual impairment in diabetes. *Ophthalmology.* 1984;91:1–8.
19. Klein R, Klein BEK, Moss SE, et al. Prevalence of diabetes mellitus in Southern Wisconsin. *Am J Epidemiol.* 1984;119:54–61.
20. Klein R, Klein BEK, Moss SE, et al. The Wisconsin Epidemiologic Study of Diabetic Retinopathy. VI. Diabetic macular edema. *Ophthalmology.* 1987;94:754–760.
21. Klein R, Klein BEK, Moss SE, et al. The Wisconsin Epidemiologic Study of Diabetic Retinopathy. IX. Four-year incidence and progression of diabetic retinopathy when age of diagnosis is less than 30 years. *Arch Ophthalmol.* 1989;107: 237–243.
22. Kohner EM. The evolution and natural history of diabetic retinopathy. *Int Ophthalmol Clin.* 1978;18(4):1–16.
23. Lee CM, Olk RJ. Modified grid laser photocoagulation for diffuse diabetic macular edema: Long-term visual results. *Ophthalmology.* 1991;98:1594–1602.
24. Mainster MA. Wavelength selection in macular photocoagulation: Tissue optics, thermal effects, and laser systems. *Ophthalmology.* 1986;93:952–958.
25. McDonald HR, Schatz H. Grid photocoagulation for diffuse macular edema. *Retina.* 1985;5:65–72.
26. McMeel JW, Trempe CL, Franks EB. Symposium: Current status of photocoagulation of macular disease: Diabetic maculopathy. *Trans Am Acad Ophthalmol Otolaryngol.* 1977;83:476–487.
27. Moss SE, Klein R, Klein BEK. The incidence of vision loss in a diabetic population. *Ophthalmology.* 1988;95: 1340–1348.
28. Olk RJ. Modified grid argon (blue-green) laser photocoagulation for diffuse diabetic macular edema. *Ophthalmology.* 1986;93:938–950.
29. Olk RJ. Argon-green vs krypton-red modified grid laser photocoagulation for diffuse diabetic macular edema. In: Gitter KA, Schatz H, Yannuzzi LA, et al., eds. *Laser Coagulation of Retinal Disease.* San Francisco, CA: Pacific Medical Press; 1988:75–81.
30. Olk RJ. Argon green (514 nm) versus krypton red (647 nm) modified grid laser photocoagulation for diffuse diabetic macular edema. *Ophthalmology.* 1990;97:1101–1113.
31. Sigelman J. Diabetic macular edema in juvenile and adult-onset diabetes. *Am J Ophthalmol.* 1980;90:287–296.
32. Striph GG, Hart WM, Olk RJ. Modified grid laser photocoagulation for diabetic macular edema. The effect on the central visual field. *Ophthalmology.* 1988;95:1673–1679.
33. Wallow IH. Repair of the pigment epithelial barrier following photocoagulation. *Arch Ophthalmol.* 1984;102: 126–135.
34. Welter J, Zuckerman R. The influence of the photoreceptor-RPE complex on the inner retina. An explanation for the beneficial effects of photocoagulation. *Ophthalmology.* 1980;87:1133–1139.

CHAPTER 6

New Treatment Modalities

TRIAMCINOLONE

Intravitreal Triamcinolone and Vitrectomy

Intravitreal triamcinolone is used for visual demarcation of the vitreous at the time of vitrectomy. Kumagai and Burk[1,2] performed this technique using 40 mg of triamcinolone in a 3-mL syringe, connected to a three-way joint (Millipore filter), which in turn is connected to a 10-mL syringe containing balanced salt solution (BSS) (Alcon laboratories, Fort Worth, TX). The aqueous phase of the triamcinolone solution is discarded through the filter, leaving the particulate matter of the triamcinolone in the 3-mL syringe. Triamcinolone particles are mixed and washed in the 3-mL syringe. This is done three times, discarding, mixing, and washing. The final volume of 0.1 mL of desired 3-mL triamcinolone solution is suspended in the BSS and then injected into the vitreous cavity. The triamcinolone particles are trapped in the vitreous gel and enable visualization of the vitreous.[1,2]

Kumagai and Burk[1,2] used 0.2-mL triamcinolone acetonide (40 mg/mL), which was filtered through a 5-μm filter and rinsed with 2 mL of BSS and resuspended and recaptured; this was repeated for a total of three times before it was injected into the eye.[1,2] Furino et al.[3] used triamcinolone acetonide (40 mg/mL), which was injected in midvitreous to visualize the posterior hyaloid once core vitrectomy is performed. They used 0.1 to 0.2 mL of triamcinolone acetonide to visualize the retinal surface's epiretinal membranes. No adverse reactions were observed with the use of triamcinolone acetonide without the use of the BSS.

Triamcinolone acetonide has been considered for use in the treatment of diabetic macular edema.[4] Triamcinolone acetonide has been used without surgery and found to improve the macular edema in 28 eyes of 20 patients. Jonas et al.[5] found no adverse glaucomatous side effects and reported improved visual acuity after 7 months of follow-up.

The use of triamcinolone acetonide in vitrectomy surgery serves as an aid for visualization during complete vitrectomy in cases of macular edema. In addition, triamcinolone acetonide reduces postsurgical inflammation which may exacerbate macular edema.[6] Matsumoto et al.[7] have found that intravitreal triamcinolone improves the removal of posterior vitreous hyaloid by using electron microscopy to examine the surgical specimens. Intravitreal triamcinolone acetonide decreased blood ocular barrier breakdown and improved visual acuity postoperatively in eight diabetic macular edema eyes and ten proliferative diabetic retinopathy eyes of patients who underwent pars plana vitrectomy.[8] They used an anterior chamber laser flare detector to study the side effects.

Intravitreal Triamcinolone Acetonide and Diabetic Macular Edema

Intravitreal triamcinolone is used for the treatment of refractory diabetic macular edema. The treatment has its origins in 2002 when clinically significant diabetic macular edema eyes failed to respond to previous laser photocoagulation sessions. After 6 months of initial laser therapy, the response is measured by OCT and clinical examination.

If central macular thickness of 300 μm is attained (normals 200 μm), 4 mg of intravitreal triamcinolone acetonide is injected. In one small study, 16 patients were evaluated, and the average increase in Snellen visual acuity was two lines of visual improvement and a mean of 50% decrease of thickness on OCT scans.[4] Vitreous vascular endothelial growth factor (VEGF) and stromal-derived factor-1 levels were measured by enzyme linked immunosorbent assay in samples obtained immediately before and 1 month after the injection of intravitreal triamcinolone.[9,10]

In a Phase III, multicenter, randomized study, the Diabetic Retinopathy Clinical Research Network (DRCR.net) investigated the safety and efficacy of preservative-free intravitreal triamcinolone acetonide (1 and 4 mg) and compared these treatments with standard ETDRS focal/grid photocoagulation for the treatment of diabetic macular edema. The study enrolled 840 eyes divided into three treatment arms. After a 2-year follow-up, the authors concluded that the focal/grid photocoagulation treatment was more effective and displayed fewer side effects than either the 1- or 4-mg doses of preservative-free triamcinolone acetonide for diabetic macular edema patients. Thus, focal/grid photocoagulation is still the benchmark against which other treatments are compared in diabetic macular edema studies.[11]

VEGF INHIBITORS

VEGF is a potent enhancer of vascular permeability and a key inducer of angiogenesis. VEGF is identified in tumor models as a vasopermeability factor and an initiator of angiogenesis upregulated by hypoxia. VEGF is the strongest endothelial mitogen and can also induce the expression of plasminogen activator in vascular endothelial cells, which, in turn, are important in the extracellular proteolysis necessary for capillary formation and breakdown of blood retinal barrier.[12] VEGF, also known as VEGF-A or VEGF-1, is expressed as five mRNA splice variants: isoforms 121, 145, 165, 189, and 206.[13] VEGF isoform 165 is a critical isoform for both developmental and pathologic retinal angiogenesis. VEGF is expressed by retinal endothelial cells and retinal pigment epithelial cells in vitro and is upregulated by hypoxia.[14,15] Other modulators of VEGF expression are hypoglycemia, beta-estradiol, and rod outer segments.[16–19]

Clinical studies have demonstrated that VEGF plays a role in ischemic retinal diseases. Vitreous from surgical specimens show increased VEGF levels in patients with proliferative disease from diabetes or retinal vein occlusion.[20,21] VEGF protein levels decrease after successful laser retinal ablation.[22]

PEGAPTANIB (MACUGEN)

Pegaptanib, a novel RNA aptamer, originally used in the treatment of AMD, binds and inactivates VEGF isoform 165. In animal models, the VEGF isoform 165 can induce diabetes-like ocular pathology. Pegaptanib has been shown in animal models to reverse the blood retinal barrier breakdown associated with diabetes. Aptamers are short nucleic acid sequences of a specific strand shape and length, which can bind to their target polypeptides and change their final form.[23] Target polypeptides can be RNA or DNA which are chemically synthesized through a process, named systemic evolution of ligands by exponential enrichment.[24,25] In pegaptanib, a large library of RNA sequences ranging from 10^{14} to 10^{15} are incubated with the target molecule, VEGF isoform 165. The unbound sequence is washed away, and the target molecule, VEGF isoform 165, is uncoupled from the candidate strands; this process is repeated 8 to 15 times.[24,25] The end product has increased specificity of the aptamer for the target, VEGF isoform 165. The molecule is selectively binding only to VEGF isoform 165. The binding of the pegaptanib aptamer to VEGF isoform 165 lasts 6 weeks.

In the course of evaluating the properties of VEGF, two are particularly relevant in the pathogenesis of diabetic retinopathy. VEGF is upregulated by hypoxia and thus creates neovascularization as a response to hypoxia. Secondly, VEGF is a potent inducer of vascular permeability, 50,000 times more potent than histamine. VEGF causes fenestrations in the endothelium, dissolution of tight junctions, induction of leukostasis, and subsequent injury to the endothelium.[26] These characteristics of VEGF support a direct involvement of VEGF in the diabetic macular edema, a form of diabetic retinopathy.

These observations were the basis of the Phase II clinical trial involving pegaptanib and diabetic macular edema.[27] Participants had the best corrected visual acuity of 20/50 to 20/320 in the study eye with diabetic macular edema involving the center of the macula, for whom the investigator judged laser photocoagulation could be safely withheld for 16 weeks. Intravitreal pegaptanib was injected at the onset of study, week 6, and week 12 with additional injections and/or focal photocoagulation as needed for another 18 weeks. Final assessments were done at week 36. Outcome measures were visual acuity and central subfield thickness measurements using OCT. A total of 172 patients were enrolled in the study. Compared to sham injections, the patients given 0.3 mg had a better visual acuity (20/50) versus sham treated patients (20/63). Mean central thickness of the retina as measured by OCT showed mean reduction of 68 μm in retinal thickness in the 0.3 mg-treated group versus an increase of 4 μm in the sham-treated group at week 36. Thus, early data showed that pegaptanib may have a beneficial role in the treatment of diabetic macular edema.[27]

VEGF also plays a role in neovascularization leading to evaluation of pegaptanib for the treatment of proliferative diabetic retinopathy. Using the patient information from the Phase II clinical trial of pegaptanib and diabetic macular edema,[27] data were retrospectively analyzed to discern the effects of pegaptanib on retinal neovascularization.[28] Patients in the analysis had the best corrected vision of 20/50 to 20/320 and had received a sham injection or intravitreal pegaptanib (0.3, 1, or 3 mg) at onset, week 6, and week 12. Changes in neovascularization were assessed by fundus photography and fluorescein angiography. Of the 172 original study patients, 19 had retinal neovascularization in the study eye at baseline. One of these 19 patients was excluded because he had scatter laser photocoagulation 13 days before randomization; two others were excluded because fundus photographs were not available. The median age of the remaining 16 patients was 55.5 years. Eight of the thirteen patients in the pegaptanib-treatment group showed regression documented by fundus photographs or fluorescein angiography at 36 weeks versus none in the sham group. No fellow (nonstudy) eyes showed regression of neovascularization at 36 weeks on fundus photographs or fluorescein angiography. This small study showed that pegaptanib treatment can lead to regression of diabetic neovascularization.[27,28]

BEVACIZUMAB (AVASTIN)

Bevacizumab is a mouse-derived monoclonal antibody to all isoforms of VEGF. In animal studies using tumor cell lines and models with ocular neovascularization, bevacizumab was effective against primary permeability and proliferative effects of VEGF. It has a molecular weight of 148 kDa, and it is a larger molecule than ranibizumab with 48 kDa.

There have been small studies evaluating bevacizumab and proliferative diabetic retinopathy. Forty-five eyes of 32 patients with retinal and/or iris neovascularization secondary to diabetes were given intravitreal 6.2 μg to 1.25 mg. All of the patients showed regression of neovascularization as seen with fluorescein angiography within 1 week. About 73% had complete resolution of disc neovascularization; 82% of the eyes had resolution of iris neovascularization. Follow-up was 11 weeks (Figs. 6-1 and 6-2).[29–31]

Two patients with proliferative diabetic retinopathy and vitreous hemorrhage were given intravitreal avastin.[30] Both patients manifested regression of retinal neovascularization after 1 month of follow-up. Vitreous hemorrhage in each patient showed partial resolution at 1 week and nearly complete regression in 1 month.[30]

These were the earliest studies of bevacizmab—in the treatment of proliferative diabetic retinopathy in 2006 when the drug was just being released for the treatment of age-related macular degeneration.

Since that time, bevacizumab (Avastin) has been used by retinal surgeons in the United States to great success, despite being a non–FDA-approved drug for diabetic retinopathy.

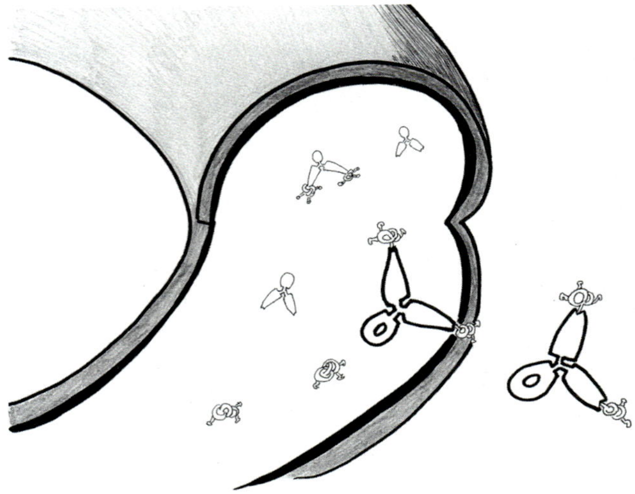

FIGURE 6-1. Monoclonal antibody blocking VEGF.

In another study, bevacizumab treatment of patients with diabetic macular edema yielded better visual outcome than laser photocoagulation.[31] Twelve weeks of follow-up was done in 37 eyes treated with bevacizumab versus 33 eyes treated with laser. Combination therapy of bevacizumab and triamcinolone eyes had a beneficial effect at 6 weeks but not at 12 weeks. Thus, bevacizumab alone was found to be more efficacious in this small study.[31]

The Pan American Collaborative Retina Study Group evaluated 78 eyes of 64 patients with a follow-up of 6 months, from six centers from six countries.[32] The patients were treated with at least one intravitreal injection of 1.25 or 2.5 mg of bevacizumab and were tested using ETDRS vision testing, OCT, and fluorescein angiography at baseline and follow-up visits. Sixteen eyes needed a second injection at a mean of 13.8 weeks (range was 4 to 28 weeks); six eyes needed a third injection at a mean of 11.5 weeks (range was 5 to 20 weeks). Final best corrected visual acuity analysis by subgroups showed that 41.1% of the eyes remained stable and 55.1% improved or had greater than or equal to two ETDRS

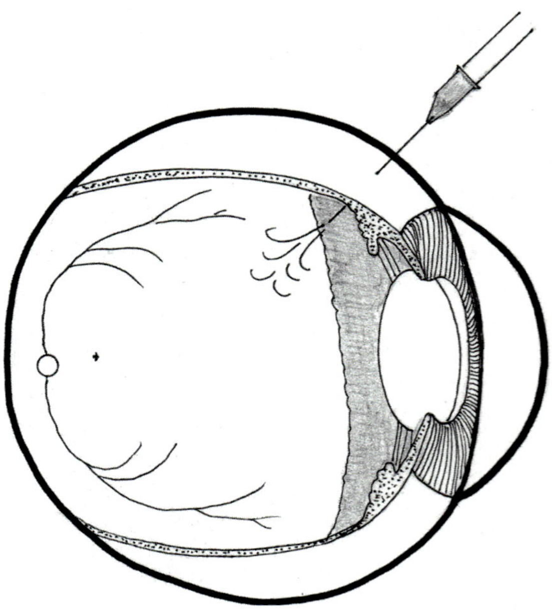

FIGURE 6-2. Intravitreal injection, cross- sectional view.

lines of visual acuity improvement. Mean central macular thickness at baseline OCT was 387.0 ± 182.8 μm and decreased to a mean 275.7 ± 108.3 μm at the end of follow-up. The authors concluded that primary intravitreal bevacizumab at doses of 1.25 and 3.5 mg provided stable or improved vision at 6 months of follow-up, using outcome measures of visual acuity, OCT, and fluorescein angiography.[32]

RANIBIZUMAB (LUCENTIS)

Ten patients were studied; five patients received 0.3 mg and five patients received 0.5 mg of ranibizumab intravitreally. At month 3, four of ten patients gained ≥10 letters of visual acuity, and eight of the ten patients gained ≥1 letter. At month 3, the mean decrease in OCT retinal thickness measurements was 45.3 ± 196.3 μm for the low-dose group and 197.8 ± 85.9 μm for the high-dose group.[33]

Ranibizumab is the antigen binding portion of the monoclonal antibody directed against VEGF. This monoclonal antibody fragment weighs 48 kDa and effectively blocks increased fluorescein leakage after laser in animal eyes. Ranibizumab is not FDA approved for diabetic macular edema, and ongoing studies at the time of this writing are being performed for the treatment of diabetic retinopathy and diabetic macular edema.[33]

A multicenter clinical trial sponsored by Juvenile Diabetes Research Foundation, named the READ Trial, is currently ongoing. READ-2 Study (Ranibizumab for Edema of the Macula in Diabetes) had its beginnings in 2006. Its purpose is to evaluate ranibizumab in diabetic patients with DME. Phase I of the study involved 20 patients with DME treated with repeated intravitreal injections of 0.5 mg of ranibizumab at baseline, months 1, 2, 4, and 6. Results showed that at month 7, the median reduction of excess of foveal thickness was 97% and a median improvement of ten letters (Fig. 6-3).[34]

Phase II of the READ Study enrolled 126 diabetic patients, with an average age of 62 years, with documented macular edema at enrollment; 115 patients had completed the trial at 6 months. Patients were included in the study if they had at least 250 μm on OCT scan of central macular thickness. Previous treatment was allowed if it had been given at least 3 months prior to the onset of the study. The majority had 20/80 average vision at enrollment. The subjects received ranibizumab 0.5 mg alone or with focal laser treatment or laser alone. At 6 months, improvement in visual acuity was noted to be the mean of 8 letters in the ranibizumab group, 3.8 letters improvement in the combination group of

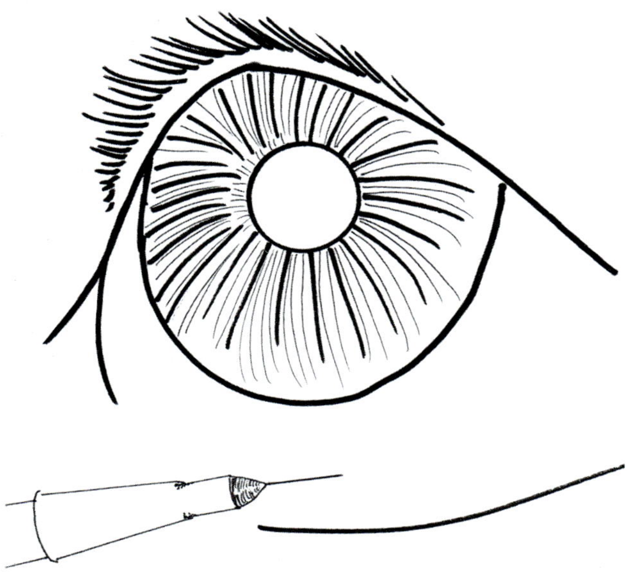

FIGURE 6-3. Intravitreal injection, external view.

ranibizumab and laser, and 1 letter loss in the laser-only group. The OCT showed 56% decrease in excess retinal thickness in the ranibizumab-treated group versus 11% reduction in those who received laser alone or laser and ranibizumab.[34–36]

Acetazolamide

Carbonic anhydrase inhibitors (CAI) have been known to work on retinal fluid absorption for the past two decades. Initial observations were based on experimental data which suggested that acetazolamide can increase fluid absorption across the retinal pigment epithelium (RPE). CAI have direct effects on retinal and retinal pigment epithelial cell function by inducing an acidification of the subretinal space, a decrease in the standing potential as well as an increase in retinal adhesion. It is thought that acidification of the subretinal space is responsible for the increase in fluid resorption from the retina through the RPE into the choroid.[37]

A normal clinical dose of CAI of 500 mg per day should be continued for 1 month to see an effect. The dose may be reduced by the patient over the course of the therapy. Metaphylaxis to the drug may occur with a rebound of edema despite continuation of treatment.[37–41]

NONSTEROIDAL ANTI-INFLAMMATORY DRUGS (NSAIDS)

Nonsteroidal Anti-inflammatory Eye Medications

Bromfenac (Xibrom ISTA) and nepafenac (Nevanac) are now available for diabetic macular edema, age-related macular degeneration, and cystoid macular edema. The prodrug formulation of the new NSAID such as nepafenac is thought to be more effective than the older generation of flurbiprofen 0.03% (Ocufen), ketorolac 0.5% (Acular), and diclofenac 0.1% (Voltaren).[42–44]

The older generation drugs, Ketorolac and Diclofenac, are FDA approved for the treatment of macular edema after cataract surgery. They have been used for the treatment of diabetic macular edema as well. Since diabetic macular edema is often refractory in diabetic patients with poor glycemic control, NSAIDs have been used along with topical prednisolone acetate and steroid injections in the vitreous such as triamcinolone.[4]

PHARMACOTECHNOLOGY

Intravitreal Implants and Drug Delivery Systems

Intravitreal implant, Iluvien, previously known as Medidur FA (Alimera Sciences, Alpharetta, GA) is a nonerodable insert. Iluvien is in Phase III clinical trials for the delivery of fluocinolone acetonide in patients with diabetic macular edema. Iluvien is 3.5 mm long and 0.37 mm in diameter. A 25-gauge insertion system facilitates intravitreal delivery in the office setting. The insert, once inside the globe, delivers an initial daily release rate of either 0.23 or 0.45 μg of fluocinolone acetonide, lasting 36 months. By October 2007, 956 patients were enrolled for a follow-up of 24 months, with a final analysis after 36 months. This is the FAME study, Fluocinolone Acetonide in Diabetic Macular Edema.[45–47]

CORTICOSTEROIDS

Fluocinolone Acetonide (Retisert)

Fluocinolone acetonide is a nonbiodegradable intravitreal corticosteroid implant. It is designed to release slowly over a 3-year time period. Retisert was originally designed for noninfectious uveitis affecting the posterior segment, affecting 175,000 people in the United States. On April 11, 2005, the FDA approved the use of Retisert for the treatment of chronic noninfectious uveitis affecting the posterior segment of the eye. The most common side effects are eye pain, cataract progression, and intraocular pressure elevation.[48]

Currently, Retisert has enrolled 80 patients who are randomized to receive either an implant 0.5 or 2.0 mg, or standard of care macular laser, or observation. These patients had refractory macular edema. At 12 months of follow-up, 49% of the eyes that are treated with 0.5-mg implant had resolution of the macular edema compared to 25% of the standard of care group ($p < 0.5$). More patients in the standard of care group had worsening diabetic retinopathy at 12 months than the 0.5-mg-implant group (30% vs. 5%). Serious ocular adverse events include increased intraocular pressure and vitreous hemorrhage, and cataract formation is significantly higher in the implant group (59%) than in the standard of care group (11%). This is an ongoing trial.[49]

Another steroid drug delivery system now being investigated is the biodegradeable dexamethasone in a posterior segment delivery system, Posurdex (Allergan, Irvine, CA). Posurdex is being evaluated for patients with diabetic macular edema, vein occlusions, pseudophakia, and uveitis. The implant is designed to last 37 days.[50]

In the Phase II trial, 306 patients were randomized to receive a 350-μg or 700-μm implant or observation. The eyes were divided as follows: 165 diabetic macular edema, 102 retinal vein occlusion, 25 Irvine Gass syndrome, and 14 uveitis. The average pretreatment vision was 20/80 to 20/85. At the 6-month endpoint, 36% of the 700-μg group and 27% in the 350-μg group had at least a two-line improvement of vision, as compared to the observation group which had 19% with two or more lines of improved vision. In the 700-μg group, 19% of patients had three or more lines of improvement, which was statistically significant compared to the 8% of the observation group who had the same improvement. The average change in retinal thickness was 142 μm for the 700-μg group and a decrease in retinal thickness of 61 μg in the 35-μg group. There was an increase of 11 μm in the central retinal thickness in the observation group.[50–52]

Another fluocinolone acetonide implant is Medidur. Medidur is a narrow 3 mm long micro-cylinder containing fluocinolone acetonide to be injected intravitreally in the office setting, using a 25-gauge injector. Its indications are being codeveloped by pSivida (Watertown, MA) and Alimera Sciences (Alpharetta, GA). Medidur has completed its initial 20-patient safety trial, and it is currently enrolling patients. The 20 patients were on a low dose of 0.23 μg a day and 17 patients on a high dose, approximately 0.45 μg a day. The 3-month results showed that 20% of the low-dose patients and 18% of the high-dose patients improved compared to controls.[53]

Another drug delivery system, I-Vation (Surmodics, Eden Prairie, MN), has been tested in a 30-patient Phase I study, with the delivery of triamcinolone acetonide in patients with diabetic macular edema. I-Vation requires surgical implantation at the pars plana region, under the conjunctiva, for rapid retrieval if needed. The Phase I study found that 100% of the patients either maintained or improved vision at 6 months. Eighty-seven percent or 26/30 patients who were treated with I-Vation triamcinolone acetonide had either the same or an improved vision. Forty-three percent or 13/30 patients achieved visual acuity of 20/40 or better compared to 20% or 6/30 patients at time of entry into the study. Mean retinal thickness decreased 164 μm or 37% and excess retinal thickness decreased 63% from baseline retinal thickness.[54]

Topical Eyedrops

CoMentis, Inc. (South San Francisco, CA) is interested in ATG-3 (mecamylamine), for the treatment of diabetic macular edema. ATG-3 works by inhibiting angiogenesis mediated by VEGF. This drug would be considered an adjunct to intravitreal ranibizumab.[45] The drug, ATG-3, is in the Phase II clinical trial. It is an antagonist of the nicotinic acetylcholine receptor pathway that may counter the vascular leakage and angiogenesis mediated by VEGF.[45]

TG100801 (tetrahydrozoline HCL) is another drug for diabetic macular edema. Its manufacturer is TargeGen, currently sponsoring Phase II clinical trials at the time of this writing. Tetrahydrozoline HCL is designed to suppress VEGF-mediated leakage associated with inflammation, edema, and angiogenesis of diabetic macular edema.[55]

Sirolimus is rapamycin, a macrolide immunosuppressive agent. It has been used to prevent coronary restenosis in the coating of coronary stents for angioplasty. Sirolimus has a target, mTOR, a protein kinase that regulates cell growth and metabolism in response to the presence of growth factors or other changes in the environment. Cell processes such as protein synthesis and nutrient transport are upregulated by mTOR.[56]

In addition, sirolimus has immunosuppressive, antiangiogenic, and antiproliferative properties. It inhibits VEGF by decreasing the endothelial cell response to VEGF activation through down-regulation of intracellular signaling. The inhibition of mTOR inhibits the activity of HIF-1 alpha which decreases VEGF production and inhibits VEGF-induced endothelial cell proliferation. For all of these properties, sirolimus is thought to have the potential in treating neovascularization in diabetic retinopathy.[56]

Sirolimus (Rapamune, Wyeth) is in a Phase I study for diabetic macular edema.[56,57] In its Phase 1 trial of 50 patients, the results showed improvements in visual acuity. Patients on the two lowest doses of sirolimus showed greater than or equal to 7.4 letters from baseline. Foveal thickness improved for 180 days after a single dose of sirolimus. One focus of the study is on the intravitreal or subconjunctival route as an effective method of drug delivery.

CLINICAL CORRELATIONS

Patient complaints: Loss of vision in one eye or sudden loss of vision, despite having had macular laser photocoagulation.

Caveats: Loss to follow-up with ophthalmologist, relocation to another city, and interruption of medical care

Case Study (Figs. 6-4–6-11)

8–22–08: JM is a 62-year-old Filipino male who has poorly controlled Type 2 diabetes for 5 years. He has relocated to California but has not had regular visits to his internist or endocrinologist in the past. However, 3 months ago, he did see an ophthalmologist who "lasered his eye." Now, he has trouble reading and working on his computer. He feels that the laser made his vision worse and states that he does "not want more laser."
Fasting blood glucose = 138 mg/dL, HbA1c = 5.9%, cholesterol = 226 mg/dL, LDL = 148 mg/dL.

V 20/60
20/20
Slit lamp examination
Cornea: Clear OU
Anterior chamber: Deep and quiet OU
Iris: Normal OU, no rubeosis OU
Lens: 1 + nuclear sclerosis OU
Applanation tonometry = 14/14 mm Hg (12:00 PM)
Gonioscopy: Open 360 degrees OU, no rubeosis OU

Dilated funduscopic examination:

Right eye: Clinically significant macular edema with previous laser
Left eye: Clinically significant macular edema with previous laser

Comment

In summary, this is nonproliferative diabetic retinopathy in a 62-year-old man with Type 2 diabetes and moderate glycemic control. After a lengthy discussion about risks and benefits of laser, the ETDRS results

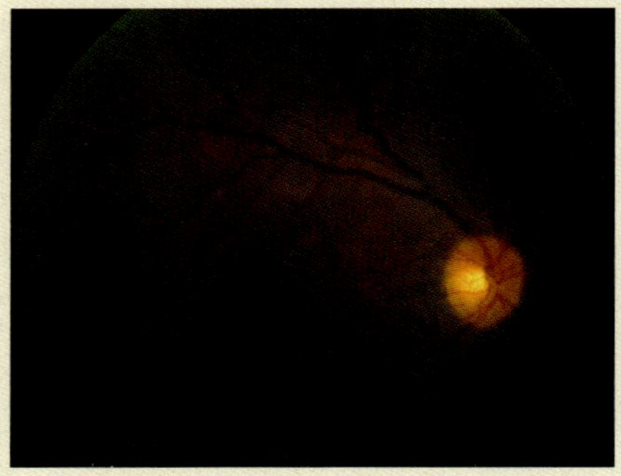

FIGURE 6-4. Photo OD, venous tortuosity, microaneurysms.

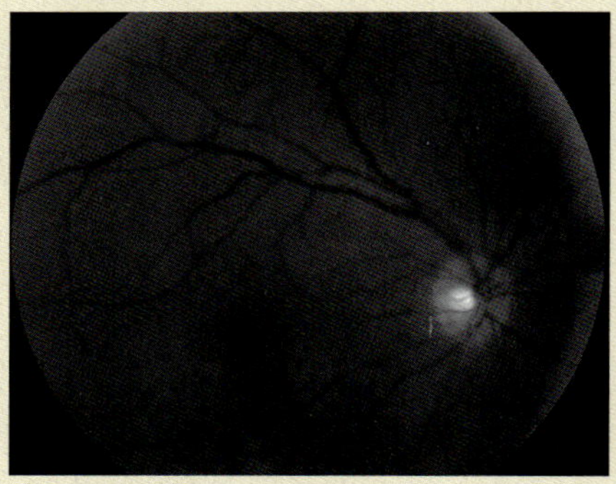

FIGURE 6-5. Red-free photo OD: abnormal, superior nerve fiber layer.

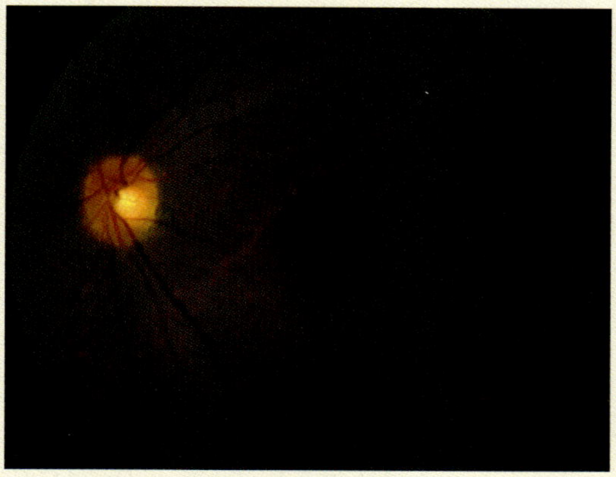

FIGURE 6-6. Photo OS: Note the straightening of arterioles OS versus OD, and the venous tortuosity at the optic nerve.

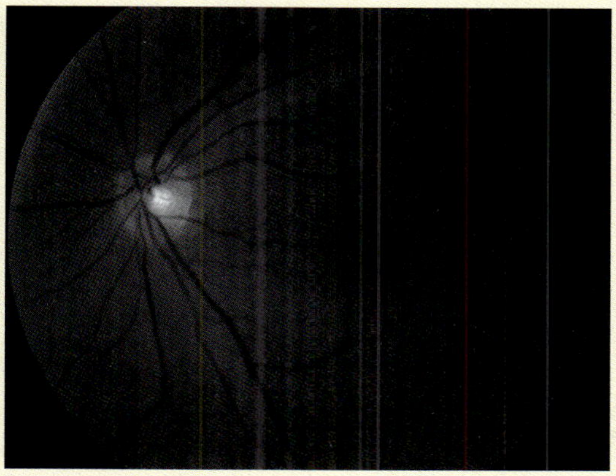

FIGURE 6-7. Red-free photo OS: abnormal nerve fiber layer.

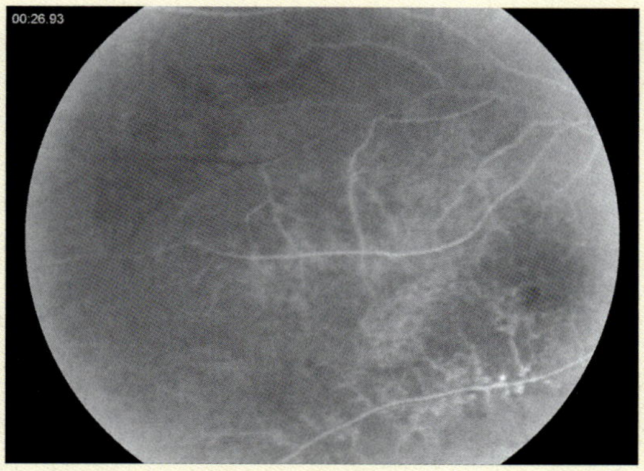

FIGURE 6-8. Fluorescein angiogram OD: (26 seconds transit) capillary nonperfusion at the fovea.

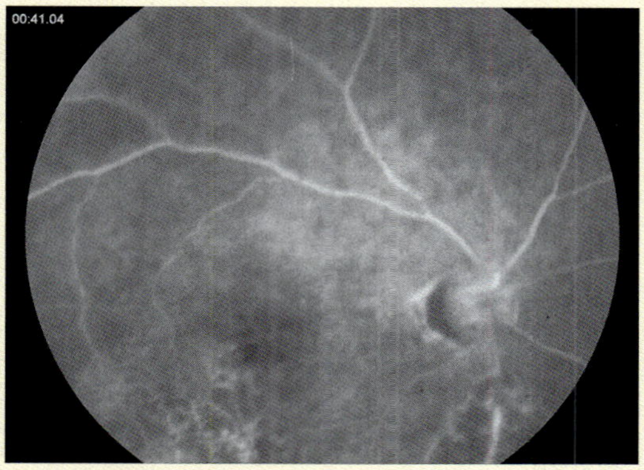

FIGURE 6-9. Fluorescein angiogram OD: (41 seconds transit) macular edema.

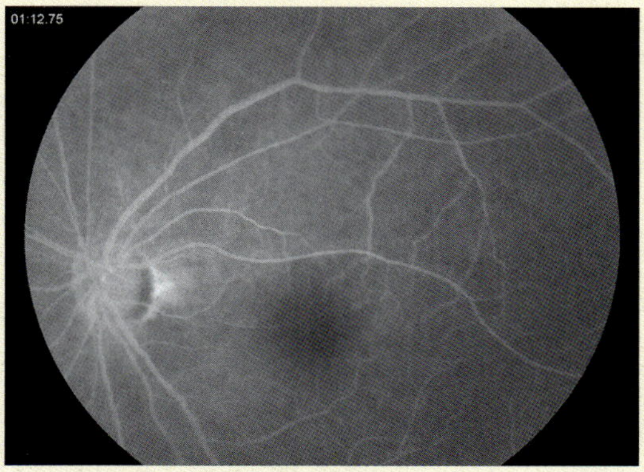

FIGURE 6-10. Fluorescein angiogram OS: (1 minute 12 seconds transit) capillary nonperfusion, top of the photo, macular edema.

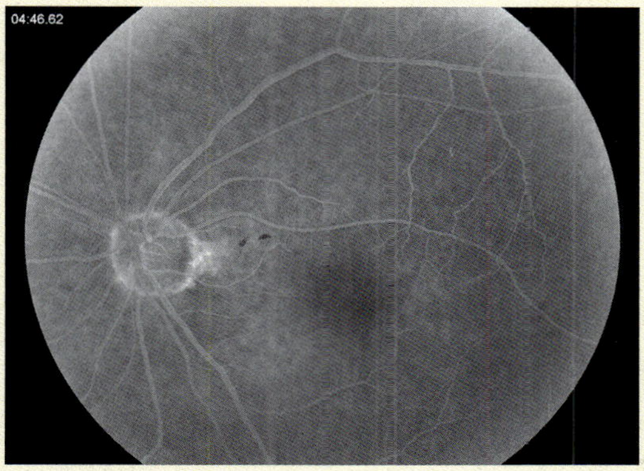

FIGURE 6-11. Fluorescein angiogram OS: (4 minutes 46 seconds transit) diffuse macular edema.

and that laser is still the benchmark for the treatment of diabetic macular edema, the patient understands that he received appropriate care in the past. He is offered intravitreal bevacizumab. He is a candidate for bevacizumab because he has had laser photocoagulation, and the residual macular edema may be responsive to bevacizumab. He is also told that there are ongoing clinical trials with DRCR.net about macular edema and bevacizumab (see Chapters 3 and 6).

CLINICAL CORRELATIONS

Patient complaints: Loss of vision.

Caveats: Loss to follow-up with ophthalmologist

Case Study (Figs. 6-12–6-15)

11–5–2008: SC is a 62-year-old Caucasian female who has poorly controlled Type 2 diabetes for 12 years, with decreased vision. Fasting blood glucose = 138 mg/dL, HbA1c = 6.4%, cholesterol = 226 mg/dL, LDL = 148 mg/dL.

V 20/50
20/50
Slit lamp examination
Cornea: Clear OU
Anterior chamber: Deep and quiet OU
Iris: Normal OU, no rubeosis OU

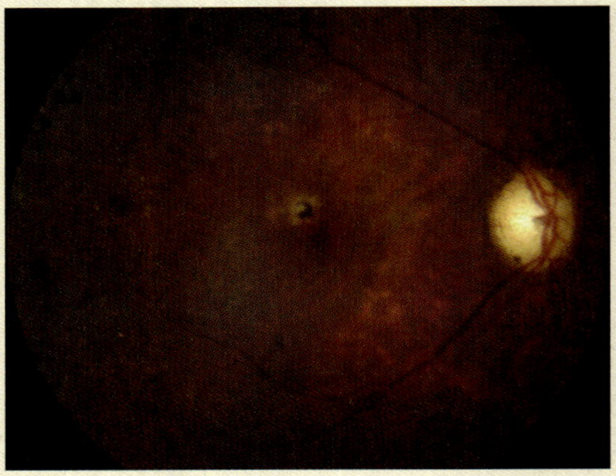

FIGURE 6-12. Photo OD: s/p previous laser, macular edema inferotemporal to the center of the fovea.

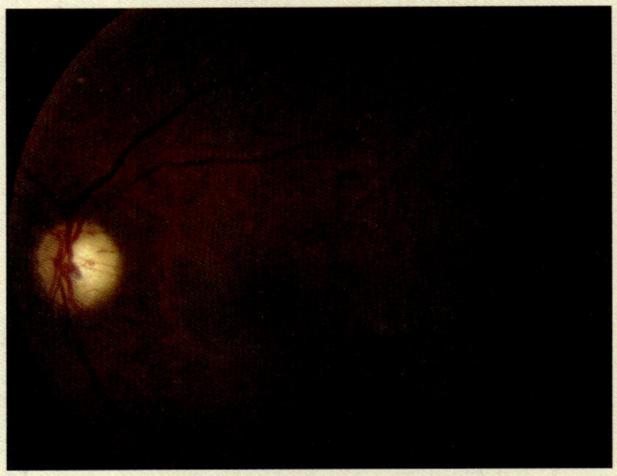

FIGURE 6-13. Photo OS: s/p previous laser, dot blot hemorrhages.

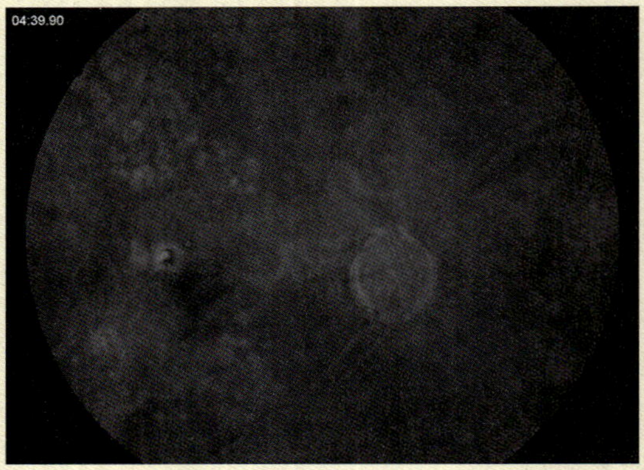

FIGURE 6-14. Fluorescein angiogram OD: (4 minutes 39 seconds transit) residual macular edema.

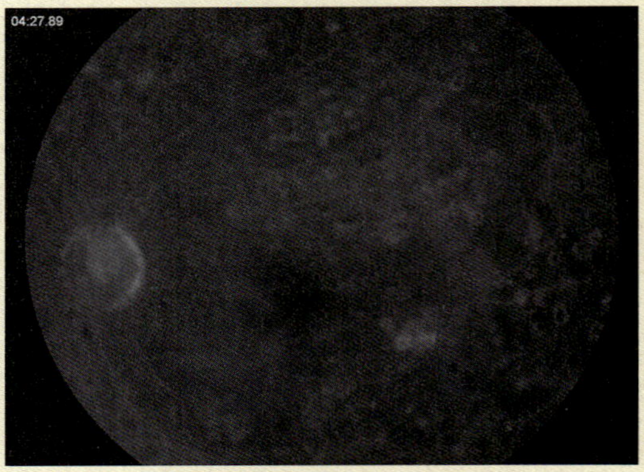

FIGURE 6-15. Fluorescein angiogram OS: (4 minutes 27 seconds transit) residual macular edema inferonasal to the foveal avascular zone. There is 3:00, 5:00 hyperfluorescence at the edge of the foveal avascular zone.

Lens: Intraocular lens implant OU
Applanation tonometry = 14/14 mm Hg (12:00 PM)
Gonioscopy: Open 360 degrees OU, no rubeosis OU

Dilated funduscopic examination:

Right eye: Clinically significant macular edema with previous laser
Left eye: Clinically significant macular edema with previous laser

Comment

In summary, this is nonproliferative diabetic retinopathy in a 68-year-old female with moderate glycemic control. She is offered intravitreal bevacizumab because she has had laser photocoagulation, and the residual macular edema may be responsive to bevacizumab. She is informed about the ongoing clinical trials with DRCR.net about macular edema and bevacizumab (see Chapters 3 and 6).

REFERENCES

1. Kumagai K. Introduction of a new method for the preparation of triamcinolone acetonide solution as an aid to visualization of the vitreous and the posterior hyaloid during pars plana vitrectomy. *Retina.* 2003;23:881–882.
2. Burk SE, DaMata AP, Snyder ME, et al. Visualizing vitreous using kenolog suspension. *J Cataract Refract Surg.* 2003;29:645–651.
3. Furino C, Micelli Ferrari T, Boscia F, et al. Triamcinolone assisted pars plana vitrectomy for proliferative vitreoretinopathy. *Retina.* 2003;23:771.
4. Martidis A, Duker J, Greenberg PB, et al. Intravitreal triamcinolone for refractory diabetic macular edema. *Ophthalmology.* 2002;109:920–927.
5. Jonas JB, Kreissig I, Sofker A, et al. Intravitreal injection of triamcinolone acetonide for diffuse diabetic macular edema. *Arch Ophthalmol.* 2003;121:57–61.
6. Enaida H, Hata Y, Ueno A, et al. Possible benefits of triamcinolone assisted pars plana vitrectomy for retinal diseases. *Retina.* 2003;23:764–770.
7. Matsumoto H, Yamanake I, Hisatomi T, et al. *Retina.* 2007;27:174–179.
8. Sakamoto T, Enaida H, Noda Y, et al. Triamcinolone acetonide-assisted pars plana vitrectomy imporves surgical procedures and decreases post-operative blood ocular barrier breakdown. *Invest Ophthalmol Vis Sci.* 2002;43:abstract 651.
9. Brooks HL, Caballero S, Newell CK, et al. With diabetic retinopathy and cystoid macular edema before and after intraocular injection of triamcinolone. *Arch Ophthalmol.* 2004:122:1801–1807.
10. Starita C, Patel M, Katz B, et al. Vascular endothelial growth factor and the potential therapeutic use of pegaptanib (Macugen) in diabetic retinopathy. In: Lang GE, ed. *Developments in Ophthalmology.* Vol. 39. Basel: Karger Publications; 2007:122–131.
11. Diabetic Retinopathy Clinical Research Network. Three year follow-up of a randomized trial comparing focal/grid photocoagulation and intravitreal triamcinolone for diabetic macular edema. *Arch Ophthalmol.* 2009;127:245–251.
12. Pepper MS, Ferrara N, Orci L, et al. Vascular endothelial growth factor (VEGF) induces plasminogen activators and plasminogen activator inhibitor-1 in microvascular endothelial cells. *Biochem Biophys Res Commun.* 1991;181: 902–906.
13. Tischer E, Gospodarowicz D, Mitchell R, et al. Vascular endothelial growth factor: A new member of the platelet derived growth factor gene family. *Biochem Biophys Res Commun.* 1989;165:1198–1206.
14. Shima DT, Adamis A, Ferara N, et al. Hypoxic induction of endothelial cell growth factors in retinal cells. *Mol Med.* 1995;1:182–193.
15. Shweiki D, Itin A, Soffer D, et al. Vascular endothelial growth factor induced by hypoxia may mediate hypoxia-initiated angiogenesis. *Nature.* 1992;359:843–845.
16. Barleon B, Sozzani S, Zhou D, et al. Migration of human monocytes in response to vascular endothelial growth factor (VEGF) is mediated via the VEGF receptor flt-1. *Blood.* 1996;87:3336–3343.
17. Huang JC, Liu DY, Dawood MY. The expression of vascular endothelial growth factor isoforms in cultured human endometrial stromal cells and its regulation by 17 beta-oestradiol. *Mol Hum Reprod.* 1998;4:603–607.
18. Kuroki M, Voest EE, Amano S, et al. Reactive oxygen intermediates increase vascular endothelial growth factor expression in vitro and in vivo. *J Clin Invest.* 1996;98:1667–1675.
19. Satake S, Kuzuya M, Miura H, et al. Up-regulation of vascular endothelial growth factor in response to glucose deprivation. *Biol Cell.* 1998;90:161–168.
20. Adamis AP, Miller JW, Bernal MT, et al. Increased vascular endothelial growth factor levels in the vitreous of eyes with proliferative diabetic retinopathy. *Am J Ophthalmol.* 1994;118:445–450.
21. Aiello LP, Avery RL, Arrigg PG, et al. Vascular endothelial growth factor in ocular fluid of patients with diabetic retinopathy and other retinal disorders. *N Engl J Med.* 1994;331:1480–1487

22. Lutty GA, McLeod DS, Merges C, et al. Localization of vascular endothelial growth factor in human retina and choroid. *Arch Ophthalmol.* 1996;114:971–977.
23. Jellinek D, Green LS, Bell C, et al. Inhibition of receptor binding by high-affinity RNA ligands to vascular endothelial growth factor. *Biochemistry*: 1994;33:10450–10456.
24. El-Hashemite N, Walker V, Zhang H, et al. Loss of Tsc1 or Tsc2 induces vascular endothelial growth factor production through mammalian target of rapamycin. *Cancer Res.* 2003;63:5173–5177.
25. Eyetech Study Group. Anti-vascular endothelial growth factor therapy for subfoveal choroidal neovascularizaiton secondary to age-related macular degeneration: Phase II study result. *Ophthalmology.* 2003;110:979–986.
26. Starita C, Patel M, Katz B, et al. Vascular endothelial growth factor and the potential therapeutic use of pegaptanib (Macugen) in diabetic retinopathy. In: Lang GE, ed. *Developments in Ophthalmology*. Vol. 39. Basel: Karger Publications; 2007:54, 62–127.
27. Cunningham ET Jr, Adamis AP, Altaweel M, et al. A phase II randomized double-masked trial of pegaptanib, an anti-vascular endothelial growth factor aptamer, for diabetic macular edema. *Ophthalmology.* 2005;112:1747–1757.
28. Adamis AP, Altaweel M, Bressler NM, et al. Changesin retinal neovascularizaiton after pegaptanib (Macugen) therapy in diabetic individuals. *Ophthalmology.* 2006;113:23–28.
29. Avery RL, Pearlman J, Pieramici DJ, et al. Intravitreal bevacizumab (Avastin) in the treatment of proliferative diabetic retinopathy. *Ophthalmology.* 2006;113:1695–1705.
30. Spaide RF, Fisher YL. Intravitreal bevacizumab (Avastin) treatment of proliferative diabetic retinopathy complicated by vitreous hemorrhage. *Retina.* 2006;26:275–278.
31. Soheilian M, Ramezani A, Bijanzadeh B, et al. Intravitreal bevacizumab (Avastin) injection alone or combined with triamcinolone versus macular photocoagulation as primary treatment of diabetic macular edema. *Retina.* 2007;27:9–15.
32. Arevalo JF, Fromow-Guerra J, Quiroz-Mercado H, et al., Pan-American Collaborative Retina Study Group. Primary intravitreal bevacizumab (Avastin) for diabetic macular edema: Results from the Pan-American Collaborative Retina Study Group at 6-month follow-up. *Ophthalmology.* 2007;114:743–750.
33. Chun D, Heier J, Topping T, et al. A pilot study of multiple intravitreal injections of ranibizumab in patients with center-involving clinically significant macular edema. *Ophthalmology.* 2006;113:1706–1712.
34. Hitt E. AAO/SOE 2008: Ranibizumab shows efficacy in phase 2 trials of diabetic macular edema. http://cme.medscape.com/viewarticle/583301. Accessed 25 March 2009.
35. Schwartz L. Promising early evidence of the superior benefits of drug therapy for diabetic eye disease. http://www.eurekalert.org/pub_releases/2008-04/jdrf-pee042908.php. Accessed 24 March 2009.
36. Nguyen Q, Tatlipinar S, Shah S, et al. Vascular endothelial growth factor is a critical stimulus for diabetic macular edema. *Am J Ophthalmol.* 2006;142:961–969.
37. Wolfensberger T. The role of carbonic anhydrase inhibitors in the management of macular edema. *Doc Ophthalmol.* 1999;97:387–397.
38. Ober, MD, Klais CM, Cunningham ET. Management options for macular edema. *Rev Ophthalmol.* 2005 (October 2005 issue) http://www.revophth.com/index.asp?page = 1_835.htm. Accessed 4 Jan 2009.
39. Milch FA, Yannuzz LA. Medical and surgical treatment of aphakic cystoid macular edema. *Int Ophthalmol Clin.* 1987;27:205–217.
40. Cox SN, Hay E, Bird AC. Treatment of chronic macular edema with acetazolamide. *Arch Ophthalmol.* 1988;106: 1190–1195.
41. Giusti C, Forte R, Vingolo EM, et al. Is acetazolamide effective in the treatment of diabetic macular edema? A pilot study. *Int Ophthalmol.* 2001;109:79–88.
42. Joussen AM, Poulaki V, Mitsiades N, et al. Nonsteroidal anti-inflammatory drugs prevent early diabetic retinopathy via TNF-alpha suppression. *FASEB J.* 2002;16:438–440.
43. Hariprasad, Seenu M. Pharmacotechnology: Novel methods to deliver ocular drugs to improve efficacy and durability. *Retinal Physician.* Nov 2008: http://www.retinalphysician.com/article.aspx?article = 102296. accessed 4 January 2009.
44. Almeida D, Johnson D, Hollands H, et al. Effect of prophylactic nonsteroidal anti-inflammatory drugs on cystoid macular edema assessed using optical coherence tomography quantification of total macular volume after cataract surgery. *J Cat Refract Surg.* 2008;34:64–69.
45. http://athenagen.com/index.php?/athenagen/pipeline/amd. Accessed 4 Jan 2009.
46. http://www.redorbit.com/news/health/1017335/targegen_initiates_multicenter_phase_ii_clinical_trial_of_tg100801_a/index.html. Accessed 4 Jan 2009.
47. pSivida reports positive interim results form diabetic macular edema study. Pharmaceutical Business Review Clinical Trials. http://clinicaltrials.pharmaceutical-business-review.com/news/psivida_reports_positive_interim_results_from_diabetic_macular_edema_study_160309. Accessed 28 March 2009.
48. Jaffe GJ, Martin D, Callanan D, et al. Fluocinolone Acetonide Uveitis Study Group. Fluocinolone acetonide implant (Retisert) for noninfectious posterior uveitis: Thirty-four week results of a multicenter randomized clinical study. *Ophthalmology.* 2006;113:1020–1027.
49. Analysis of 12 month data from diabetic macular edema clinical trial. http://www.thefreelibrary.com/Analysis+of+12-Month+Data+form+Diabetic+Macular+Edema+Clinical+Trial...-a0101341360. Accessed 26 March 2009.
50. Kupperman BD, Blumenkranz MS, Haller JA et al. Randomized controlled study of an intravitreous dexamethasone drug delivery system in patients with persistent macular edema. *Arch Ophthalmol.* 2007;125:309–317.
51. Bethke W. Present and future retinal implants. http://www.revophth.com/index.asp?page=1_990.htm. Accessed 26 March 2009.
52. Oculex announces positive clinical results for Posurdex®. http://www.prnewswire.com/cgi-bin/stories.pl?ACCT=104&STORY=/www/story/05-08-2003/0001942910&EDATE. Accessed 15 March 2009.
53. http://www.ausbiotech.org/data/downloads/pSivida%20-%20interim%20results%20on%20Human%20PK%20Medidur%20FA%20Study,%2027%20June20%2008.pdf. Accessed 26 March 2009.
54. SurModics I-vation™ intravitreal implant six month clinical study data. http://www.thefreelibrary.com/SurModics+I-vation(TM)+Intravitreal+Implant+Six+Month+Clinical+Study...-a0151257428. Accessed 26 March 2009.
55. http://www.redorbit.com/news/health/1017335/targegen_initiates_multicenter_phase_ii_clinical_trial_of_tg100801_a/index.html. Accessed 4 Jan 2009.
56. Blumenkranz MS. Sirolimus and mTOR inhibition in ocular disease: An update. http://www.retinatoday.com/Html%20Pages/0507/0507_macula_blumenkranz.html. Accessed 12 December 2008.
57. http://www.medicalnewstoday.com/articles/84208.php. Accessed 21 January 2009.

SUGGESTED READINGS

1. Antcliff RJ, Marshall J. The pathogenesis of edema in diabetic maculopathy. *Semin Ophthalmol.* 1999;14:223–232.
2. Avery RL, Pearlman J, Pieramici DJ, et al. Intravitreal bevacizumab (Avastin) in the treatment of proliferative diabetic retinopathy. *Ophthalmology.* 2006;113:1695.e1–e15.
3. Avery RL, Pieramici DJ, Rabena MD, et al. Intravitreal bevacizumab (Avastin) for neovascular age-related macular degeneration. *Ophthalmology.* 2006;113:363–372.
4. Bakri SJ, Donaldson MJ, Link TP. Rapid regression of disc neovascularization in a patient with proliferative diabetic retinopathy following adjunctive intravitreal bevacizumab. *Eye.* 2006;20:1474–1475.
5. Ferrara N. Vascular endothelial growth factor: Basic science and clinical progress. *Endocr Rev.* 2004;25:581–611.
6. Ferrara N, Hillan KJ, Gerber HP, Novotny W. Discovery and development of bevacizumab, an anti-VEGF antibody for treating cancer. *Nat Rev Drug Discov.* 2004;3:391–400.
7. Funatsu H, Yamashita H, Ikeda T, et al. Vitreous levels of interleukin-6 and vascular endothelial growth factor are related to diabetic macular edema. *Ophthalmology.* 2003;110:1690–1696.
8. Funatsu H, Yamashita H, Sakata K, et al. Vitreous levels of vascular endothelial growth factor and intercellular adhesion molecule 1 are related to diabetic macular edema. *Ophthalmology.* 2005;112:806–816.
9. Iturralde D, Spaide RF, Meyerle CB, et al. Intravitreal bevacizumab (Avastin) treatment of macular edema in central retinal vein occlusion: A short-term study. *Retina.* 2006;26:279–284.
10. Kumar A, Sinha S. Intravitreal bevacizumab (Avastin) treatment of diffuse diabetic macular edema in an Indian population. *Indian J Ophthalmol.* 2007;55:451–455.
11. Ladewig MS, Ziemssen F, Jaissle G, et al. Intravitreal bevacizumab for neovascular age-related macular degeneration. *Ophthalmology.* 2006;103:463–467.
12. Malecaze F. Clamens S, Simorre-Pinatel V, et al. Detection of vascular endothelial growth factor messenger RNA and vascular endothelial growth factor-like activity in proliferative diabetic retinopathy. *Arch Ophthalmol.* 1994;112: 1476–1182.
13. Manzano RP, Peyman GA, Khan P, Kivilcom M. Testing intravitreal toxicity of bevacizumab (Avastin). *Retina.* 2006;26:257–261.
14. Mason JO, Albert MA Jr, Mays A, Vail R. Regression of neovascularization iris vessels intravitreal injection of bevacizumab. *Retina.* 2006;26:839–841.
15. Maturi RK, Bleau LA, Wilson DL. Electrophysiologic findings after intravitreal bevacizumab (Avastin) treatment. *Retina.* 2006;26:270–274.
16. Michels S, Rosenfeld PJ, Puliafito CA, et al. Systemic bevacizumab (Avastin) therapy for neovascular age-related macular degeneration: Twelve-week results of an uncontrolled open-label clinical study. *Ophthalmology.* 2006;112:1035–1047.
17. Oshima Y, Sakaguchi H, Gomi F, Tano Y. Regression of iris neovascularization after intravitreal injection of bevacizumab in patients with proliferative diabetic retinopathy. *Am J Ophthalmol.* 2006;142:155–158.
18. Rich RM, Rosenfeld PJ, Puliafito CA, et al. Short-term safety and efficacy of intravitreal bevacizumab (Avastin) for neovascular age-related macular degeneration. *Retina.* 2006;26:495–511.
19. Shahar J, Avery RL, Heilweil G, et al. Electrophysiologic and retinal penetration studies following intravitreal injection of bevacizumab (Avastin). *Retina.* 2006;26:262–269.
20. Shan PK, Narendran V, Tawansy KA, Raghuram A, Narendran K. Intravitreal bevacizumab (Avastin) for post laser anterior segment ischemia in aggressive retinopathy of prematurity. *Indian J Ophthalmol.* 2007;55:75–76.
21. Spaide RF, Laud K, Fine HF, et al. Intravitreal bevacizumab treatment of choroidal neovascularization secondary to age-related macular degeneration. *Retina.* 2006;26:383–390.
22. Spandau UH, Ihloff AK, Jonas JB. Intravitreal bevacizumab treatment of macular oedema due to central retinal vein occlusion. *Acta Ophthalmol Scand.* 2006;84:555–556.
23. Tolentino MJ, McLeod DS, Taomoto M, et al. Pathologic features of vascular endothelial growth factor-induced retinopathy in the nonhuman primate. *Am J Ophthalmol.* 2002;133:373–385.
24. Tolentino MJ, Miller JW, Gragoudas ES, et al. Intravitreous injections of vascular endothelial growth factor produce retinal ischemia and microangiopathy in an adult primate. *Ophthalmology.* 1996;103:1820–1828.

CHAPTER 7

Management of Nonproliferative Diabetic Retinopathy

DIAGNOSIS

Physical Examination

Nonproliferative diabetic retinopathy (NPDR) is also known as background diabetic retinopathy in the internal medicine literature. While the term, "nonproliferative" suggests a nonprogressive condition to the diabetic patients and the nonophthalmic physicians, NPDR is not a benign or safe condition. As we are all aware, diabetic retinopathy is progressive and can be relentless in its course. Thus, it is vitally important that patients and the medical community understand that blindness can still occur if the patient is noncompliant with his diabetic treatment plan.

The pathologic processes of NPDR include the formation of capillary microaneurysms, vascular permeability, and capillary closure.

Microaneurysms are red, round dots, measuring 15 to 60 μm, most commonly found in the posterior pole. The mechanism for the formation of microaneurysms is unknown. It may be that there is a release of vasoproliferative factor with endothelial cell proliferation.

NPDR is classified into four levels of severity: mild, moderate, severe, and very severe. The extent of IRMA (intraretinal microvascular abnormalities), venous abnormalities, and retinal hemorrhages are the determining factors of mild, moderate, severe, and very severe NPDR.

Mild to moderate NPDR (also formerly known as background diabetic retinopathy) has few intraretinal hemorrhages and microaneurysms and minimal venous changes.

Severe NPDR (formerly known as preproliferative diabetic retinopathy) shows increasing ischemia and can be seen by examining the four quadrants for these characteristics: (i) severe intraretinal hemorrhages and microaneurysms in four quadrants, greater or equal to standard photograph 2A, (Fig. 7-1); (ii) venous beading in two or more quadrants; or (iii) moderate IRMA in at least one quadrant, greater than or equal to standard photograph 8A, (Fig. 7-2). This is the 4–2–1 rule.

Very severe NPDR is defined when two of the above characteristics are present. The retinopathy level of "very severe NPDR" is associated with rapid worsening of diabetic retinopathy to proliferative diabetic retinopathy (PDR).

Chief Complaint

The patient may complain of minimally decreased vision or may not have any visual complaints. The patient may be referred to the ophthalmologist for routine "screening" examination for diabetic retinopathy.

Patient History and Review of Systems

In taking the patient history, one can assess if the patient is knowledgeable or cognizant of the consequences of his diabetes. His responses to simple questions about duration of diabetes, history of postprandial blood sugar readings, fasting blood sugar (FBS)

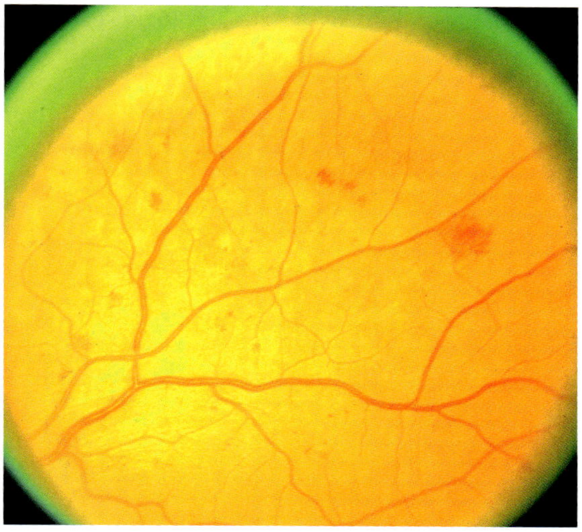

FIGURE 7-1. Standard photograph 2A intraretinal hemorrhages and microaneurysms. (Courtesy of the Fundus Reading Center, Madison, WI.)

readings, and knowledge of blood sugar medications demonstrate his health literacy and compliance. Many times, the patient is referred to a specialist, but the patient thinks that he is there for a "baseline examination." However, in reality, the patient has significant diabetic retinopathy or systemic manifestations of diabetes.[1] Thus, the ophthalmologist and retinal specialist play the role of an educator who educates patients about diabetic retinopathy and diabetic eye disease.

If the patient cannot remember the name of his medication or how long he has had the disease, he must be newly diagnosed or his diabetes has not affected his activities of daily living. Or he could be in denial. In any case, the ophthalmologist is the diplomatic educator who tells the patient about the need for compliance in diabetes.[2] In addition, the patient must understand the need for a "team" approach to diabetes: the patient and the medical doctors are a "team." If the patient follows the instructions of his team of doctors, he will have a good treatment outcome. However, if the patient does not follow the treatment regimen for his diabetes, the treatment outcome may be disappointing.[3] Consequently, the patient may suffer accelerated and severe vision loss along with systemic complications involving the heart and kidneys.[3]

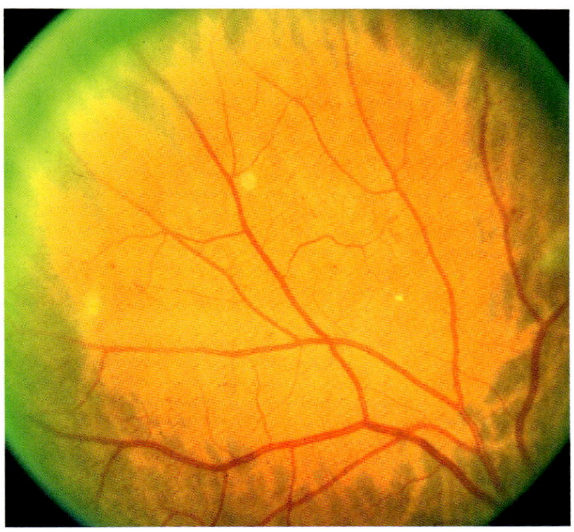

FIGURE 7-2. Standard photograph 8A IRMA. (Courtesy of the Fundus Reading Center, Madison, WI.)

Similarly, in asking about the review of systems, the ophthalmologist gains an understanding of the patient's level of cardiovascular health, hypertension, and lipid metabolism.[4] All these factors play a role in taking care of the patient. Weight issues and obesity play a role in diabetes and cardiovascular disease. It is estimated that 33.3% of men and 35.3% of women are obese.[5,6] Smoking plays an adverse role in the development of diabetes.[7] Smoking has been associated in the development of NPDR.[8]

Lastly, excessive alcohol intake can hamper the compliance of an ADA diet unless the patient takes into account that each glass of wine is 150 cal. Alcoholism in diabetic patients can result in loss of optic nerve function and thus, loss of vision over time.[9,10]

It is thought that the increase of obesity in the United States parallels the increase in cases of diabetes. Roughly, one third of adults in the United States are obese. In patients with diabetes, cardiovascular disease is a comorbid risk factor: the diagnosis of cardiovascular disease has been reported by 38.1% of adults with diabetes.[11–13] Heart disease and stroke are responsible for 68% of deaths in diabetic patients. Diabetic adults have a two- to fourfold increase in heart disease death rates compared to nondiabetic adults.[13]

The metabolic syndrome is a constellation of interrelated risk factors of metabolic origins that appear to promote the development of atherosclerotic cardiovascular disease and increased risk of developing Type 2 diabetes mellitus.

The metabolic risk factors are atherogenic dyslipidemia, elevated blood pressure and elevated plasma glucose, or FBS. Thus, patients with the metabolic syndrome are at increased risk of developing diabetes. The history and physical examination will reveal these risk factors since they will play a role in the patient's diabetes and diabetic retinopathy. The systemic risk factors, such as heart disease and elevated blood pressure, all are a part of the metabolic syndrome. These risk factors play a role in the development of retinal abnormalities such as "copper wiring" or "silver wiring" changes in hypertension, decreased blood flow in cardiovascular disease, or embolic phenomena in cardiovascular disease. While these retinal lesions are unrelated to diabetic retinopathy, they can decrease retinal function and cause visual disturbances, as well.

Family History

Patients with family history of severe diabetic retinopathy serve as a red flag for all ophthalmologists. Family history of death related to diabetes implies that the patient may have a genetic predisposition to severe diabetes and its complications.

Epidemiology

Certain ethnic groups are more prone to an accelerated course of diabetic retinopathy such as Pima Indians, Asians, and Native Americans. African Americans are more liable for hypertensive complications. When African Americans are diagnosed with diabetes, it may rapidly progress to severe diabetic retinopathy. Poor health literacy of chronic diseases such as diabetes is common among racial and ethnic minorities which may affect clinical diabetes outcomes[2] (see Chapter 1). Similarly, obese individuals, who are Type 2 diabetics, may be at risk for rapid worsening of their diabetic retinopathy, as well. Certain ethnic groups, Asian Americans and Pacific Islanders are at a higher risk for diabetes than their Caucasian counterparts (Table 7-1).

TABLE 7.1 Nonproliferative Diabetic Retinopathy

1. Ask about comorbid associations: obesity, hypertension, cardiovascular disease, hyperlipidemia, and metabolic syndrome.
2. If comorbid conditions exist, diabetic retinopathy can be more severe and deteriorate quickly.
3. Ask that the patient's laboratory results be sent to your office as well.

TABLE 7.2 Mild NPDR

Visual acuity: 20/20 to 20/40

1. If compliant and no comorbid conditions, see an ophthalmologist once a year.
2. Ask that the patient's laboratory results be sent to your office as well.
3. If noncompliant, no comorbid conditions, see twice a year.
4. Ask that the patient's laboratory results be sent to your office as well.
5. If noncompliant and with comorbid conditions, see three times a year or more if Amsler grid changes occur with home monitoring.
6. Ask that the patient's laboratory results be sent to your office as well.
7. Be sure to emphasize to the patient that if visual loss occurs, he should come see the retinal specialist before their scheduled 4-month visit.

Examination

Patients with Visual Acuity of 20/20 to 20/40

Visual acuity, slit lamp examination and retinal examination are the standard examination techniques. These patients with NPDR usually present with visual acuity of 20/20 to the 20/40 range. These patients may or may not have abnormalities on Amsler grid testing. However, upon closer questioning, they will notice problems with driving at night more frequently than their nondiabetic counterparts with similar visual acuity. These patients note loss of visual acuity with reading or at the computer terminal.

If the visual acuity is <20/20, the ophthalmic exam will most likely reveal macular edema upon slit lamp biomicroscopy and some microaneurysms in the posterior pole. These patients may or may not need fluorescein angiography depending on their level of visual loss. Small changes in the internal limiting membrane at the fovea will lead to minor changes in visual acuity.

If the patient has background diabetic retinopathy with <30 microaneurysms, monitor the patient and tell him to continue to be vigilant with diet and medications. Follow the patient's lipid profiles, FBS, and hemoglobin A1c (HbA1c). See the patient twice a year if he is compliant; otherwise, see him more frequently if patient experiences unexpected visual loss (Tables 7-2 and 7-3).

Patients with Visual Acuity of 20/50 to 20/80

These patients will probably have macular edema, dot blot hemorrhages, hard exudates, and cotton-wool spots. Their macular edema can present as mild or moderate, and the cotton-wool spots can occur in the area of the equator. Fluorescein angiography is needed for further evaluation and management of their macular edema. The Early Treatment Diabetic Retinopathy Study (ETDRS) classification can be used for treatment guidelines.[14] Laser photocoagulation can be offered to these patients with clinically significant macular edema (CSME). OCT monitoring of the macular edema is useful for follow-up in these patients.

Patients with Visual Acuity of 20/100 to 20/400

While these NPDR patients do not have neovascularization, these patients can present with either severe macular edema with associated hard exudate rings or severe capillary nonperfusion at the retina. This type of patient is at a higher risk for developing PDR

TABLE 7.3 Moderate to Severe NPDR

Visual acuity: 20/20 to 20/40

1. Ask that the patient's laboratory results be sent to your office as well.
2. See ophthalmologist twice a year if diabetes is the only disease and the patient has no comorbid conditions.

if he has risk factors such as obesity, dyslipidemia, hypertension, poor eating habits, and poorly controlled diabetes.

These patients' prognosis for full recovery of vision to the 20/20 or 20/30 level will be guarded. However, recovery to the 20/40 level can be attained with laser treatment, treatment with anti-VEGF monoclonal antibodies such as bevacizumab, and medical treatment of their systemic disease of diabetes and hypertension. If obesity is an issue, diet and exercise must be addressed in the medical and ophthalmic rehabilitation of the patient.

Documentation

Fundus Photography, Fluorescein Angiography, or OCT

Documentation of the retinal findings is important not only for medicolegal reasons but for the patient education process. Fundus photography and fluorescein angiography are part of the standard of care for the diabetic eye patient. The fluorescein angiogram would reveal capillary nonperfusion to the clinician and thus enable more precise classification of the patient's diabetic retinopathy. Neovascularization elsewhere can be difficult to see in the periphery in an uncooperative or anxious retinal patient, but fluorescein angiography can show areas of severe capillary nonperfusion in the equatorial region. The angiographic picture of neovascularization would lead the clinician to be more concerned about rapid acceleration to PDR. The subsequent treatment plans would be different if the patient had neovascularization versus no neovascularization. There would be a need for closer follow-up appointments in the person with areas of severe capillary nonperfusion.

The OCT can record the thickness of the macular retina with a scan of the retina's anatomy in that region. In addition, the OCT provides a numerical reading of the actual thickness of the macula which can be followed over time. Lastly, there is a documentation of the change in Henle layer with the evolution of the patient's macular edema.

SEVERE NONPROLIFERATIVE DIABETIC RETINOPATHY

Patients with Visual Acuity of 20/50 and Worse Vision

These patients with severe NPDR require monitoring of their FBS and HbA1c with an internal medicine and endocrinology colleague. By the time the patient reaches this stage of retinopathy, the patient will have an abnormal HbA1c and fasting blood glucose in the mid 150 to 200 range. Or in some instances, these patients have been lost to follow-up

TABLE 7.4 Moderate to Severe NPDR

Visual acuity: 20/50 and worse + good glycemic control
Compliant with medications, diet, and exercise.
Ask that the patient's laboratory results be sent to your office as well.
No comorbid conditions, see ophthalmologist three times a year.

Visual acuity: 20/50 and worse + poor glycemic control
Noncompliant.
Cardiovascular disease, hypertension, obesity, and lipid abnormalities.
Ask that the patient's laboratory results be sent to your office as well.
See ophthalmologist three times a year or more if noncompliant and with comorbid conditions.

TABLE 7.5 Clinically Significant Macular Edema

1. Usually comorbid conditions exist at this point.
2. Ask that the patient's laboratory results be sent to your office as well.
3. Ask that the patient's laboratory results be sent to your office as well.
4. Use Amsler grid home testing.

with their internist for several years. To rehabilitate a patient with severe NPDR requires a team approach. The team would include an internist, endocrinologist, nutritionist, and a nephrologist.

This type of patient will have more obvious macular edema in that he will complain about loss of vision at near. It is at this visual acuity threshold of 20/50 and beyond that the patient needs to be seen more frequently. Home monitoring of the Amsler grid is suggested to the patient. At the first sign of change or deterioration of vision, the patient should return for an ophthalmic examination.

If the patient has hypertension, cardiovascular issues, and hyperlipidemia, his macular edema may be difficult to treat if he is noncompliant. However, with laser treatment, the patient's vision can be restored to a level of 20/40 or better vision.

Cotton-wool spots and areas of capillary nonperfusion and macular edema may require close monitoring. The patient can be seen at 1-month intervals especially in a patient with a history of noncompliance with diabetic medications.

In NPDR patients with only cotton-wool spots, watch the patient and tell him to continue to be vigilant with diet and medications. Follow patient's lipid profiles, FBS, and HbA1c. See the patient every 4 months a year if he is compliant; otherwise, see him more frequently if the patient experiences unexpected visual loss (Table 7-4).

MACULAR EDEMA

Depending on the severity of macular edema, there can be a choice of monitoring the progress versus laser photocoagulation (Tables 7-5 and 7-6).

Patients with Visual Acuity of 20/20 to 20/30

In asymptomatic patients with the visual acuity of 20/20 to 20/30, the ophthalmic exam may or may not show CSME according to the ETDRS guidelines.[14] This patient who is asymptomatic may only need patient education if there is no CSME.

TABLE 7.6 Metabolic Syndrome

Diagnosis by any three of the following characteristics:

1. Men: waist circumference $\geq$102 cm ($\geq$40 in.) in men; $>$90 cm in Asian men.
2. Women: waist circumference $\geq$88 cm ($\geq$35 in.) in women; $\geq$80 cm in Asian women.
3. Triglycerides $\geq$150 mg/dL.
4. HDL cholesterol (HDL-C) $<$40 mg/dL (men).
   HDL-C $<$50 mg/dL (women).
5. Systolic blood pressure $\geq$130 mm Hg or diastolic blood pressure $\geq$85 mm Hg.
6. Fasting plasma glucose or FBS $\geq$100 mg/dL.
7. Patients receiving drug therapy to reduce triglycerides, raise HDL-C, lower blood pressure, or decrease glucose levels are considered to have a corresponding component of the metabolic syndrome.

Source: Grundy SM, Cleeman JI, Daniels SR, et al. Diagnosis and management of the metabolic syndrome: An American Heart Association/National Heart, Lung, and Blood Institute Scientific Statement. *Circulation.* 2005;112:2735–2752.

If there is CSME with good visual acuity of 20/20 to 20/30 level, the patient is a candidate for laser treatment after he understands the ramification of treatment versus no treatment using the ETDRS guidelines.[14] Informed consent is important for this group of patients.

Patients with Visual Acuity of 20/40

The visual acuity of 20/40 is a threshold for treatment for many patients since 20/40 is the visual acuity level needed to pass the driving test in many states. This group of patients is very motivated to see better. However, if this 20/40 patient opts for no treatment, the clinician can monitor him and ask him to check with the Amsler grid once a week. The patient needs to understand fully that the laser will preserve his vision in the long term, but in the short term, results may be some minor and immediate changes of vision as can be seen on Amsler grid testing. Informed consent is extremely important in this group of patients with relatively good visual acuity of 20/20 to 20/40.

Patients with Visual Acuity of 20/50 to 20/80

However, if the macular edema is 20/50 or worse and there is CSME on slit lamp biomicroscopy, laser photocoagulation can be offered. OCT and fluorescein angiogram are usually helpful to see the abnormal foveal net or areas of microaneurysms not seen by slit lamp biomicroscopy. With these patients, it is important that the clinician understands the ramification of treatment versus no treatment using the ETDRS guidelines.[14] In addition, in patients who have 20/40 vision but are "asymptomatic," or feel that they "see fine," be careful in doing laser because they may see the scotoma postlaser and may be very unhappy postoperatively. For these patients who need to have macular laser, a preoperative visual field may be useful to map the central scotoma, and careful informed consent is necessary. The demonstration of macular edema on OCT and/or fluorescein angiography may be necessary in the informed consent stage.

Patients with Visual Acuity of 20/100 or Worse

These patients usually present with poor vision and have associated poor compliance with their medical treatment and/or obesity. Typically, these patients have the metabolic syndrome, have abnormal FBSs in the 150 range, and have HbA1c levels of >6.5%.

Previous Laser

These patients who have had previous macular laser will have residual macular edema. They need fluorescein angiography and OCT evaluations of their macula. From the fluorescein angiogram, the clinician will be looking for areas of capillary nonperfusion and areas of abnormal foveal capillary net. From the OCT, the ophthalmologist will be looking at the macular thickness measurement and the abnormalities of Henle layer.

These previously treated eyes are candidates for additional laser or bevacizumab intravitreal injection. It is important to warn these patients about a prolonged course of recovery. It must be emphasized that their diabetes must be under control during this time of visual rehabilitation.

No Previous Laser

In those patients who present for the first time to the ophthalmologist's office with diabetic macular edema at the visual acuity level of 20/100 or worse, fluorescein angiography and OCT are needed to determine if there is focal or diffuse leakage.

They are a candidate for macular laser using the ETDRS guidelines.[15] The fluorescein angiogram will identify hundreds of additional microaneurysms not seen on regular fundus photography of the macular region. If this is the case, focal laser treatment can be performed. If upon OCT testing there are large foveal cysts, grid laser and bevacizumab may be offered together.

Glaucoma

Glaucoma is a blood flow problem for the optic nerve in some diabetic patients. Low-tension glaucoma can be seen in diabetic patients. In addition, glaucoma is difficult to diagnose in patients who have had previous panretinal photocoagulation, and therefore, their visual field will be abnormal. These patients will need more sophisticated testing such as Heidelberg retinal tomography or OCT documentation of the optic nerve. Gonioscopy is essential to look for rubeosis iridis at each follow-up visit. Central corneal thickness measurement can be used to calibrate Goldmann tonometry readings. They may have to come back for a few readings of the intraocular pressure in the mornings and in the late afternoons to establish the diurnal curve of their intraocular pressure. These patients may need provocative testing as well. Lastly, if the patient complains of visual disturbance not related to macular edema seen on OCT or fluorescein angiography, he may need a consultation with a glaucoma specialist.

MANAGEMENT OF NONPROLIFERATIVE DIABETIC RETINOPATHY

The treatment strategies for NPDR are based on the results of the Diabetic Retinopathy Study (DRS) and the ETDRS. The treatment of NPDR depends on the severity of retinopathy and the presence or absence of CSME which can be present at any stage of diabetic retinopathy.

The DRS has evaluated patients with severe NPDR or PDR and visual acuity of 20/100 or better. The DRS shows 50% reduction in severe visual loss in eyes that have received photocoagulation compared with eyes that have not received photocoagulation. Laser photocoagulation is designated as scatter or focal photocoagulation. Severe visual loss is defined as visual acuity of 5/200 or worse at two or more consecutively completed follow-up visits scheduled at 4-month intervals.

The ETDRS shows that for severe or very severe NPDR or early PDR, early scatter photocoagulation is effective in reducing severe visual loss in patients with Type 2 diabetes.[16] For mild to moderate NPDR, the rates of severe visual loss between the early treatment group and deferred treatment groups were insignificant; thus, any reductions in severe visual loss do not seem sufficient to compensate for the unwanted side effects of scatter photocoagulation.[17]

Scatter Photocoagulation

The technique of a standard “full scatter” laser photocoagulation is 1,200 to 1,600 burns of moderate intensity. The spot size is approximately 500 μm. Green laser can be used with a Goldmann type contact lens. For the Goldmann contact lens, the power density is usually 300 to 500 MW for a 500 μm spot size. The different intensity strengths are proportional to the lens' changes or pigmentation of the fundus.

There are a variety of lenses which allow for full scatter. In using a Rodenstock contact lens where the lens optics provide a wide-field view which is minified, the laser settings would be a 200-μm spot size with an appropriate power density. One could start with 200 MW power and increase the power until a yellow-white burn is achieved.

CLINICAL CORRELATIONS: Nonproliferative Diabetic Retinopathy 20/20 to 20/40

Patient complaints: Occasional difficulty in reading.

Caveats: This may be a screening examination only. The patient may need patient education and work toward attaining "health literacy."

Case Study (Figs. 7-3 and 7-4)

1–28–2009: AV is a 43-year-old South Asian male who is diagnosed with "borderline diabetes." His father, mother, paternal grandparents, and maternal grandparents have Type 2 diabetes. He is here for his first visit to an ophthalmologist. He has previously seen optometrists once a year. Fasting blood glucose = 112. He is 30 lb overweight.

V 20/20
20/30 PH 20/20
Slit lamp examination
Cornea: Clear OU
Anterior chamber: Deep and quiet OU
Iris: Normal OU, no rubeosis OU
Lens: No lens opacity OU. Y sutures seen OU
Applanation tonometry = 12/12 mm Hg (10:00 AM)
Gonioscopy: Open 360 degrees OU, no rubeosis OU

Dilated funduscopic examination:

Right eye: No diabetic retinopathy (NDR), cup-to-disc ratio = 0.6, peripapillary atrophy (see Fig. 7-3).
Left eye: NDR, tilted disc, cup-to-disc ratio = 0.6, peripapillary atrophy (see Fig. 7-4).

Comment

In summary, this is NPDR in a 43-year-old male with blood sugar that is borderline normal. He has NDR, but he has a strong family history for Type 2 diabetes. He is asked to see us once a year unless his metabolic state changes or his blood sugars become higher. An Amsler grid is given to the patient. Information about the American Diabetes Association Web site and the local chapter of the American Diabetes Association are given to the patient.

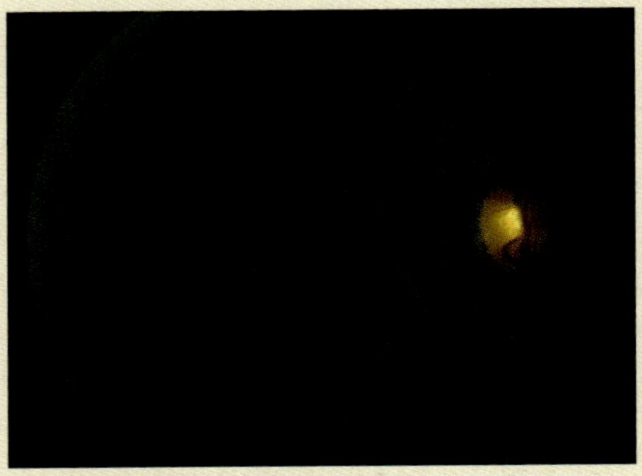

FIGURE 7-3. Forty-three-year-old South Asian male with borderline Type 2 diabetes and 30 lb overweight. He has a family history of Type 2 diabetes in his mother, father, and both paternal and maternal grandparents. V 20/20 OD; V 20/30 NIPH OS. Fundus photographs were requested by the patient to send to his ophthalmologist in India, where he travels several months each year. Photo OD, NDR.

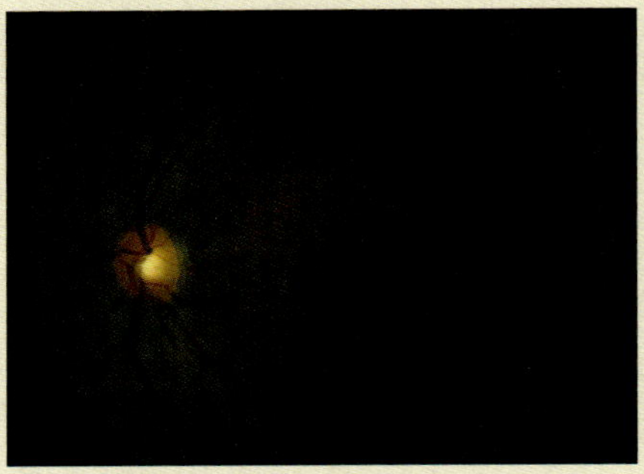

FIGURE 7-4. Photo OS, NDR.

CLINICAL CORRELATIONS: Nonproliferative Diabetic Retinopathy 20/20 to 20/40

Patient complaints: Occasional difficulty in reading. This is not a bothersome problem to the patient. However, some patients may notice a "central spot" when reading which is "annoying."

Caveats: The patient's ability to articulate the minor disturbance in vision tells the clinician how precise is the patient's need for vision. For example, a patient who is an architect, accountant, physicist, or engineer will want to see the smallest numbers, figures, and graphs in great detail. If the patient is not bothered about his vision, he may not be very demanding in his need for precise vision, and he may have a high tolerance for poor vision. Consequently, he may have a high tolerance for poor health and its sequelae. This latter type of patient may be noncompliant and seek ophthalmic care only when he experiences severe vision loss.

Case Study (Figs. 7-5–7-9)

3–26–2009: AA is a 57-year-old Caucasian male who was diagnosed with Type 2 diabetes 5 years ago. He is here for his first visit to an ophthalmologist. He has previously seen optometrists once a year.

V 20/30 PH 20/25
 20/30 PH 20/25
M −0.50 → 20/25 + 1
 −0.50 → 20/25 + 1
Slit lamp examination
Cornea: Clear OU
Anterior chamber: Deep and quiet OU
Iris: Normal OU, no rubeosis OU

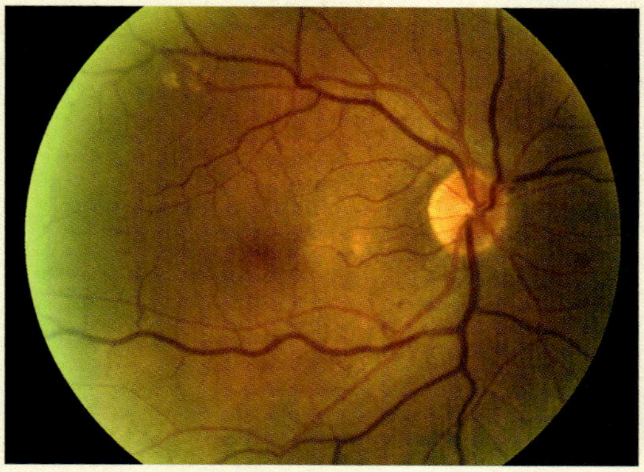

FIGURE 7-5. Fifty-seven-year-old Caucasian male, diagnosed with Type 2 diabetes 5 years ago. V20/25 OD; V 20/25 OS. Photo OD, hard exudates seen at 12:00, 1:00, 4:00, 6:00, and 9:00 at the edge of the foveal avascular zone. In addition, at the macula at 1:00, 2:00, 3:00, there are additional hard exudates. At the temporal arcade, there are hard exudates. Dot blot hemorrhage is seen as area nasal to optic disc and at 7:00 inferotemporal to the optic disc.

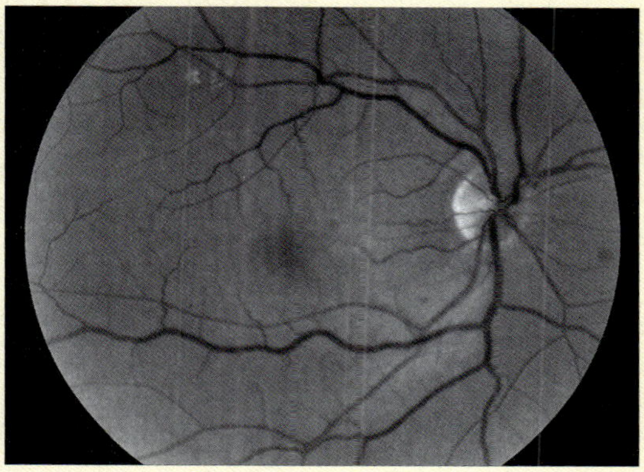

FIGURE 7-6. Red-free photograph OD, hard exudates seen at 12:00, 1:00, 4:00, 6:00, and 9:00 at the edge of the foveal avascular zone can be seen as white specks. In addition, at the macula at 1:00, 2:00, 3:00, they are better seen in the black and white contrast of the red-free photograph. At the temporal arcade, the hard exudates are seen as white dots. Dot blot hemorrhage seen as an area nasal to optic disc and at 7:00 inferotemporal to the optic disc is seen as black.

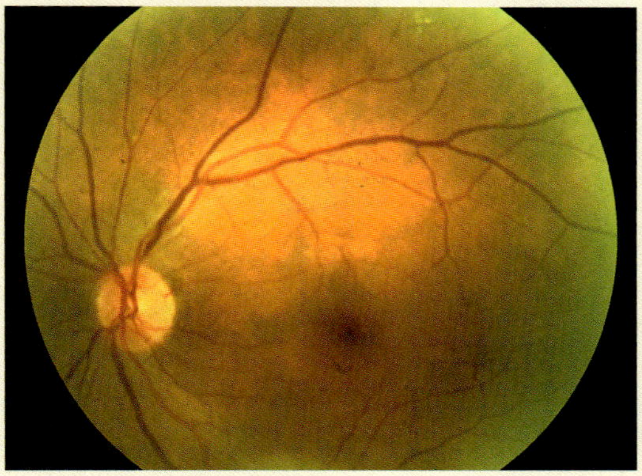

FIGURE 7-7. Photo OS, area of hard exudates seen superotemporally, at the top right corner of the photograph. There is venous tortuosity seen as the vessels emanate from the optic disc. Small hard exudate seen in the edge of the foveal avascular zone at 2:00.

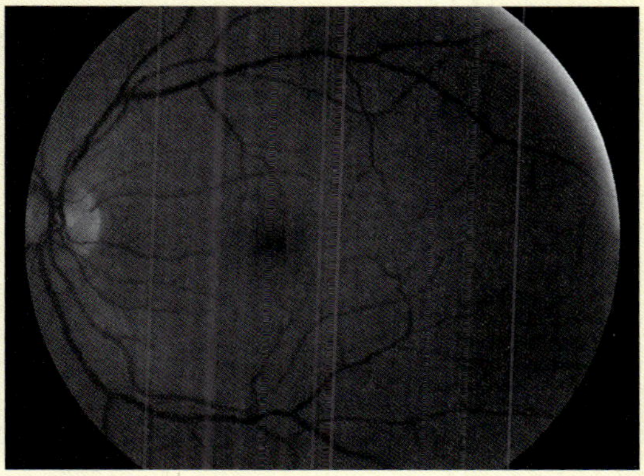

FIGURE 7-8. Red-free photograph OS, hard exudates are seen as white dots, very subtle at the edge of the foveal avascular zone at 2:00.

Lens: 1 + nuclear sclerosis OU
Applanation tonometry = 14/14 mm Hg (10:00 AM)
Gonioscopy: Open 360 degrees OU, no rubeosis OU

Dilated funduscopic examination:
Right eye: Microaneurysms, but dot blot hemorrhage, superior temporal arcade, hard exudates, cup-to-disc ratio = 0.4 (see Figs. 7-5 and 7-6).
Left eye: Microaneurysms, hard exudates superotemporally, cup-to-disc ratio = 0.4 (see Figs. 7-7 and 7-8).
OCT: OD central subfield thickness: 261 μm. The OCT scan shows hard exudates of the outer plexiform layer (see Fig 7-9).
OCT: OS central subfield thickness: 255 μm

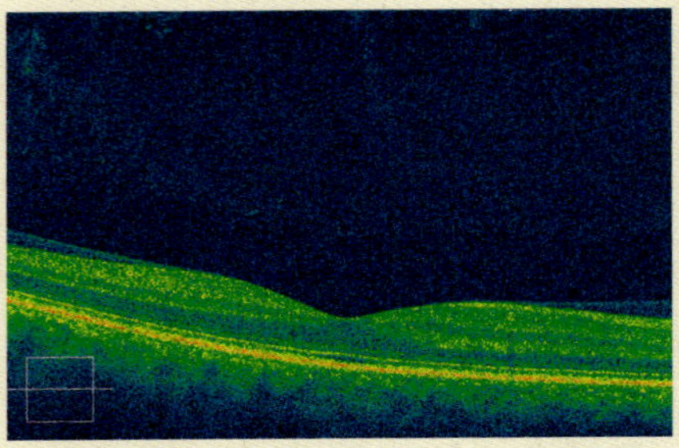

FIGURE 7-9. OCT OD, there are hard exudates seen in the outer plexiform layer corresponding to the fundus photograph, temporal to the foveal avascular zone at 9:00.

Comment
In summary, this is NPDR in a 57-year-old man with good glycemic control. He has some microaneurysms and dot blot hemorrhages placing him in the NPDR category, the mild form. On OCT, there is some mild abnormality of the central subfield thickness in the right eye. He will continue to do well if he takes care of his diabetes. We will watch his OCT in the future if he develops more macular edema. Amsler grid is given for the patient to do home testing. He is instructed to return if his vision becomes abnormal.

CLINICAL CORRELATIONS: Nonproliferative Diabetic Retinopathy 20/50 to 20/80

Patient complaints: Decreased vision at near and at distance.

Caveats: Poor glycemic control. She may have multisystem organ involvement with her diabetes. Look for abnormal lipid profiles and renal insufficiency which will point to a poor prognosis for long-term visual rehabilitation.

Case Study (Figs. 7-10–7-24)

3–10–2009: CG is a 58-year-old Caucasian female who was diagnosed with Type 2 diabetes 3 years ago. She has been compliant recently. She did not have time previously because she was a working, single mother trying to raise her children.

V 20/25
20/40
Slit lamp examination
Cornea: Clear OU
Anterior chamber: Deep and quiet OU
Iris: Normal OU, no rubeosis OU
Lens: 1 + nuclear sclerosis OU
Applanation tonometry = 18/18 mm Hg (1:00 PM)
Gonioscopy: Open 360 degrees OU, no rubeosis OU

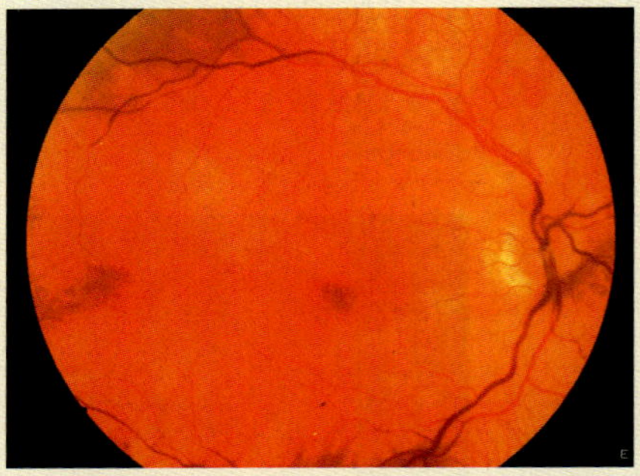

FIGURE 7-10. Fifty-eight-year-old Caucasian female. Diagnosis: CSME OU. V20/25 OD; V 20/40 OS, photo OD, CSME is seen.

Dilated funduscopic examination:
Right eye: CSME, hard exudates, superotemporal to macula, microaneurysms in macula.
Fundus photograph OD: CSME is seen; retinal thickening is seen in a wedge-shaped area, filled with small hard exudates and hemorrhages, from the superior fovea to superior macula, pushing into the area of the superior arcades. Some hard exudates and hemorrhages are seen in the area inferior to the macula, as well. There is an unexplained area of white discoloration at 10:00 from the macula (Fig. 7-10).

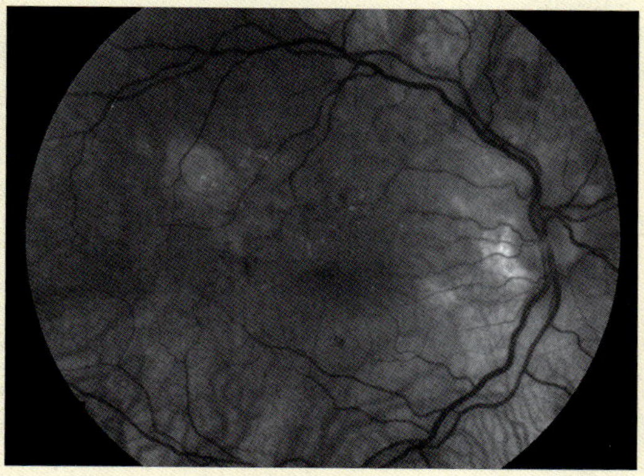

FIGURE 7-11. Red-free photograph OD, hemorrhages are seen as black, and the hard exudates are seen as white specks. The 10:00 area temporal to the macula shows hypopigmentation, and it needs a fluorescein angiogram for diagnosis.

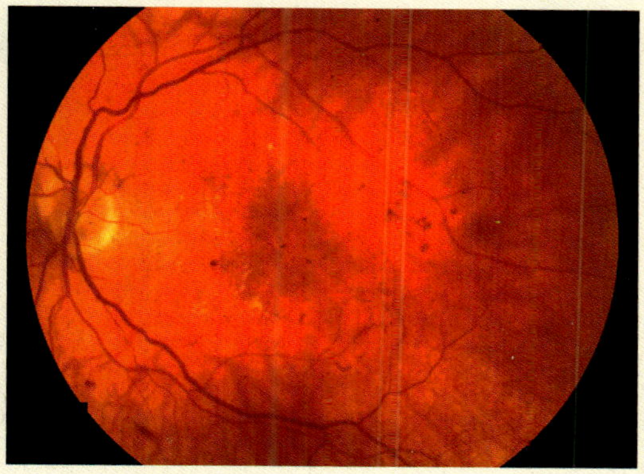

FIGURE 7-12. Photo OS, numerous small hard exudates, flame-shaped hemorrhage inferotemporally along the arcade are present. Hemorrhages are seen as well.

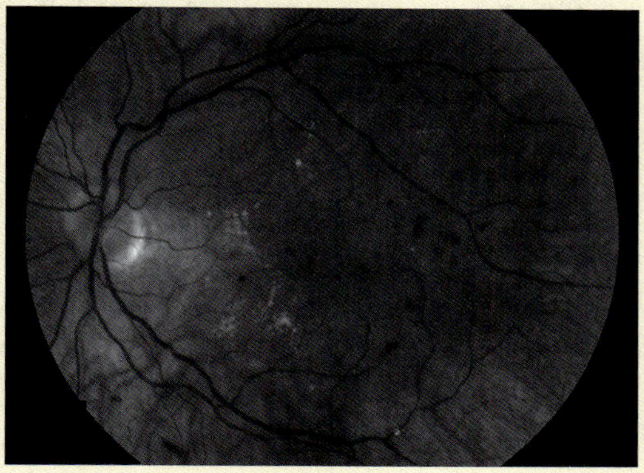

FIGURE 7-13. Red-free photograph OS, hemorrhages are seen clearly as black specks, and the hard exudates are clearly seen as white specks.

FIGURE 7-14. Fluorescein angiogram OD at 15 seconds of transit.

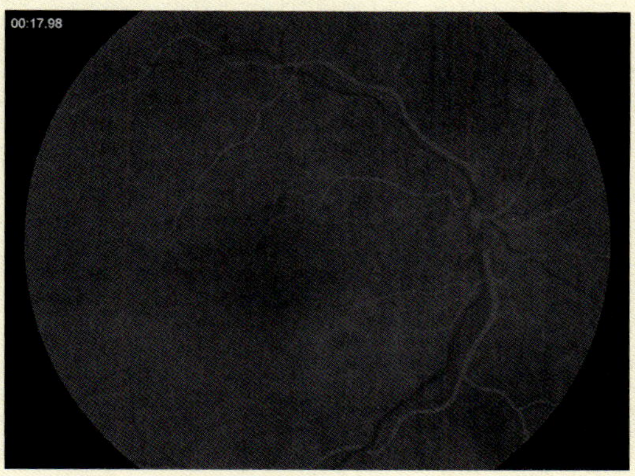

FIGURE 7-15. Fluorescein angiogram OD at 17 seconds of transit.

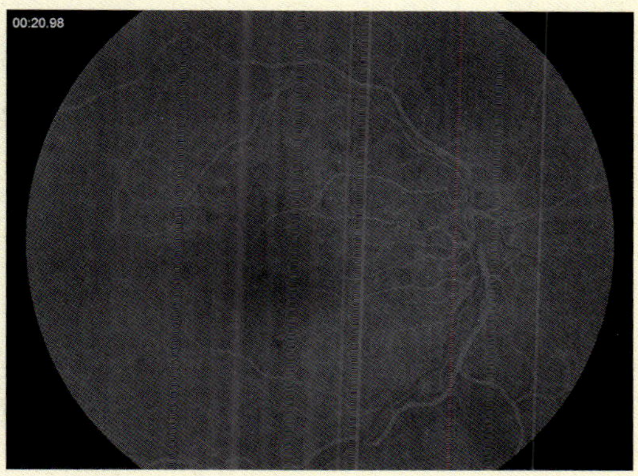

FIGURE 7-16. Fluorescein angiogram OD at 20 seconds of transit, multiple microaneurysms are seen.

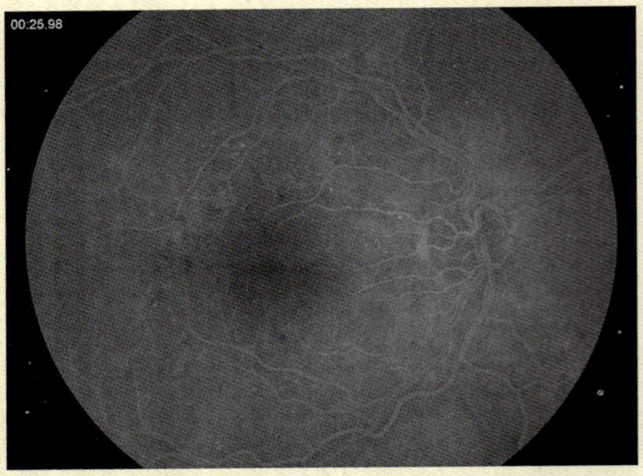

FIGURE 7-17. Fluorescein angiogram OD at 25 seconds of transit, multiple microaneurysms.

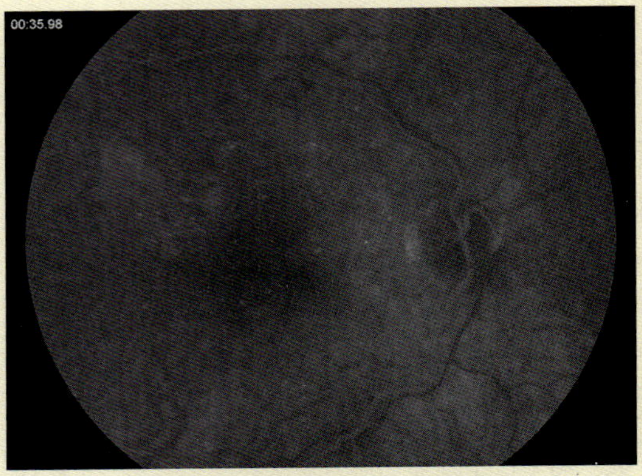

FIGURE 7-18. Fluorescein angiogram OD at 35 seconds of transit, macular edema.

FIGURE 7-19. Fluorescein angiogram OD at 46 seconds of transit.

FIGURE 7-20. Fluorescein angiogram OS at 1 minute 27 seconds of transit, hyperfluorescence of the fluorescein dye at the macula.

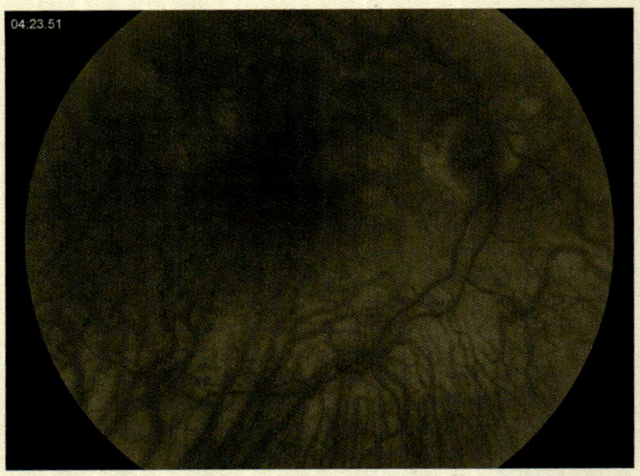

FIGURE 7-21. Fluorescein angiogram OD at 4 minute 23 seconds of transit, hyperfluorescence denoting macular edema.

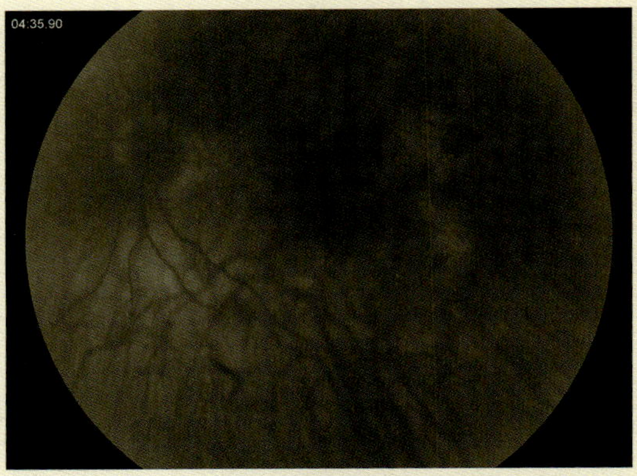

FIGURE 7-22. Fluorescein angiogram OS at 4 minute 35 seconds of transit, hyperfluorescence of the fluorescein dye representing macula edema.

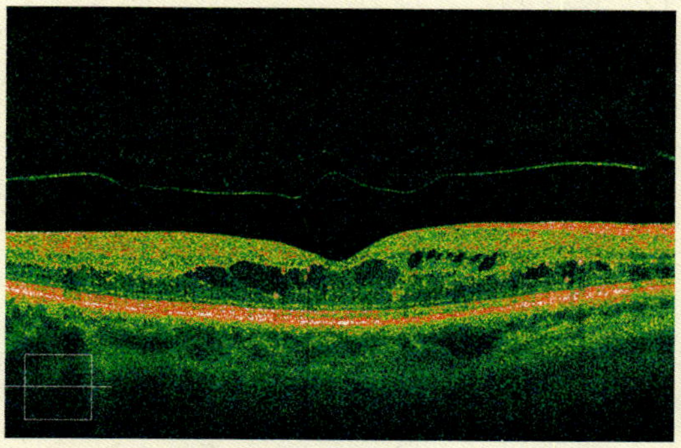

FIGURE 7-23. OCT OD, massive cyst formation in the outer plexiform layer, Henle layer.

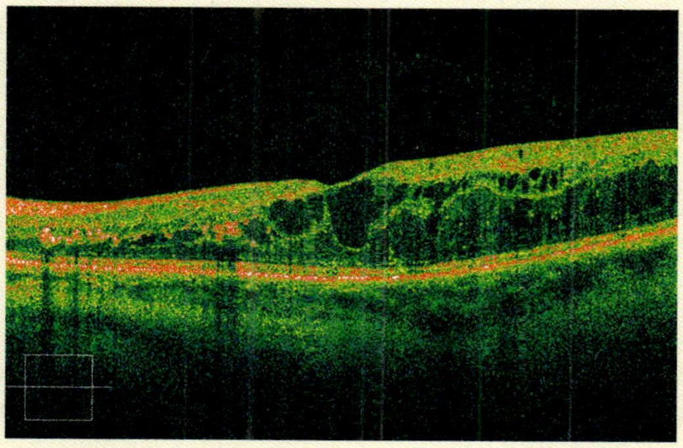

FIGURE 7-24. OCT OS, massive cyst formation in the outer plexiform layer, Henle layer.

Red-free photograph shows hard exudates in black (Fig. 7-11).

Left eye: CSME, hard exudates in macula, microaneurysms in macula, dot blot hemorrhages in macula with color photograph OS and associated red-free photograph OS (Figs. 7-12 and 7-13).

Fluorescein angiogram OD at 15 seconds of transit, there is uneven filling of the choroidal circulation. The 10:00 area of temporal to the macula remains unclear to the viewer. This is the beginning of the AV phase, and we expect slightly more delineation of the arterioles and venules by 15 seconds. The slight delay in transit is seen in out of control diabetic patients (Fig. 7-14).

Fluorescein angiogram OD at 17 seconds of transit, hyperfluorescence is seen in the macular area, and the foveal avascular zone is not circular or symmetrical but irregular in shape suggesting macular edema. The area in question at 10:00 does not reveal itself on fluorescein until 35 seconds of transit (Fig. 7-15).

Fluorescein angiogram OD at 20 seconds of transit, multiple microaneurysms can be seen in great detail (Fig. 7-16).

Fluorescein angiogram OD at 25 seconds of transit, multiple microaneurysms can be seen. Finally, there is full perfusion of the arteriovenous system. This is delayed in this patient (Fig. 7-17).

Fluorescein angiogram OD at 35 seconds of transit, the 10:00 area temporal to the macula is seen as capillary nonperfusion, thus, explaining its abnormal coloration on fundus photograph and indirect ophthalmolscopy. This corresponds to macular edema (Fig. 7-18).

Fluorescein angiogram OD at 46 seconds of transit, there is a suggestion of an additional area of capillary nonperfusion at 12:00, at the top of the photograph. Thus, this patient has areas at 12:00 that need to be monitored (Fig. 7-19).

Fluorescein angiogram OS at 1 minute 27 seconds of transit, hyperfluorescence of the fluorescein dye at the macula confirms the clinical picture of macular edema (Fig. 7-20).

Fluorescein angiogram OD at 4 minute 23 seconds of transit, hyperfluorescence of the fluorescein dye at the macula confirms the extent of the macular edema in the right eye (Fig. 7-21).

Fluorescein angiogram OS at 4 minute 35 seconds of transit, hyperfluorescence of the fluorescein dye at the macula demonstrates the edema (Fig. 7-22).

OCT OD shows massive cyst formation in the outer plexiform layer, Henle layer. Note that the macular cystic spaces are almost a mirror image, with the foveola in the center (Fig. 7-23).

OCT OS shows massive cyst formation in the outer plexiform layer, Henle layer, but the cysts are more irregular. The extent of the edema correlates with the patient's visual acuity of 20/40 (Fig. 7-24).

Comment

In summary, this is NPDR in a 58-year-old female with poor glycemic control. She has not had any medical care for a number of years. The first step is to send her to an internist and endocrinologist. She needs laboratory workup such as a lipid profile, complete blood count, electrolytes, FBS, and HbA1c. She needs focal macular laser photocoagulation OU.

CLINICAL CORRELATIONS: Nonproliferative Diabetic Retinopathy 20/50 to 20/80

Patient complaints: Decreased vision suddenly but the vision "returned after 15 minutes." Cannot pass the drivers' license test. He wants to use Viagra.

Caveats: Expect to find a history of poor glycemic control. The patient may not have adequate health education about diabetes. He may not be health literate.

Case Study (Figs. 7-25–7-30)

12–16–2008: FC, an 81-year-old Caucasian male, presents with "red eye" OD, who was diagnosed with "borderline diabetes" last year. He lost vision for 15 minutes 2 weeks ago and loss of vision returned yesterday. He used tadalafil (Cialis) this past week. He has no history of hypertension. He does not worry about his diet. He owns a stone masonry company. FBS = 114 mg/dL (normal = 99)

V 20/40 PH 20/25
20/25 NIPH
Slit lamp examination
Conjunctiva: Subconjunctival hemorrhage inferiorly OD; clear OS
Cornea: Clear OU
Anterior chamber: Deep and quiet OU
Iris: Normal OU, no rubeosis OU
Lens: 1 + nuclear sclerosis OU
Applanation tonometry = 18/18 mm Hg (1:00 PM)
Gonioscopy: Open 360 degrees OU, no rubeosis OU

Dilated funduscopic examination:

Right eye: Depigmented retinal pigment epithelial foci superotemporally; venous engorgement where the normal vein-to-artery ratio is 3:1, and in this patient, the ratio is increased.

Venous caliber changes are noted on fundus photograph OD. The vein-to-artery ratio is greater than 3:1. A few pinpoint areas of retinal pigment epithelial depigmentation in the fovea (Fig. 7-25).

Left eye: Depigmented retinal pigment epithelium superior temporally; venous engorgement as in the right eye.

Fundus photograph OS shows attenuated arterioles noted with respect to the veins. The vein-to-artery ratio is greater than 3:1. Larger areas of retinal pigment epithelial depigmentation are seen in the center of the fovea (Fig. 7-26).

Fluorescein angiography: There is delayed filling at the arteriovenous phase at 2 minutes instead of the normal 15 seconds. The vascular filling pattern is abnormal and irregular. There is no presence of emboli or capillary nonperfusion. The patient's history describes a transient ischemic attack, which needs further evaluation.

Fluorescein angiogram OD at transit time of 23 seconds, there is incomplete arteriovenous filling of fluorescein dye which would usually occur at 15 seconds. The patient is demonstrating significant delay of AV filling. In addition, there is abnormal choroidal filling. Note the irregular areas of hypofluorescence mixed with the background of fluorescence in the posterior pole (Fig. 7-27).

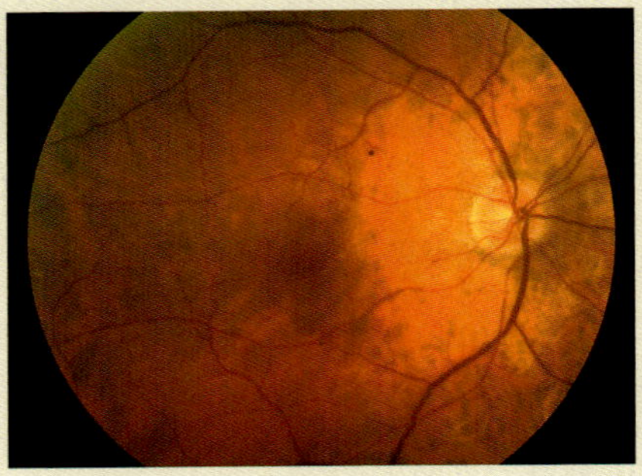

FIGURE 7-25. Photo OD, venous caliber and vein-to-artery ratio changes are noted.

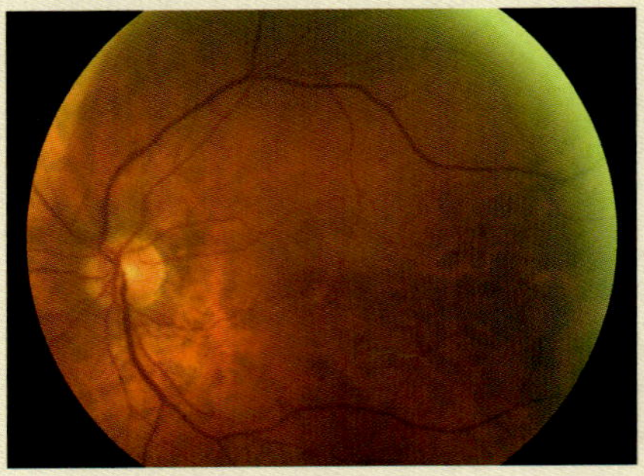

FIGURE 7-26. Photo OS, attenuated arterioles noted with respect to the veins.

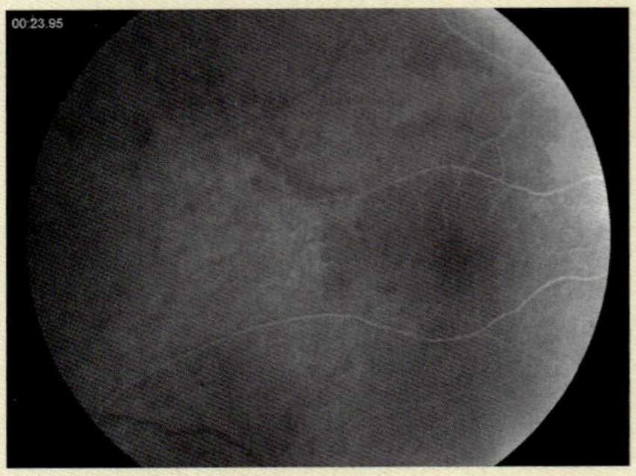

FIGURE 7-27. Fluorescein angiogram OD at transit time of 23 seconds, there is incomplete arteriovenous filling.

Fluorescein angiogram OD at transit time of 38 seconds, there is abnormal retinal pigment epithelium showing small window defects throughout the posterior pole suggesting ischemic RPE in the setting of diabetes or mild ocular ischemia (Fig. 7-28).

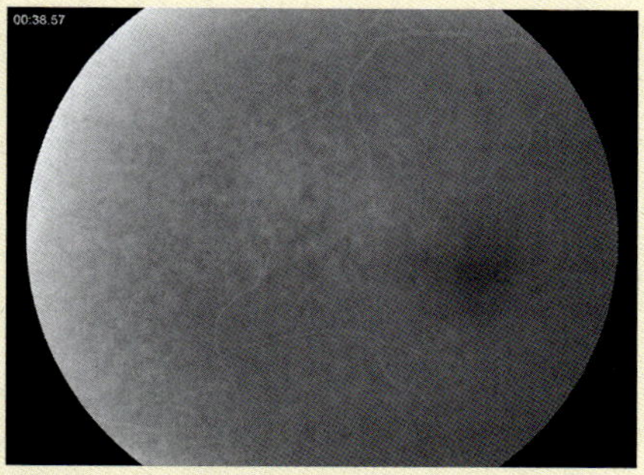

FIGURE 7-28. Fluorescein angiogram OD at transit time of 38 seconds, there is abnormal retinal pigment epithelium.

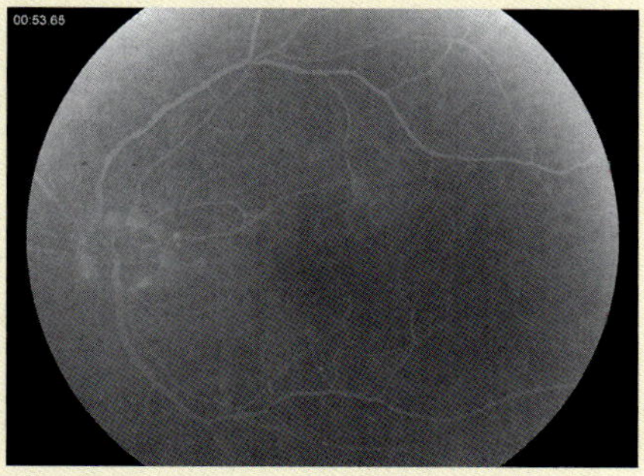

FIGURE 7-29. Fluorescein angiogram OD at transit time of 53 seconds, macular edema.

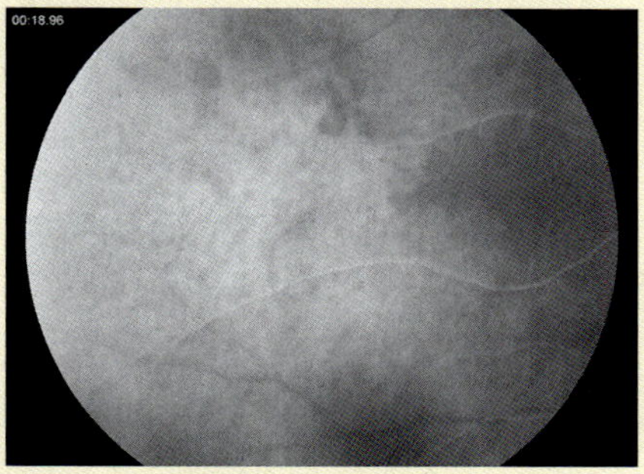

FIGURE 7-30. One month later, fluorescein angiogram OD at transit time of 18 seconds, his blood flow to the eye has improved.

Fluorescein angiogram OD at transit time of 53 seconds, some hyperfluorescence seen superotemporally suggesting macular edema (Fig. 7-29).

One month later, fluorescein angiogram OD at transit time of 18 seconds, the patient reaches this same phase as in last month's angiogram 5 seconds earlier, approaching a normal time for this transit of dye to occur. His blood flow to the eye has improved with treatment with aspirin, timolol maleate 1/2% BID OU, and NSAID eyedrops to decrease inflammation (Fig. 7-30).

Comment

In summary, this is NPDR in a 68-year-old male with the diagnosis of "borderline diabetes" and a transient ischemic attack. The designation of NPDR is based on the venous caliber engorgement and the subtle filling defects in the early transit of the fluorescein angiogram. While there is not the presence of microaneurysms or dot blot hemorrhages, there is subtle flow abnormalities which suggests vasculopathic abnormalities. There is the need to obtain last lab records to see what "borderline diabetes" implies to his internist. Does "borderline diabetes" serve as a euphemism for Type 2 diabetes? If the patient does not have recent laboratory work within the past 6 months, he needs new laboratory workup such as a lipid profile, complete blood count, electrolytes, FBS, and HbA1c. The HbA1c is important in assessing his glucose control over time.

Does the patient have a transient ischemic attack and needs a cardiology evaluation? He would then need a cardiac ECHO, carotid ultrasound, carotid MRA scan, ECG, and Holter monitoring. He may need to be placed on aspirin while he awaits his cardiology appointment.

The patient's use of tadalafil (Cialis) for erectile dysfunction can be a problem in diabetic patients. Tadalafil is the only one with 36-hour effectiveness and can be taken daily, as needed. This group of drugs, tadalafil, sildenafil (Viagra), and vardenafil (Levitra), is phosphodiesterase type 5 (PDE5) enzyme inhibitors. Sildenafil was FDA approved on March 27, 1998, vardenafil on August 19, 2003, and tadalafil on November 21, 2003. In May 2005, the FDA found that there was vision impairment and nonarteritic anterior ischemic optic neuropathy related to the use of these drugs. Most of the patients with visual complaints and PDE5 use had vascular risk factors such as low cup-to-disc ratio (crowded disc appearance), age over 50, diabetes, hypertension, and coronary artery disease. It is thought that sildenafil and this group of PDE5 compounds impair retinal function at the level of the photoreceptors but affect the neuronal network of the inner retina, at the bipolar cell level. Using an isolated superfused vertebrate retina, ERG testing shows that the B-wave amplitude is extinguished after infusion of sildenafil and remains extinguished despite a washout of technique after 240 minutes. Thus, it is postulated that there is inhibition of the phototransduction cascade by sildenafil via phosphodiesterase 6.[18]

Follow-up

1–7–2009: The patient's cardiac ECHO is normal, no ECG abnormalities, and no carotid USG abnormalities to warrant surgery. He is placed on aspirin. After cessation of tadalafil (Cialis), 3 months later, the patient's fluorescein angiogram returns to normal, showing the AV phase at 15 seconds which is within normal limits. The abnormal filling defects have spontaneously resolved.

CLINICAL CORRELATIONS: Nonproliferative Diabetic Retinopathy 20/100 to 20/400

Patient complaints: Decreased vision for 6 months.

Caveats: Poor glycemic control. Ask about new infections, foot ulcers or foot infections, or hand infections. Look for abnormal lipid profiles, renal insufficiency, metabolic syndrome, smoking history, and cardiovascular disease which will point to a poor prognosis for long-term visual rehabilitation.

Case Study (Figs. 7-31–7-36)

A 75-year-old Caucasian male with decreased vision was referred by local optometrist. He has had 10 years duration of diabetes, now taking insulin for the past 2 years. He has been in poor glycemic control. HbA1c = 9.3% but his fasting blood glucose is 111. He has had 10 years of hypertension as well. He lives alone and has a foot ulcer. He is currently using a wheelchair. His neighbor occasionally helps him and brings him to doctors' appointments. He has a son who lives nearby.

V 20/100
20/100
Slit lamp examination
Cornea: Clear OU
Anterior chamber: Deep and quiet OU
Iris: Normal OU, no rubeosis OU
Lens: 2 + nuclear sclerosis OU
Applanation tonometry = 16/16 mm Hg (9 AM)
Gonioscopy: 360 degrees OU, no rubeosis OU

Dilated funduscopic examination:

Right eye: CSME, with hard exudates, areas of edematous retina along the superior arcade. There is a discoloration of the retina seen along the superior arcade. There are hemorrhages seen temporal to the macula. The cup-to-disc ratio shows 0.8 cupping with abnormal optic nerve vessels at 11:00. Venous engorgement is noted along the superior temporal arcade (Fig. 7-31). Hemorrhages are seen as black in the red-free photograph (Fig. 7-32).

Left eye: Small cotton-wool spot at the first bifurcation of the veins superior to the optic disc margin. The cup-to-disc ratio is 0.8 as well. Venous engorgement is seen in the superior and inferior arcades (Fig. 7-33). The red-free photograph (Fig. 7-34) shows the venous abnormality very clearly.

Fluorescein angiogram OD at 23.96 seconds, showing delayed arteriovenous transit time. There is macular edema and dilated capillaries at the foveal avascular zone. There are microaneurysms (Fig. 7-35).

Fluorescein angiogram OS at 4 minutes 34 seconds transit time, late phase angiogram, there is macular edema at the superior aspect of the macula and macular edema in the foveal region. The cotton-wool spot shows some hyperfluorescence at this late transit suggesting reactive edema as well as ischemia (Fig. 7-36).

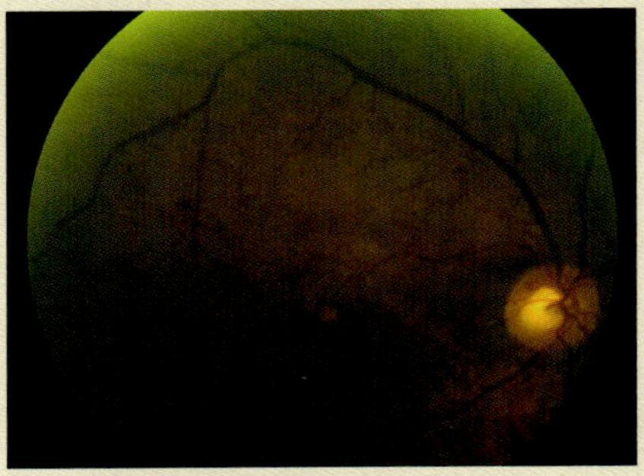

FIGURE 7-31. Photo OD, CSME.

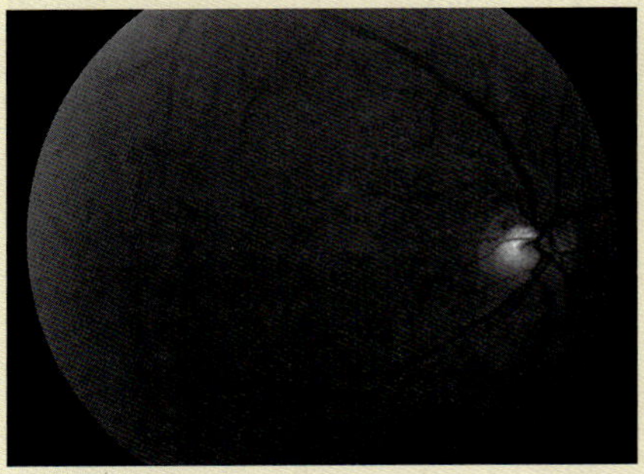

FIGURE 7-32. Red-free photograph OD, hemorrhages are seen.

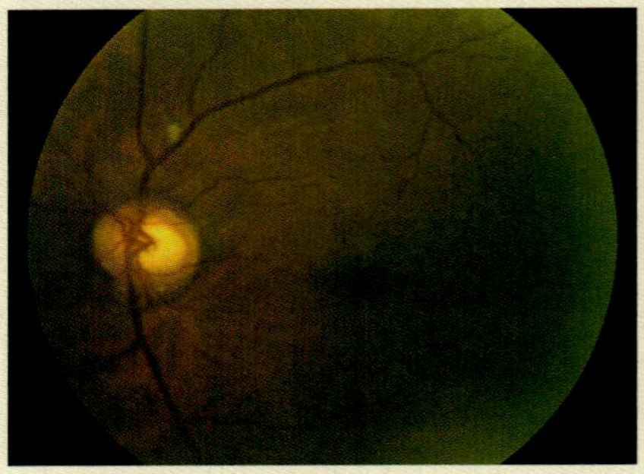

FIGURE 7-33. Photo OS, small cotton-wool spot at the margin.

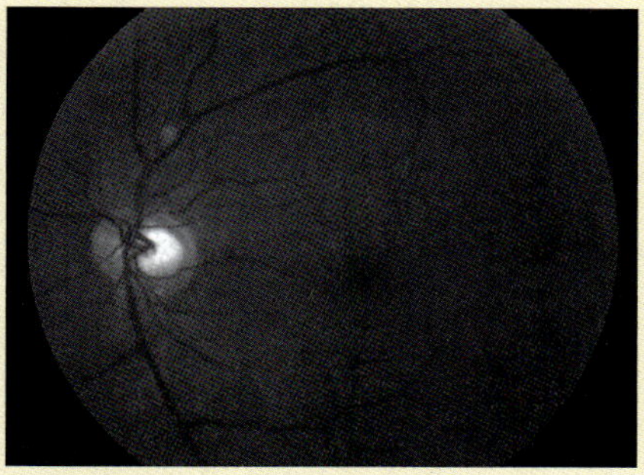

FIGURE 7-34. Red-free photograph OS, some features of the venous engorgement are seen.

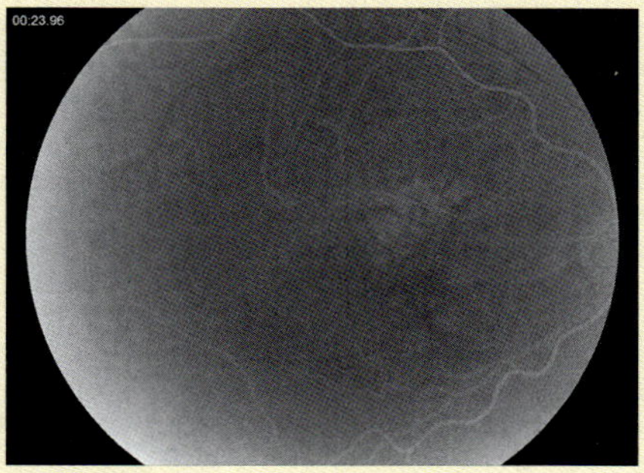

FIGURE 7-35. Fluorescein angiogram OD at 23.96 seconds, macular edema.

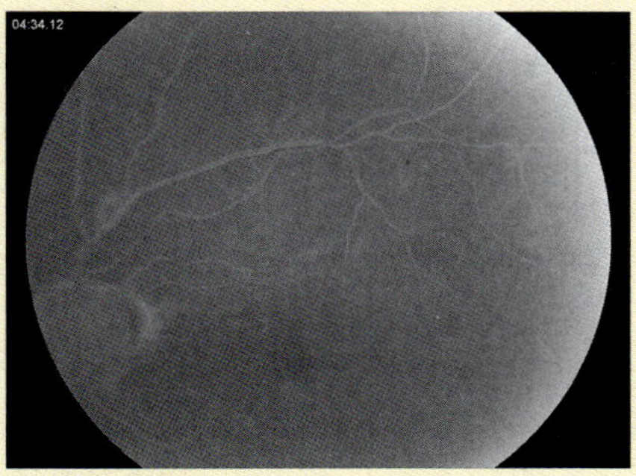

FIGURE 7-36. Fluorescein angiogram OS at 4 minutes, 34 seconds transit time, late phase angiogram, macular edema.

Comment

In summary, this is severe NPDR and CSME in an elderly male who has a foot ulcer and is wheelchair bound. He has been noncompliant for many years because his HbA1c is very elevated (9.3%). In addition, his foot ulcer makes his diabetes hard to control. He needs a fluorescein angiogram to ascVertain the extent of capillary nonperfusion and the future risk of PDR. In addition, the fluorescein angiogram will delineate if previous macular laser was already performed. Is this residual macular edema or an eye that has never received any laser treatment?

His optic nerve is abnormal, and he may have chronic open-angle glaucoma which needs further evaluation with a visual field.

This patient will need social worker intervention since he is wheelchair bound, lives alone, and has severe NPDR with CSME. He needs to have follow-up care once the ophthalmologist initiates laser treatment according to the ETDRS protocol if this eye has never previously had laser. Or, if the patient has had recent laser treatment, it is important to offer him options such as additional laser, bevacizumab with laser, or bevacizumab alone. It is important to establish rapport with the patient and have the patient understand the health issues involved in this level of diabetic retinopathy. He needs to have made a decision about his treatment options before signing informed consent. At this point, it may be helpful to contact his family members in order for everyone to be informed about his care. He will need follow-up every 2 to 3 months because of his diagnosis of severe NPDR with CSME.

The next step is to send him to his internist and endocrinologist for laboratory evaluation for lipid profiles, complete blood count, electrolytes, FBS, and HbA1c.

REFERENCES

1. Buse JB, Ginsburg HN, Bakris GL, et al. Primary prevention of cardiovascular disease in people with diabetes melloitus: A scientific statement for the American Heart Association and American Diabetes Association. *Diabetes Care.* 2007;30:162–172.
2. Schillinger D, Grumbach D, Piette J, et al. Association of health literacy with diabetes outcomes. *JAMA.* 2002;288: 475–482.
3. Coffey JT, Brandle M, Zhou H, et al. Valuing health-related quality of life in diabetes. *Diabetes Care.* 2002;25: 2238–2243.
4. St-Pierre J, Lemieux I, Perron P, et al. Relation of the "hypertriglyceridemic waist" phenotype to earlier manifestations of coronary artery disease in patients with glucose intolerance and type 2 diabetes mellitus. *Am J Cardiol.* 2007;99: 369–373.
5. Buse JB, Ginsburg HN, Bakris GL, et al. Primary prevention of cardiovascular disease in people with diabetes mellitus: A scientific statement for the American Heart Association and American Diabetes Association. *Diabetes Care.* 2007;30:162–172.
6. Centers for Disease Control and Prevention. National Center for Chronic Disease Prevention and Helath Promotion. http://www.cdc.gov/nccdphp/dnpa/obesity/. Accessed 21 February 2009.
7. Rimm EB, Chan J, Stampfer MJ, et al. Prospective Study of Cigarette Smoking, alchohol use, and the risk of diabetes in men. *Br Med J.* 1995;310:555–559.
8. Muhlhauser K, Sawicki P, Berger M. Cigarette Smoking as a risk factor for macroproteinuria and proliferative retinopathy in Type 1 (insulin- dependent) diabetes. *Diabetologia.* 1986;29:500–502.
9. Marshall G, Garg SK, Jackson WE, et al. Factors influencing the onset and progression of diabetic retinopathy in subjects with insulin-dependent diabetes. *Ophthalmology.* 1993;100:1133–1139.
10. Young RJ, McCulloch DK, Prescott RJ, et al. Alcohol: Another risk factor for diabetic retinopathy? *BMJ* 1984;288: 1035–1037.
11. Centers for disease control and Prevention. National Center for Chronic Disease Prevention and Health Promotion. http://www.cdc.gov/nccdphp/dnpa/obesity/. Accessed 21 February 2009.
12. http://www.cdc.gov/diabetes/statistics/prev/national/tablebysex.htm. Accessed 10 February 2009.
13. Centers for disease control. National Center for Chronic Disease Prevention and Health Promotion website. http://www.cdc.gov/diabetes/pubs/factsheet07.htm. Accessed 21 February 2009.
14. Early Treatment Diabetic Retinopathy Study Research Group. Photocoagulation for diabetic macular edema. Early Treatment Diabetic Retinopathy Study report number 1. *Arch Ophthalmol.* 1985;103:1796–1806.
15. Grundy SM, Cleeman JI, Daniels SR, et al. Diagnosis and management of the metabolic syndrome: An American Heart Association/National Heart, Lung, and Blood Institute Scientific Statement. *Circulation.* 2005;112:2735–2752.
16. Ferris F. Early photocoagulation in patients with either Type I or Type II diabetes. *Trans Am Ophthalmol Soc.* 1996;94:505–537.
17. ETDRS Research Group. Early photocoagulation for diabetic retinopathy report no 9. *Ophthalmology.* 1991;98: 767–785.
18. Luke M, Szurman P, Schneider T, et al. The effects of phosphodiesterase type V inhibitor sildenafil on human and bovine retinal function in vitro. *Graefe's Arch Clin Exp Ophthalmol.* 2007;245:1211–1215.

SUGGESTED READINGS

1. Aaberg TM. Clinical results in vitrectomy for diabetic traction retinal detachment. *Am J Ophthalmol.* 1979;88: 246–253.
2. Aaberg TM. Pars plana vitrectomy for diabetic traction retinal detachment. *Ophthalmology.* 1981;88:639–642.
3. Aaberg TM, Abrams GW. Changing indications and techniques for vitrectomy in management of complications of diabetic retinopathy. *Ophthalmology.* 1987;94:755–779.
4. Aaberg TM, Maggiano JM. Choroidal edema associated with retinal detachment repair. Experimental and clinical correlation. *Mod Probl Ophthalmol.* 1979;20:6.
5. Abrams GW, Williams GA. "En bloc" excision of diabetic membranes. *Am J Ophthalmol.* 1987;103:302–308.
6. Blankenship G. Management of vitreous cavity hemorrhage following pars plana vitrectomy for diabetic retinopathy. *Ophthalmology.* 1986;93:34–44.
7. Blankenship G, Cortez, R, Machemer R. The lens and pars plana vitrectomy for diabetic retinopathy complications. *Arch Ophthalmol.* 1979;97:1263.
8. Blankenship GW, Flynn HW, Kokame GT. Posterior chamber intraocular lens insertion during pars plana lensectomy and vitrectomy for complications of proliferative diabetic retinopathy. *Am J Ophthalmol.* 1980;108:1–5.
9. Blankenship GW, Machemer R. Long-term diabetic vitrectomy results. Report of 10 year follow-up. *Ophthalmology.* 1985;92:503–506.
10. Charles S. *Vitreous Microsurgery.* Baltimore, MD: Williams & Wilkins; 1981:107–120.
11. Charles S, Flinn CE. The natural history of diabetic extramacular traction retinal detachment. *Arch Ophthalmol.* 1981;99:66–68.
12. Cohan HB, McMeel JW, Franks EP. Diabetic traction detachment. *Arch Ophthalmol.* 1979;97:1268.
13. Davis MD. Vitreous contraction in proliferative diabetic retinopathy. *Arch Ophthalmol.* 1965;74:741.
14. Davis MD. Proliferative diabetic retinopathy. In: Ryan SJ, ed. *Retina.* Vol. 2. St Louis, MO: CV Mosby Co; 1989: 367–402.
15. DeBustros S, Thompson JT, Michels RG, Rice TA. Vitrectomy for progressive proliferative diabetic retinopathy. *Arch Ophthalmol.* 1987;104:196–199.
16. Diabetic Retinopathy Vitrectomy Study Research Group. Report no 1. Two-year course of visual acuity in severe proliferative diabetic retinopathy with conventional management. *Ophthalmology.* 1985;92:492–502.

17. Diabetic Retinopathy Vitrectomy Study Research Group. Report no 2. Early vitrectomy for severe vitreous hemorrhage in diabetic retinopathy. Two-year results of a randomized trial. *Arch Ophthalmol.* 1985;103:1644–1652.
18. Diabetic Retinopathy Vitrectomy Study Research Group. Report no 3. Early vitrectomy for severe proliferative diabetic retinopathy in eyes with useful vision. Results of a randomized trial. *Ophthalmology.* 1988;95:1307–1320.
19. Diabetic Retinopathy Vitrectomy Study Research Group. Report no 4. Early vitrectomy for severe proliferative diabetic retinopathy in eyes with useful vision. Clinical application of results of a randomized trial. *Ophthalmology.* 1988;95:1321–1334.
20. Diabetic Retinopathy Vitrectomy Study Research Group. Report no 5. Early vitrectomy for severe vitreous hemorrhage in diabetic retinopathy. Four-year results of a randomized trial. *Arch Ophthalmol.* 1990;108:958–964.
21. Hutton WL, Pesicka GA, Fuller DG. Cataract extraction in the diabetic eye after vitrectomy. *Am J Ophthalmol.* 1987;104:1.
22. Lewis H, Abrams GW, Foos RY. Clinicopathologic findings in anterior hyaloidal fibrovascular proliferative after diabetic vitrectomy. *Am J Ophthalmol.* 1987;104:614.
23. Lewis H, Abrams GW, Foos RY. Clinicopathologic findings in anterior hyaloidal fibrovascular proliferation after diabetic vitrectomy. *Am J Ophthalmol.*1987;104:614–618.
24. Lewis H, Abrams GW, Williams GA. Anterior hyaloidal fibrovascular proliferation after diabetic vitrectomy. *Am J Ophthalmol.* 1987;104:607–613.
25. Lewis H, Han D, Williams GA. Management of fibropupillary block glaucoma after pars plana vitrectomy with intravitreal gas injection. *Am J Ophthalmol.* 1987;103:180.
26. Liggett PE, Lean JS, Barlow WE, Ryan SJ. Intraoperative argon endophotocoagulation for recurrent vitreous hemorrhage after vitrectomy for diabetic retinopathy. *Am J Ophthalmol.* 1987;103:146–149.
27. Machemer R, Blankenship G. Vitrectomy for proliferative diabetic retinopathy associated with vitreous hemorrhage. *Ophthalmology.* 1981;88:643–646.
28. Machemer R, Buettner H, Norton EWD, et al. Vitrectomy: A pars plana approach. *Trans Am Acad Ophthalmol Otolaryngol.* 1971;75:813–820.
29. Meredith TA, Kaplan HJ, Aaberg TM. Pars plana vitrectomy techniques for relief of epiretinal traction by membrane segmentation. *Am J Ophthalmol.* 1980;89:408.
30. Michels RG, Rice TA, Rice EF. Vitrectomy for diabetic vitreous hemorrhage. *Am J Ophthalmol.* 1983;95:12–21.
31. Murphy RP, Egbert PR. Regression of iris neovascularization following panretinal photocoagulation. *Arch Ophthalmol.* 1979;97:700.
32. O'Hanley GP, Canny CLB. Diabetic dense premacular hemorrhage. *Ophthalmology.* 1985;92:507–511.
33. Pendergast SD, Margher RR, Williams, GA, Cox MS. Vitrectomy for diffuse diabetic macular edema associated with a taut premacular posterior hyaloid. *Am J Ophthalmol.* 2000;130:178–186.
34. Ramsay RC, Knoblock WH, Cantrill HL. Timing of vitrectomy for active proliferative diabetic retinopathy. *Ophthalmol.* 1986;93:283–289.
35. Rice TA, Michels RG, Maguire MG, Rice EF. The effect of lensectomy on the incidence of iris neovascularization and neovascular glaucoma after vitrectomy for diabetic retinopathy. *Am J Ophthalmol.* 1983;95:1–11.
36. Rice TA, Michels RG, Rice EF. Vitrectomy for diabetic rhegmatogenous retinal detachment. *Am J Ophthalmol.* 1983;95:34–44.
37. Rice TA, Michels RG, Rice EF. Vitrectomy for diabetic traction retinal detachment involving the macula. *Am J Ophthalmol.* 1983;95:22–33.
38. Sebestyen JG. Fibrinoid syndrome; a severe complication of vitrecomy surgery in diabetics. *Ann Ophthalmol.* 1982;14:853–856.
39. Shea M. Early vitrectomy in proliferative diabetic retinopathy. *Arch Ophthalmol.* 1983;101:1204–1205.
40. Smiddy WE, Stark WJ, Michels RG, et al. Cataract extraction after vitrectomy. *Ophthalmology.* 1987;94:483.
41. Thompson JT, Auer CL, DeBustros S, et al. Prognostic indicators of success and failure in vitrectomy for diabetic retinopathy. *Ophthalmology.* 1986;93:290–295.
42. Thompson JT, deBustros S, Michels RG, et al. Results and prognostic factors in vitrectomy for diabetic traction detachment of the macula. *Arch Ophthalmol.* 1987;105–497.
43. Thompson JT, deBustros S, Michels RG, et al. Results and prognostic factors in vitrectomy for diabetic traction-rhegmatogenous retinal detachment. *Arch Ophthalmol.* 1987;105:503.
44. Williams DF, Williams GA, Hartz A, et al. Results of vitrectomy for diabetic traction retinal detachments using the en bloc excision technique. *Ophthalmology.* 1989;96:752–758.

CHAPTER 8

Management of Clinically Significant Macular Edema or Diabetic Macular Edema

DIAGNOSIS

Diabetic macular edema is the most frequent cause of visual loss in patients with nonproliferative diabetic retinopathy. Approximately 50,000 people in America have diabetic macular edema.[1] The ETDRS show that the 3-year risk of moderate visual loss for patients with foveal or perifoveal macular edema was 24% for the control group and 12% for the photocoagulation treated group.[2] However, only 2% of the treated group had three or more lines of improved visual acuity. The limitation of the laser may be the development of small focal scotomas, choroidal neovascularization, macular ischemia, and macular scarring. Often patients have refractory or residual macular edema after several focal or grid laser photocoagulation treatments.

Metamorphopsia on Amsler grid testing can occur 2 to 5 degrees from center fixation. Microperimetry with the scanning laser ophthalmoscope can map macular scotomas in diabetic patients with clinically significant macular edema (CSME).[3–5]

There are several ways in which the patient with diabetic macular edema will present to the ophthalmologist. The first is that he or she is referred to the ophthalmologist/retina specialist after having been seen by another eye care practitioner, an optometrist, for having macular edema. A second referral route is through the patient's primary care practitioner, for an evaluation of a first eye examination. Thirdly, the patient complains of decreased vision. Lastly, the patient is asymptomatic and comes for an evaluation for a chief complaint other than his or her diabetic macular edema. Upon routine examination, the patient is found to have macular edema.

In all of these instances, it is best to document the patient's duration of diabetes, his or her type of diabetes, Type 1 or Type 2, and obtain from the patient, the latest fasting blood glucose and hemoglobin A1c (HbA1c).

If this patient is unclear about his or her diabetes status or thinks he or she is a "borderline diabetic" but presents with diabetic retinopathy, then the ophthalmologist may send him or her for a physical examination with his or her family practitioner or internist. If the patient has not seen an internist for a year, he or she should be sent for lipid profiles, CBC and electrolytes, fasting blood glucose, and hemoglobin A1c. Another ophthalmic follow-up appointment can be made after the lab values are available. Follow-up appointments with his or her internist and endocrinologist are also suggested. One third of the diabetic population does not know that they have the disease.[1] Thus, undiagnosed diabetic patients may present for a routine exam when they in fact have diabetes and diabetic retinopathy.

Health literacy is defined as a measure of the patients' ability to read, comprehend, and act on medical instructions. Patient awareness is now being studied in the medical literature. A health literacy study evaluated 114 diabetic patients presenting to general medicine clinics at two urban hospitals in Atlanta, Georgia. The authors found that 94% of the patients with functional health literacy know the symptoms of hypoglycemia versus 50% with inadequate literacy. Poor health literacy is common among racial and ethnic minorities, elderly persons, and patients with chronic conditions, particularly in public-sector settings. Thus, it is important to continue to educate the diabetic patients about their chronic disease and side effects.[6,7]

The HbA1c shows that the patient has been compliant with his or her blood sugar over the past 6 months. If the HbA1c is over 7%, there is a high risk of diabetic retinopathy. If the triglyceride is over 150 mg/dL and within the 200 mg/dL range, we would expect to see more hard exudates changes in the retina. If there is hyperlipidemia, obesity, or cardiovascular disease, we will anticipate an accelerated rate of diabetic retinopathy as we follow up the patient (Chapter 7). The HbA1c could be elevated but the fasting glucose could be normal denoting good patient compliance for 24 hours but poor long-term compliance for the past 6 months. We would expect his or her eye findings to show diabetic retinopathy depending on his or her HbA1c status.

In another study evaluating HbA1c status and health literacy, it is found that patients with inadequate health literacy are less likely than patients with adequate health literacy to achieve tight glycemic control (HbA1c ≤7.2%). Those with the lower HbA1c are more likely to achieve tight control than those patients with poor glycemic control (HbA1c ≥9.5%) and to report retinopathy.[7]

In large metropolitan areas with medical schools in the city, patients usually have more laboratory follow-up and they present to the ophthalmologist with full medical evaluations. In large, sprawling suburban or rural areas where there are no nearby medical schools or medical centers, the patient may present to the ophthalmologist with poor vision and fulminant diabetic retinopathy without even knowing that he or she has diabetes.[6,7]

Similarly, with macular edema, which can be an insidious disease affecting near vision, the patient may not have seen an eye care provider for many years because he or she "felt fine." Often, a patient with severe diabetic macular edema presents to the ophthalmologist not knowing that he or she has diabetes.

Chief Complaint

Listen to what the patient is saying. What is the patient's chief complaint? In the patient's own words, what bothers him or her? If the clinician finds macular edema but the patient's reason is his or her failing grade in the driving test, then, the clinician must answer that his or her driving test result is correlated to his or her diabetic macular edema.

Ask about his or her symptoms: Is it a gradual, painless loss of vision? Is it transient visual loss? Is the visual loss at night only? Decreased contrast sensitivity may mean the additional diagnosis of glaucoma which can be associated with diabetes. Is the visual impairment at sunset? Decreased rod function from previous laser photocoagulation for diabetic retinopathy can lead to loss of contrast sensitivity at sunset. All this time, we are taking notes so that we can ask the patient more questions after he or she finishes speaking. Let the patient tell the story.

Past Medical History

The review of systems sheet and history form filled out by the patient provides information about the duration of diabetes, treatment with insulin, without insulin, family history, hypertension, cardiovascular disease, renal disease, thyroid disease, and metabolic syndrome risk factors (Chapter 7). Their answers to the previous questions and their physical habitus may lead to further questioning about their American Diabetes Association Diet, their exercise regimen, their weight gain, eating issues involving weight gain or weight loss, and weight loss surgery.

Red flags are comorbid conditions, obesity, recent hospitalizations for stroke, heart disease, diabetic ketoacidosis, smoking, surgery for any reason, hospitalizations for infections, history of foot ulcers, and previous laser to the eyes for any reason. These mean that the patient may have accelerated diabetic retinopathy issues in the future.

We always send a referral letter to the internist or optometrist or referring ophthalmologist. If the problem is urgent, requiring laser or surgery, we call the referring doctor.

In our office, we have available handouts from the American Diabetes Association, the literature about the pathophysiology of diabetes, the epidemiology of diabetes as it affects the patient. We tailor the statistics to the patient sitting in the exam chair.

The office staff could provide Web site information and handouts about diets recommended by the American Diabetes Association, a list of cookbooks for the diabetes diet, and a list of endocrinologists whom they could see near their geographic region.

Before patients leave, we ask them to sign a medical release form so that our office can obtain their previous lab results from their internist or family care practitioner.

We ask that their future lab results be sent to our office as well as to their internist.

Physical Exam

Our approach to CSME is simple: visual acuity, Amsler grid testing, pupillary testing, slit lamp examination, and then a dilated funduscopic examination with a 90 D lens and a 20 D lens. Fundus photography and Optical Coherence Tomography (OCT) are part of the first visit.

Once we make the diagnosis of CSME, we obtain a fluorescein angiogram depending on the severity of the macular edema and level of retinopathy. Capillary nonperfusion can be documented by fluorescein angiography. Prior to macular laser, fluorescein angiography is extremely helpful in identifying microaneurysms for focal treatment.

We also assess the level of diabetic retinopathy that the patient has in terms of his or her vascular disease (optic nerve appearance, arteriolar changes, venous beading changes, vein-to-artery ratio of 3:1).

Fovea

In examining the fovea, we look for the internal limiting membrane reflex, its relationship to the posterior hyaloid face, the appearance of the fovea, smooth like normal, and whether the surface is cystic or is it irregular because of gliosis from old inflammation or chronic hypertension. This can be verified by the OCT.

Optical Coherence Tomography

When we perform the OCT examination, we look at the central subfield thickness of the fovea expressed in microns. The OCT describes the contour of the fovea and its relationship to the vitreous. This measurement can diagnose early gliosis, macular cysts, and macular edema at the Henle layer. The information is very accessible for all ophthalmologists and eye care practitioners.

ETDRS Classification of Macular Edema

Diagnosis of CSME by the ETDRS criteria is thickening of the retina at or within 500 μm of the center of the macula; hard exudates at or within 500 μm of the center of the macula, if associated with thickening of the adjacent retina (not residual hard exudates remaining after the disappearance of retinal thickening); or a zone or zones of retinal thickening of one disc area or larger, any part of which is within one disc diameter of the center of the macula[2] (Table 8-1).

The diagnosis of CSME is through slit lamp biomicroscopy and is documented with stereo fundus photography. Fluorescein angiography is required by the ETDRS only after the clinical diagnosis is made by slit lamp biomicroscopy. Thus, fluorescein angiography leakage without clinical thickening does not fulfill the definition of CSME according to the ETDRS criteria.

TABLE 8.1 ETDRS Classification of Macular Edema[2]

1. Thickening of the retina at or within 500 μm of the center of the macula
2. Hard exudates at or within 500 μm of the center of the macula
   a. if associated with thickening of the adjacent retina
   b. no residual hard exudates remaining after the disappearance of retinal thickening
3. Zone or zones of retinal thickening of one disc area or larger
   a. any part of which is within one disc diameter of the center of the macula.

Now, 20 years after the landmark ETDRS, there are clinical modifications in the retina practice. The use of the OCT is commonplace and noninvasive. Thus, the imaging of macular edema can be identified and quantified easily. The macular cysts and the amount of macular edema can be seen in cross section on OCT for each patient.

While macular edema can present at every stage of diabetic retinopathy, from background diabetic retinopathy to nonproliferative to proliferative diabetic retinopathy, the tools are the same for the diagnosis. The treatment is different depending on the severity of the disease.

Patients with Visual Acuity of 20/20 to 20/30

In asymptomatic patients with the visual acuity of 20/20 to 20/30, with CSME according to the ETDRS guidelines, these patients would be eligible for treatment.[2] However, because they are asymptomatic, these patients may not want treatment. Patient education with your nurse or assistants over several visits may prepare them for the eventuality of treatment. The emphasis is that laser will keep them at their visual acuity level.

Patients with Visual Acuity of 20/40

The visual acuity of 20/40 is a threshold for treatment for many patients since 20/40 is the driving test vision requirement. At the 20/40 level of visual acuity, the patient is usually symptomatic. The patient needs to understand fully that the laser will preserve his or her vision in the long term. For anxious patients, we perform a central visual field to map the preoperative visual scotoma from the macular edema and then proceed to laser. We make sure that the patient understands that there is always a risk for some immediate vision loss but in the long run, he or she will maintain his or her vision.

Patients with Visual Acuity of 20/50 to 20/80

At this visual acuity of 20/50 or worse, the patient is unhappy and wants treatment. OCT and fluorescein angiography are helpful in documenting the pathology for laser planning. The fluorescein angiographic photos will demonstrate the extent of the diabetic retinopathy to the patient. Patient education is important prior to informed consent.

Patients with Visual Acuity of 20/100 or Worse

Previous Laser

The most important question to ask is "why" is the vision 20/100? In eyes with previous laser, ask these questions:

1. Is the patient noncompliant with his or her diabetes treatment?
2. Is the patient obese and has the metabolic syndrome characteristics?
3. Is the patient going to be compliant in our office and follow our instructions for follow-up?
4. Does the patient have renal disease, which would cause fluid retention, and therefore have cystic macular edema?
5. Is the patient infected with a foot ulcer?
6. What are the patient's HbA1c status, FBS, and lipid profiles?
7. Does the patient have undiagnosed glaucoma? Is it open angle glaucoma or early rubeotic glaucoma?

Those patients who have had previous macular laser will have residual macular edema. They need fluorescein angiography and OCT evaluations of their macula. From the fluorescein angiogram, the clinician will be looking for areas of capillary nonperfusion, areas of abnormal foveal capillary net. Look at the time of the arteriovenous phase transit. If the transit time is significantly longer than the normal expected 15 to 16 seconds, the retina specialist might think of decreased flow to the retina, common with internal carotid disease or poor cardiovascular perfusion. If the flow is abnormal, the retina specialist might consider sending the patient to a cardiologist. The cardiologist would probably perform echocardiogram of the heart, ECG, internal carotid ultrasonography, magnetic resonance angiography, or Holter monitoring of his or her heart.

In these patients with residual macular edema with 20/100 vision of worse would lead the clinician to ask: has the previous laser caused macular scarring that has enlarged and caused additional inflammation and gliosis? Is there a functioning macula with adequate blood flow? From the OCT, the ophthalmologist will be looking at the macular thickness measurement and the abnormalities of Henle layer.

Lastly, examine the patient for glaucoma. The optic nerve, the angle, and the trabecular meshwork must be looked at carefully. Look at the patient's visual field and visual evoked potential for optic nerve function. Send the patient to a glaucoma specialist if there is no clear reason as to why the vision is decreased.

These previously treated eyes are candidates for additional laser or bevacizumab intravitreal injection. Bevacizumab may be the only treatment option if the macula shows poor perfusion and extensive derangement of foveal capillary net. It is important to warn these patients about a prolonged course of recovery. It must be emphasized that their diabetes must be under control during this time of visual rehabilitation.

No Previous Laser

In those patients who present for the first time to our office with diabetic macular edema, we order fluorescein angiography, OCT to determine if there is focal or diffuse leakage. We want to ascertain what type of leakage they have in the macula. In addition, how thick is the retinal? Is there massive cyst formation? They are a candidate for macular laser using the ETDRS guidelines.[2] The fluorescein angiogram can identify hundreds of additional microaneurysms not seen on regular fundus photography of the macular region. If this is the case, focal laser treatment can be performed. The fluorescein angiogram can reveal areas of capillary nonperfusion within the macula. If upon OCT testing there are large foveal cysts, grid laser and bevacizumab may be offered.

TREATMENT

Patients with CSME should be considered for laser surgery. While a minority of patients have improvement of vision, for the majority of cases, the goal of treatment with laser photocoagulation is the stabilization of vision. Most patients need more than one treatment session. The average number of treatment sessions is 3 to 4 separated by 2 to 4 months, for the retinal thickening to resolve.

OCT and fluoresecein angiography document the macular edema. The fluorescein angiogram is useful in delineating the abnormal derangement of the foveal avascular zone. The extent of the foveal capillary net and the fovea will allow the clinician in planning laser treatment.

Follow-up examination for post-op laser patients with CSME can be scheduled 2 to 4 months after surgery. However, if the patient notes worsening of vision, he or she should come in before the scheduled appointment.

New Treatment Modalities (See Chapter 5)

Combination of laser and triamcinolone, and laser and pegaptanib and bevacizumab, is now done throughout the United States since 2006. The newer agents which are monoclonal antibody intravitreal treatments have not had a large scale multicentered trials yet.[8,9]

TABLE 8.2 Grid Laser for Diffuse Diabetic Macular Edema

1. Aim for the area with diffuse leakage.
2. 3–4 burn widths apart (postoperatively, the small laser burn can scar and enlarge over time).
3. Try a test burn in far periphery, anterior to arcades to see the burn strength. Each patient's retina is different because of melanin pigment.
4. Aim for a lighter burn than for the focal lesion:
   100-μm spot size
   100 mW
   Argon green laser
   Goldmann lens

Treatment Options

These macular edema patients who fulfill the ETDRS criteria can be offered the treatment of laser, and the clinician can provide proof of the macular edema using the OCT and fundus photos and fluorescein angiography. However, if the patient resists treatment, the clinican can offer the Amsler grid testing and ask that they return in 6 weeks, and monitor their hemoglobin A1c and fasting blood sugars in the interim.

If the macular edema is diffuse, and the patient does not want laser or intravitreal bevacizumab, one can offer topical NSAID eye drops for treatment as a temporizing measure.[10]

Laser

If the macular edema has discrete microaneurysms with leakage seen on fluorescein, laser is used for those microaneurysms in a "focal" treatment.

For this group of patients who opt for laser, make sure the laser burn is focused on the microaneurysm and that the burn is a light "white burn." A bright white, oversized burn would mean the risk of a scotoma in the macula in a patient with pre-op visual acuity of 20/20 to 20/30. The light burn would prevent secondary macular gliosis as a secondary consequence.

The laser settings are 100 mW, argon green laser, 100 μm spot size, 0.1 seconds. If you want to use less power, you can use a 50-μm spot size with lower power. Always try a test burn in the far periphery with your desired laser settings (Tables 8-2 and 8-3).

Intravitreal Triamcinolone

Prep the cul-de-sac with topical proparacaine HCl 0.5%, 5% povidone iodine. We use topical proparacaine, instilled over the intended injection site for about 10 to 15 seconds. Continuously apply proparacaine HCl eye drops over the site, with a sterile 4×4 held against the lower eyelid to catch the runoff of the excess eye drops.

TABLE 8.3 Focal Laser for Diabetic Macular Edema

1. Fluorescein angiogram of area to be treated
2. Try a test burn in far periphery, anterior to arcades to see the burn strength. Each patient's retina is different because of melanin pigment.
3. Look at the area with microaneurysms visible on the Goldmann lens examination and initiate treatment away from the foveal avascular zone, as your first treatment spot.
4. Aim with aiming beam at the microaneurysm, using 100-μm spot size or 50-μm spot size according to the size of the microaneurysm.
5. Aim for a white-yellow burn on the lesion. Do not create a bigger than necessary burn:
   100-μm spot size
   100 mW
   0.1 sec (if using 50-μm spot size, decrease the time and power setting to get the white-yellow burn)
   Argon Green laser
   Goldmann lens

TABLE 8.4 Intravitreal Injection Supplies

Materials
5% povidone iodine
Proparacaine HCl 0.5%
30-gauge needle
Tuberculin syringe
4×4 sterile sponges
Lid speculum
Sterile gloves
Sterile caliper

Then, we apply 5% povidone iodine to the injection site. We place three drops and ask the patient to close his or her eyes and blink a few times. We wait for 3 minutes before we inject. During this 3-minute waiting period, we get ready to prep the outside of the eye with 10% povidone iodine with sterile 4 × 4 sponges (Table 8-4).

For injection, 4 mg of triamcinolone acetonide is injected intravitreally with a tuberculin syringe with a 30-gauge needle. Other authors have used 25 mg of triamcinolone acetonide intravitreally as well.[11]

Immediately postoperatively in the office, the patient receives topical timolol maleate XE ½% instilled in their cul-de-sac (Table 8-5). Postoperatively, the patients go home with instructions to use either topical moxifloxacin or gatifloxacin four times daily for 4 days, or erythromycin ophthalmic ointment four times daily for 4 days. Ointment can be used if the patients cannot put in eye drops or if they live alone. The patients are asked to instill timolol maleate XE ½% once a day for a week and then return to see us for an intraocular pressure check the next day.[1]

Risks of glaucoma and intraocular pressure usually occur by the third week. The pressure rise can be managed with topical antiglaucoma medications. Intraocular pressure rise can be as high as 21 to 35 mm Hg, all managed successfully with antiglaucoma medications.

Vitrectomy for Persistent Diffuse Diabetic Macular Edema

Removal of posterior hyaloid face in eyes with persistent macular edema has been discussed in the literature. In one study, 55 vitrectomized eyes with the refractory macular edema with average vision of 20/260 preoperatively, after vitrectomy, have an average vision of 20/80 postoperatively.[12]

TABLE 8.5 Prevention of Infection with Intravitreal Injections

1. Prep the cul-de-sac with 5% Betadine: two drops
2. Prep the orbit and eyelid with 10% Betadine
3. Always use a speculum
4. Hold sterile cotton tip applicator, presoaked with proparacaine HCl 0.5% or presoaked with 2% lidocaine, on conjunctiva, for 30 sec.
5. Wait 3 min.
6. Inject
7. Instill a drop of timolol maleate ½% postoperatively (optional)
8. Send patient home with prescription for Ocuflox QID for 4 days or erythromycin ophthalmic ointment QID for 4 days.
9. All patients are sent home with an "endophthalmitis" instruction sheet: Call the office if redness, sensitivity to light, loss of vision, pain, or any of the above.
10. Someone from the office calls and checks on them on day 3 or 4 and fills out a form which is filled in the chart.
11. Avastin/Lucentis—return for next injection/evaluation in 1 month.
12. Triamcinolone—return in 3 weeks for IOP check, since it usually takes about 3 weeks for steroid induced glaucoma/hypertension to manifest.

Primary Intravitreal Bevacizumab (Avastin) For Diabetic Macular Edema

Eighty-eight patients with 110 eyes are treated with 1.25 mg or 2.5 mg of bevacizumab, and are followed up for 6 months. About 41% eyes remain stable, and 55% of the eyes show improvement greater than or equal to two lines of ETDRS lines of best corrected visual acuity. Only 3.8% have decreased vision. OCT thickness decreases from 387.0 μm to a mean of 275.7 μm of retinal thickness. The difference is found to be statistically significant.[8]

In another study, 51 consecutive patients with diffuse diabetic macular edema are treated with intravitreal bevacizumab. All patients have failed therapy such as focal laser, full scatter PRP, vitrectomy, and intravitreal triamcinolone. These patients also show improvement after 6 weeks of follow-up.[9]

CLINICAL CORRELATIONS: Clinically Significant Macular Edema 20/20 to 20/40

Patient complaints: "Sometimes, I cannot see well to read but if I blink, I can see again."

Caveats: This patient is a candidate for Amsler grid testing.

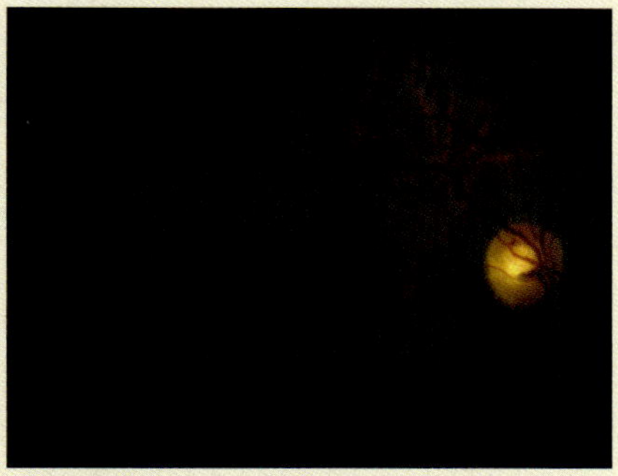

FIGURE 8-1. Photo OD, hard exudates, inferior macula.

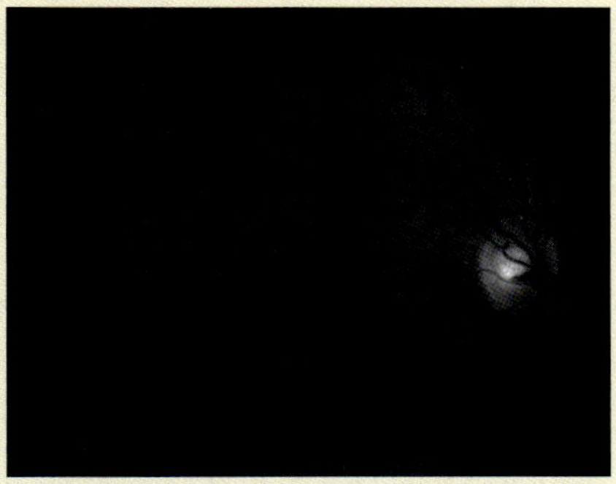

FIGURE 8-2. Red-free photograph OD, hard exudates better seen.

Case Study (Figs. 8-1–8-6)

3–6–2009: DE is a 69-year-old Caucasian male who has been diagnosed with Type 2 diabetes 3 years ago. He is here for his first visit to an ophthalmologist. He has previously seen optometrists occasionally.

V 20/25 NIPH
20/25 NIPH
Slit lamp examination
Cornea: Clear OU
Anterior chamber: Deep and quiet OU
Iris: Normal OU, no rubeosis OU
Lens: 1 + nuclear sclerosis OU
Applanation tonometry = 17/17 mm Hg (9:00 AM)
Gonioscopy: Open 360 degrees OU, no rubeosis OU
OCT central subfield thickness: OD = 277 mm
OS = 278 μm

Dilated funduscopic examination:

Right eye: Fewer than 30 microaneurysms, dulled internal limiting membrane reflex via slit lamp examination with 90 D lens. Abnormal venous tortuosity along the superior arcade. There is an abnormal course of the artery arising from the optic cup, delineating cupping of the optic nerve at 10:00 position. The arterioles are narrowed as well. The artery along the inferotemporal arcade is straightened when compared to the superotemporal arcade.

Color fundus photography OD: The abnormalities of the arteriovenous changes can be seen in the color photos and the red-free photographs. The red-free photographs highlight the abnormalities in vessel caliber because of the contrast in the photographic technique. The macula is not sharp or well delineated suggesting macular edema (Fig. 8-1).

Red-free photography OD: The optic nerve vessels are seen clearly. The optic nerve cupping is pronounced. The vascular looping at 10:00 is pronounced in the red-free photograph. This is a reminder about glaucoma follow-up in the future (Fig. 8-2).

Left eye: Fewer than 30 microaneurysms, dulled internal limiting membrane reflex via slit lamp examination with 90 D lens. Arteriovenous nicking seen along the superotemporal arcade. There is increased cupping seen in the left optic nerve but it is less pronounced than in the right optic nerve.

Color fundus photography OS: The superotemporal arcade is straightened as is the inferotemporal arcade. The macula does not look defined or crisp (Fig. 8-3).

Red-free photography OS: The optic nerve vessels are seen to be straight and going across the optic disc at 2:00. The cupping is pronounced on the red-free photograph. This eye is at risk for glaucoma in the future (Fig. 8-4).

Comment

In summary, this is nonproliferative diabetic retinopathy in a 69-year-old man with good glycemic control. While his visual acuity is excellent, he does not have CSME as seen on slit lamp biomicroscopy. He has some microaneurysms, placing him in the nonproliferative diabetic retinopathy category, the mild form. The OCT shows some macular thickening (Figs. 8-5 and 8-6).

Thus, the macula needs to be monitored despite the excellent visual acuity and lack of symptoms. He should be given an Amsler grid or be told to check his reading vision. The office staff can remind the patient to return for future examinations if his vision deteriorates while reading the fine print of a newspaper or if his glycemic control suddenly worsens. He will continue to do well if he takes care of his diabetes.

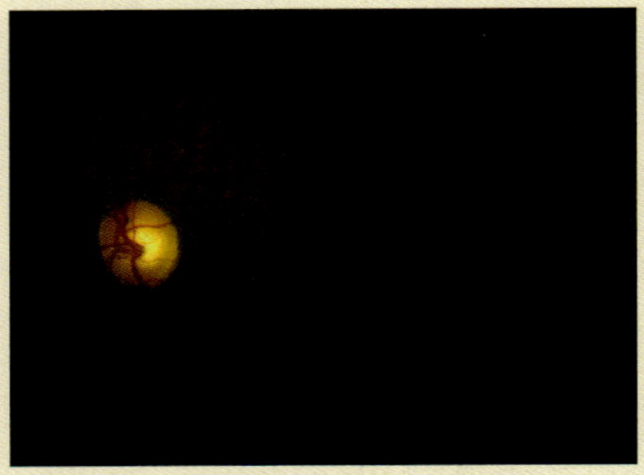

FIGURE 8-3. Photo OS, microaneurysm superonasal to disc.

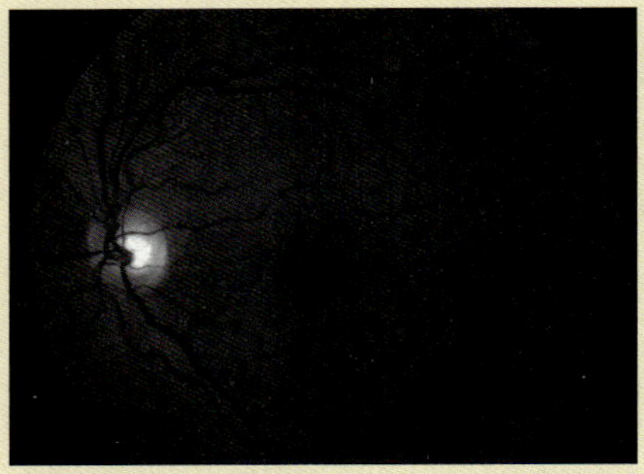

FIGURE 8-4. Red-free photograph OS, few microaneurysms.

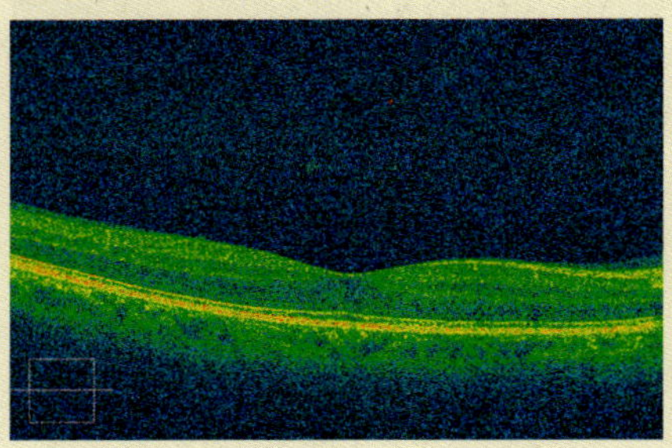

FIGURE 8-5. OCT OD, abnormal internal limiting membrane interface with vitreous, thickened external plexiform layer, early macular edema.

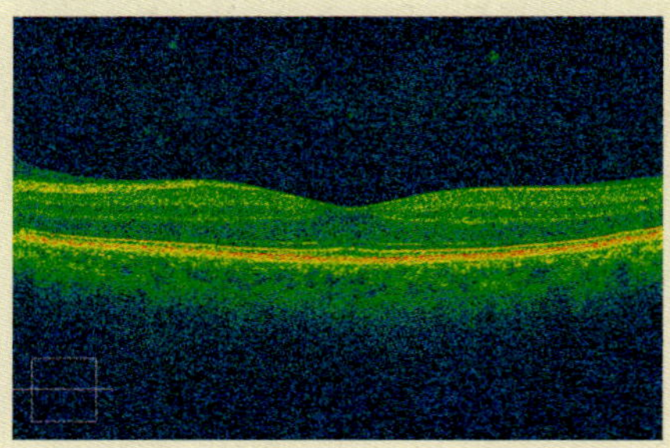

FIGURE 8-6. OCT OS, thickened external plexiform layer, early macular edema.

CLINICAL CORRELATIONS: Clinically Significant Macular Edema 20/20 to 20/40

Patient complaints: "I see a black spot sometimes when I drive in the daylight."

Caveats: This patient is a candidate for Amsler grid testing.

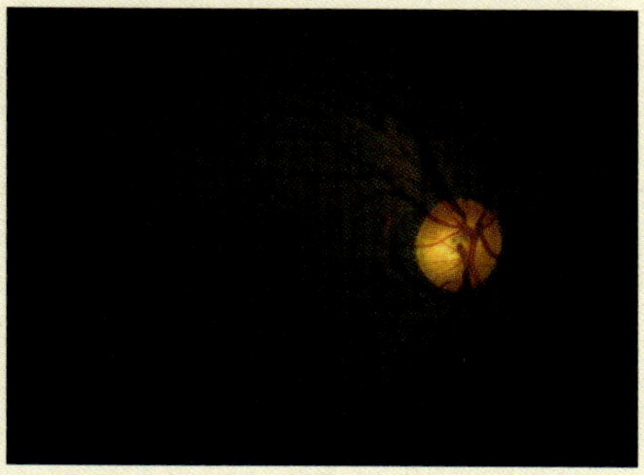

FIGURE 8-7. Photo OD, hard exudates.

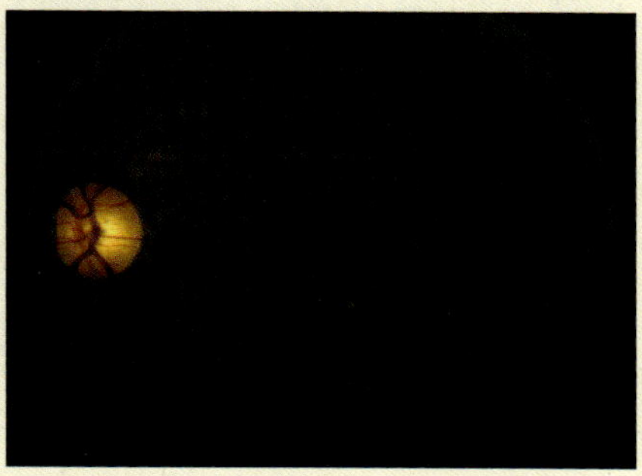

FIGURE 8-8. Photo OS, hard exudates.

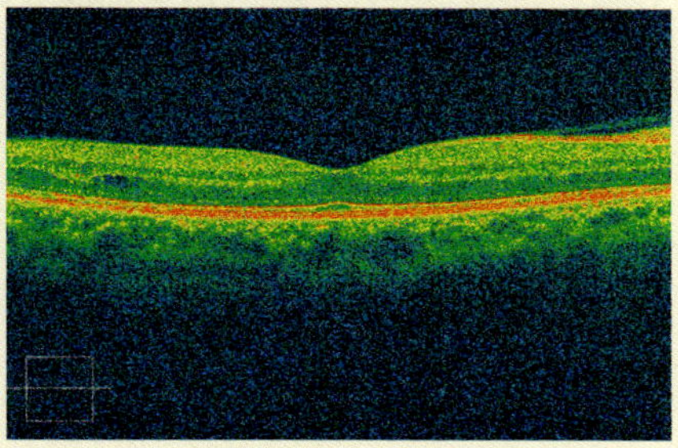

FIGURE 8-9. OCT OD.

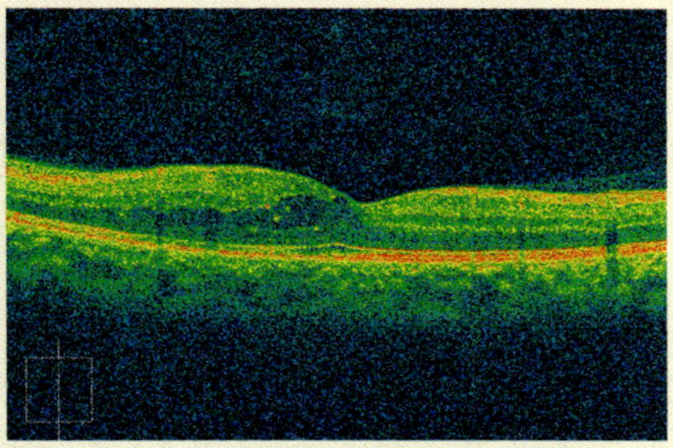

FIGURE 8-10. OCT OS.

Case Study (Figs. 8-7–8-10)

3–13–2009: FT is a 43-year-old Caucasian male who has Type 2 diabetes for the past 5 to 6 years. He is here for his first visit to an ophthalmologist. His primary care practitioner sends him to our office for an evaluation for decreased vision and poorly controlled diabetes. He works as an airport dispatcher. He denies history of hypertension. He tells us that his blood sugars are "stable at 150s range."

V 20/15
20/30
Slit lamp examination
Cornea: Clear OU
Anterior chamber: Deep and quiet OU
Iris: Normal OU, no rubeosis OU
Lens: No nuclear sclerosis OU
Applanation tonometry = 18/18 mm Hg (11:00 AM)
Gonioscopy: Open 360 degrees OU, no rubeosis OU

Dilated funduscopic examination:

Right eye: Hard exudates, dot blot hemorrhages, microaneurysms. Hard exudates are in the fovea, at edge of his foveal avascular zone at 4:00 (Fig. 8-7).

Left eye: Hard exudates, dot blot hemorrhages, microaneurysms, more hard exudates seen in the left eye than his right eye. The hard exudates extend from foveola inferiorly in a wedge shape, with base of triangle at 4:00 to 6:00 at macula (Fig. 8-8).

Comment

In summary, this is nonproliferative diabetic retinopathy in a 43–year-old man with "poor" glycemic control. He presents without any recent laboratory results. Thus, we send him for new test results. This level of diabetic retinopathy is mild nonproliferative retinopathy. We asked the patient to return after laboratory testing.

Follow-up: His new fasting blood sugar is 586 mg/dL, HbA1c = 15%, cholesterol = 227 mg/dL and triglycerides = 251 mg/dL. Thus, we asked the patient to return for a fluorescein angiogram to look for capillary nonperfusion. OCT scans would also document the extent of macular edema, as measured by central subfield thickness measurements (Figs. 8-9 and 8-10).

CLINICAL CORRELATIONS: CSME 20/20 to 20/40

Patient complaints: "I am having problems reading."

Caveats: Think about presbyopia, cataracts, obesity, and metabolic syndrome

Case Study (Figs. 8-11–8-14)

3–6–2009: GB is a 41-year-old Caucasian female, with a 2-year history of 50 lb of weight gain. She is now 3 years postpartum. She has recently been diagnosed with diabetes, as of last week. She has the history of gestational diabetes with both of her pregnancies. Fasting blood sugar is 110 mg/dL by using home testing with glucometer. Her usual fasting blood sugars are in the 150 mg/dL range usually. HbA1c = 6.5%.

V 20/25 NIPH
20/25 NIPH
Slit lamp examination
Cornea: Clear OU
Anterior chamber: Deep and quiet OU
Iris: Normal OU, no rubeosis OU
Lens: Clear OU
Applanation tonometry = 16/16 mm Hg (10:00 AM)
Gonioscopy: Open 360 degrees OU, no rubeosis OU
OCT central subfield thickness: OD = 274 mm
OS = 277 μm

Dilated funduscopic examination:

Right eye: No microaneurysms, dulled internal limiting membrane reflex via slit lamp examination with 90 D lens (Figs. 8-11 and 8-12).
Left eye: No microaneurysms, dulled internal limiting membrane reflex via slit lamp examination with 90 D lens (Figs. 8-13 and 8-14).

Comment

In summary, this is "no diabetic retinopathy" in a 41-year-old woman with borderline glycemic control with "diet control" only. While her visual acuity is excellent, she does not have CSME as seen on slit lamp biomicroscopy, but the OCT shows some macular thickening. Thus, the macula needs to be monitored despite the excellent visual acuity and lack of symptoms. Amsler grid testing should be taught to this patient. She needs weight management and nutrition counseling. More laboratory testing should be done to monitor her HbA1c.

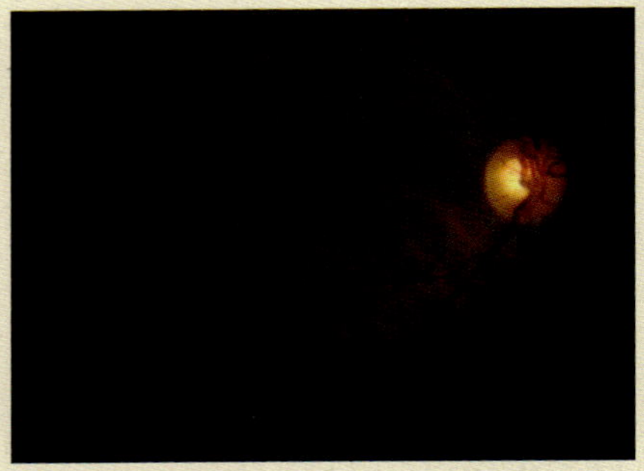

FIGURE 8-11. Photo OD: Venous engorgement and mild venous tortuosity.

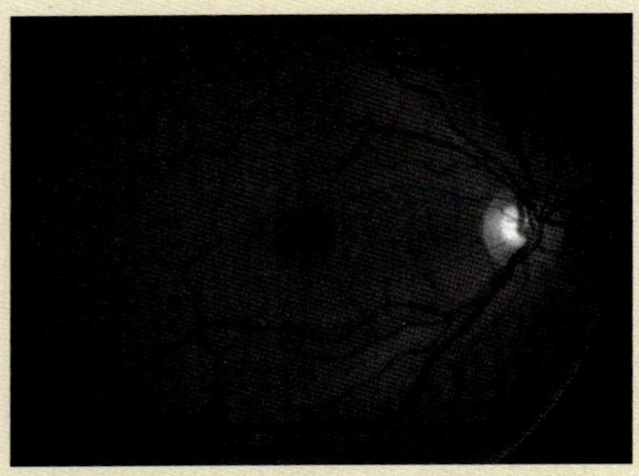

FIGURE 8-12. Red-free photograph OD.

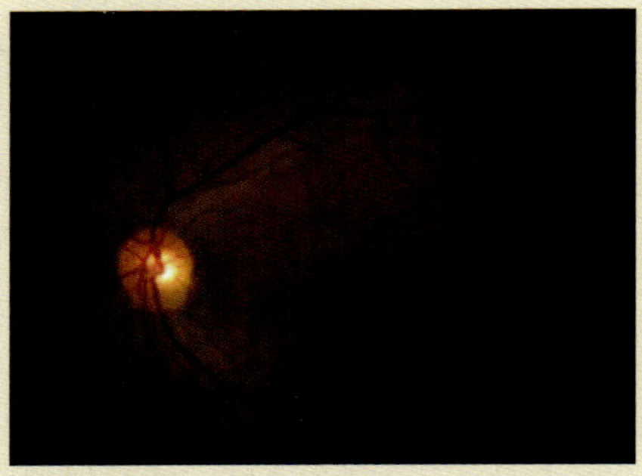

FIGURE 8-13. Photo OS: Less prominent venous engorgement and mild venous tortuosity.

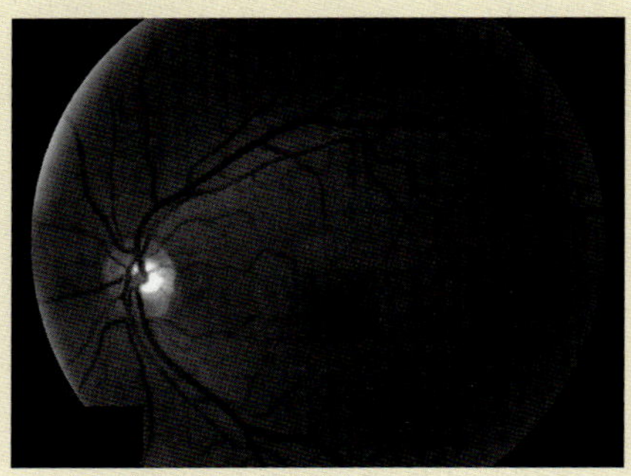

FIGURE 8-14. Red-free photograph OS.

CLINICAL CORRELATIONS: Clinically Significant Macular Edema 20/50 to 20/80

Patient complaints: "Sometimes, I cannot see well to read." "I used to be able to read but now I cannot see clearly to read."

Caveats: The patient notes a deterioration of vision. It is important to listen if the patient has had new medications for her diabetes or has changed to insulin or has just been diagnosed with diabetes.

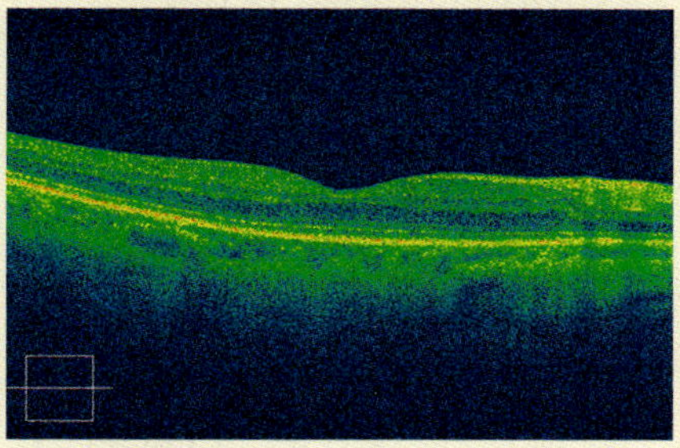

FIGURE 8-15. OCT OD, external plexiform layer swelling consistent with macular edema.

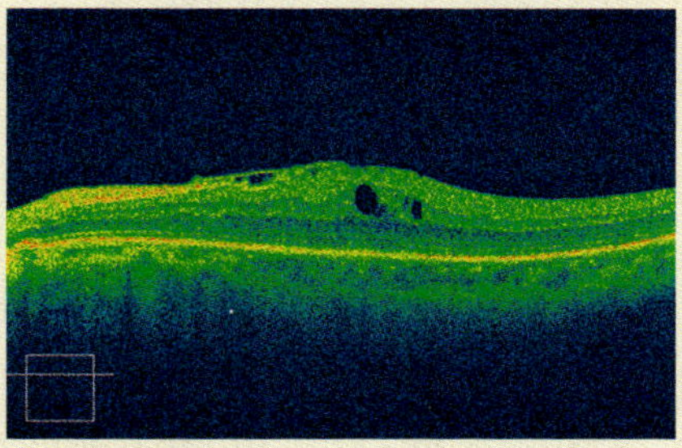

FIGURE 8-16. OCT OS, macular edema with cystic changes in foveal region.

Case Study (Figs. 8-15–8-22)

10–22–2008: NE is a 65-year-old Caucasian female diagnosed with Type 2 diabetes last week. Fasting blood sugar = 122 mg/dL, HbA1c = 6.2%. She is overweight. She has had a myocardial infarction and a stroke 3 years ago.

V 20/50 NIPH
20/50 NIPH
Slit lamp examination
Cornea: Clear OU
Anterior chamber: Deep and quiet OU
Iris: Normal OU, no rubeosis OU
Lens: 1 + nuclear sclerosis OU
Applanation tonometry = 20/20 mm Hg (9:00 AM)
Gonioscopy: Open 360 degrees OU, no rubeosis OU
OCT central subfield thickness: OD = 277μm (Fig. 8-15)
OS = 278 μm (Fig. 8-16)

Dilated funduscopic examination:

Right eye: Diabetic macular edema seen. Note the tortuosity of the 12:00 vein arising from the optic nerve. It begins its course as narrowed and then is engorged as it heads along the superotemporal arcade. Note the smaller caliber arterioles. The vein-to-artery ratio is not the normal 3:1 but rather closer to 4:1 ratio. These arteriovenous changes are consistent with her cardiovascular history of having had a myocardial infarction in the past. Look at the optic nerve and watch for changes in the future, since she may be at risk for low tension glaucoma.

Color fundus photography OD: Note the thinning of the retinal pigment epithelium at the area between the optic nerve and macula. It shows the underlying choroidal vessels (Fig. 8-17).

Red-free photography OD: The venous tortuosity and vein-to-artery ratio are more prominent in the red-free photographs. Note the abnormality of the optic nerve, shown more prominently in this photograph. This photograph serves to remind the clinician to watch for glaucoma, which can present with higher incidence in diabetics and in patients with cardiovascular disease (Fig. 8-18).

Left eye: Diabetic macular edema and gliosis are seen.

Color fundus photography OS: Note the thinning of the retinal pigment epithelium at the area between the optic nerve and macula in the direction of the inferotemporal arcades. It shows the underlying choroidal vessels, this is less prominent than that of the right eye. There are arteriovenous crossing changes seen in the color photograph starting from the optic nerve, emanating toward the superotemporal arcade. Note the straightening of the arteries along the inferotemporal arcade (Fig. 8-19).

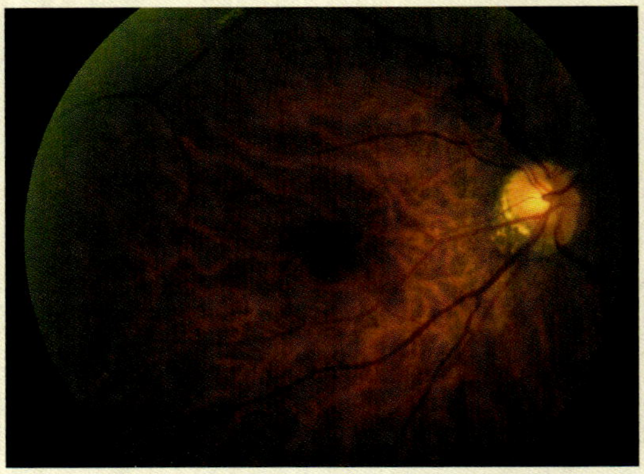

FIGURE 8-17. Photo OD, venous tortuosity superior arcade.

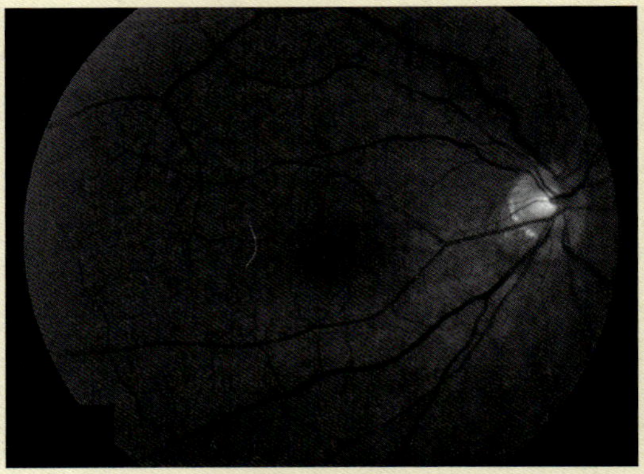

FIGURE 8-18. Red-free photograph OD, relative loss of retinal pigment epithelium inferiorly, note abnormal cup-to-disc ratio.

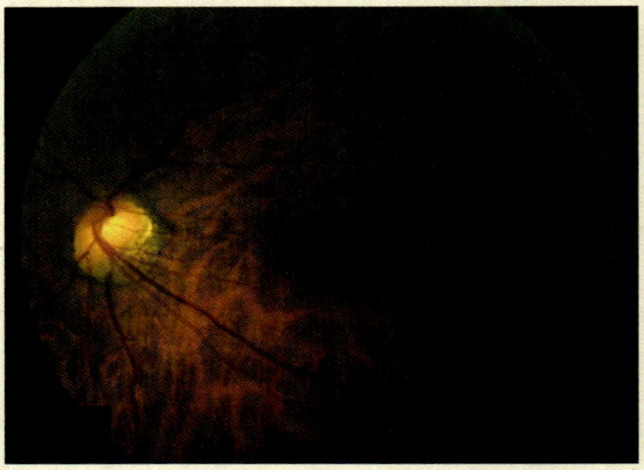

FIGURE 8-19. Photo OS, venous tortuosity less pronounced but arteriolar changes consistent with hypertension.

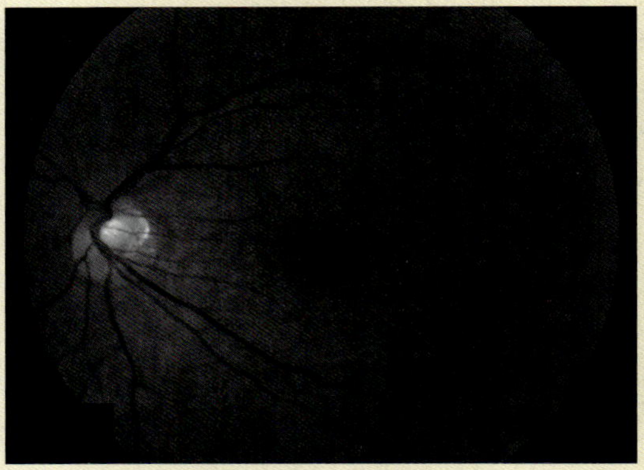

FIGURE 8-20. Red-free photograph OS, note abnormal cup-to-disc ratio.

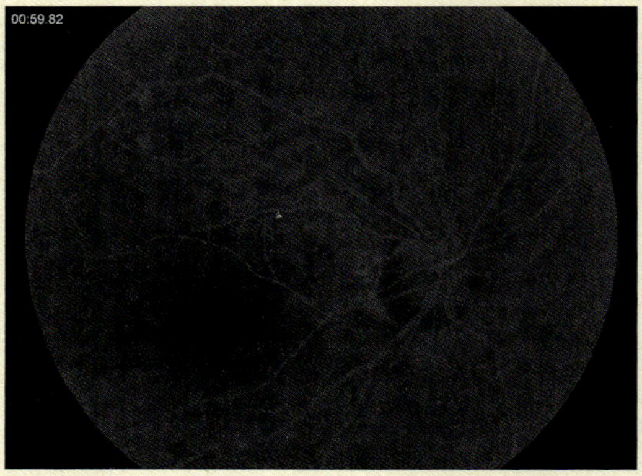

FIGURE 8-21. Fluorescein angiogram OD, 59 seconds transit, abnormal foveal avascular zone, some leakage of fluorescein around this same area, temporal to fovea.

FIGURE 8-22. Fluorescein angiogram OS, 4 minutes transit, abnormal foveal avascular zone, some leakage of fluorescein around macula arising from window defects of the retinal pigment epithelium.

Red-free photography OS: The arteriovenous nicking changes are more prominent in the red free photographs than in the color photographs. The optic nerve is tilted and has a loss of the temporal rim. The red-free photograph shows the disc abnormality more clearly than in the color photograph. Watch for glaucoma in this eye, as well (Fig. 8-20).
Fluorescein angiography: OS shows in mid transit some leakage of the macular capillaries at 4:00 (Figs. 8-21 and 8-22).

Comment

In summary, this is nonproliferative diabetic retinopathy along with diabetic macular edema in a 65-year-old Caucasian female, who is a vasculopath, having had a myocardial infarction and cerebrovascular accident 3 years ago. She is overweight and may have lipid metabolism problems as well. Look for lipid profile abnormalities. Encourage her to use the American Diabetes Association Web site. Give her the local address of the local American Diabetes Association chapter.

CLINICAL CORRELATIONS: Clinically Significant Macular Edema 20/50 to 20/80

Patient complaints: "I have trouble seeing to do my work. I work on the computer all the time as a secretary."

Caveats: This is a patient where the duration of diabetes is important, as well as, the fasting blood sugar, HbA1c, lipid profiles, hypertension, cardiovascular risks, kidney function.

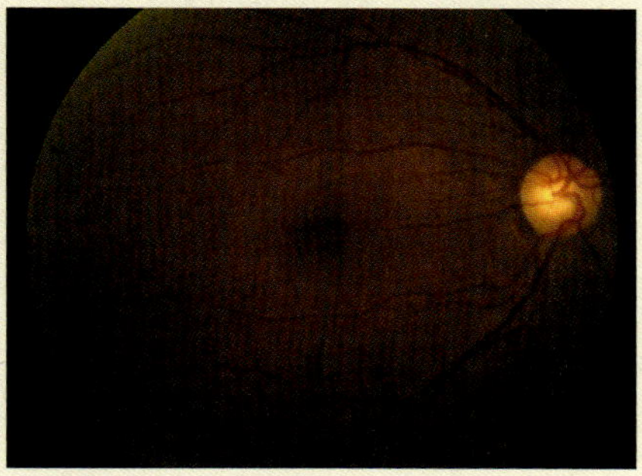

FIGURE 8-23. Photo OD, arteriolar straightening but note tortuosity of veins at superior arcade.

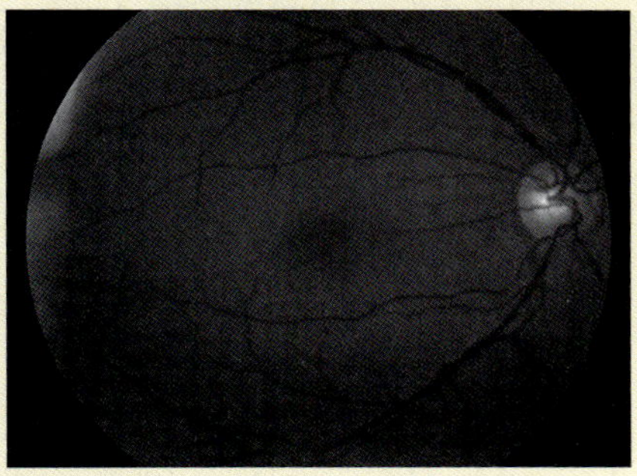

FIGURE 8-24. Red-free photograph OD, cup-to-disc ratio is 0.7, small venous loop in the optic cup.

Case Study (Figs. 8-23–8-29)

A 48-year-old Caucasian female complaining of decreased vision for 6 months. She has a fasting blood sugar of 215, HbA1c = 8.8%, which she says has improved from previous lab testing. She was referred by her new internist for an evaluation of her retina. She admits to poor control. She enjoys cheeseburgers and French fries.

V 20/80
20/40
Slit lamp examination
Slit lamp examinat ion
Cornea: Clear OU
Anterior chamber: Deep and quiet OU
Iris: Normal OU, no rubeosis OU
Lens: 1 + nuclear sclerosis OU
Applanation tonometry = 12/12 mm Hg (2 PM)
Gonioscopy: 360 degrees OU, no rubeosis OU

Dilated funduscopic examination:

Right eye: CSME, with arteriolar narrowing. Cup-to-disc ratio is 0.6 (Fig. 8-23).

Color photograph shows the blunting of the macular reflex (see Fig. 8-23).

Red-free photograph demonstrates the cup-to-disc ratio of 0.7 with a small venous loop in the optic cup. There is optic nerve vessel tortuosity at 6:00 in the optic cup, suggesting abnormality of a vascular pattern consistent with hypertension (Fig. 8-24).

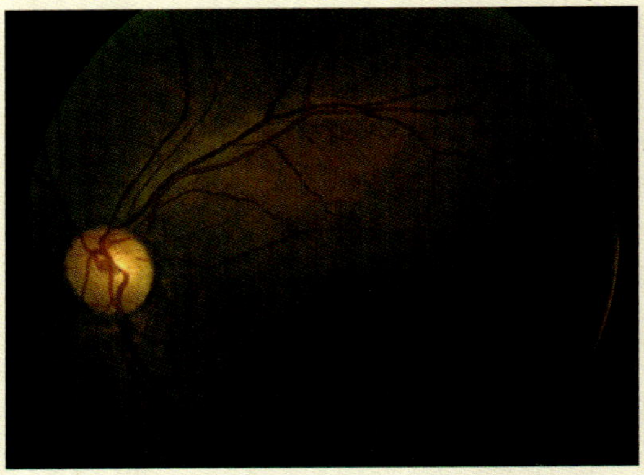

FIGURE 8-25. Photo OS, arteriolar straightening, abnormal light reflex at macula.

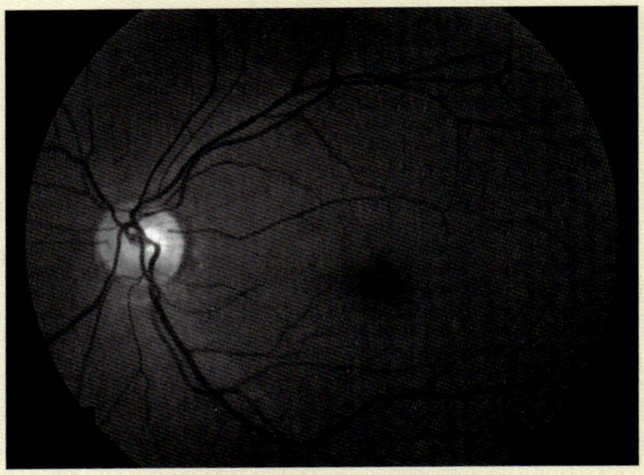

FIGURE 8-26. Red-free photograph OS, abnormal light reflex is prominent in this photo. Abnormal nerve fiber layer superiorly.

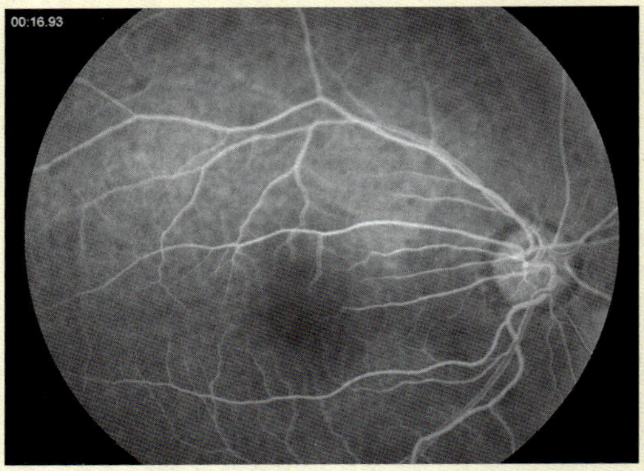

FIGURE 8-27. Fluorescein angiogram OD, 16 seconds transit, abnormal foveal avascular zone.

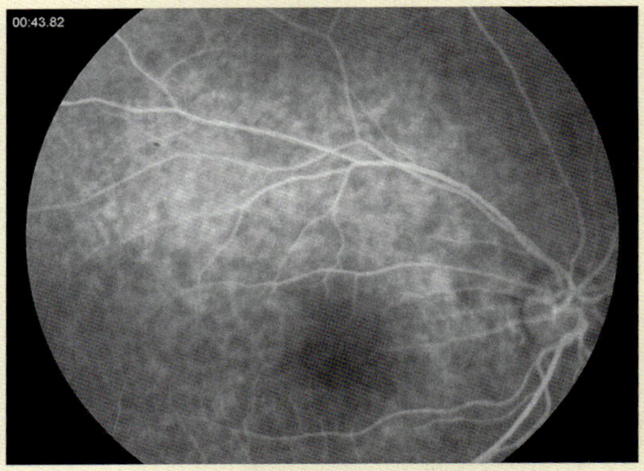

FIGURE 8-28. Fluorescein angiogram OD, 43 seconds transit, macular edema seen as fluorescein hyperfluorescence in the foveal area.

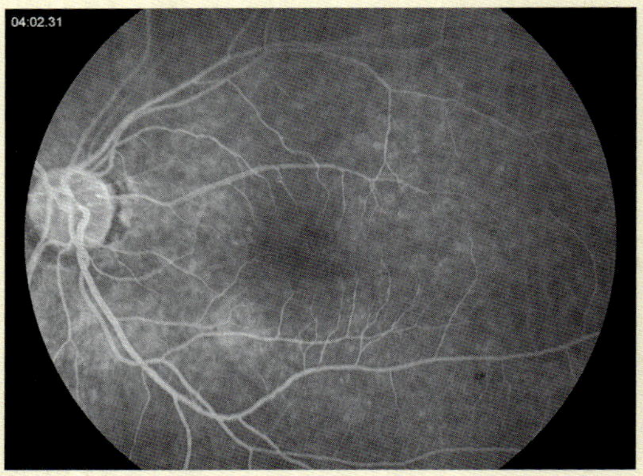

FIGURE 8-29. Fluorescein angiogram OS, 4 minutes transit, macular edema seen as fluorescein hyperfluorescence in the foveal area.

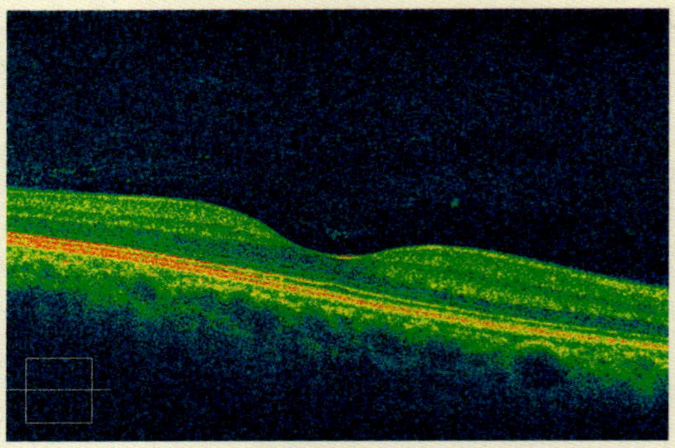

FIGURE 8-30. OCT OD, edema under fovea, in the external plexiform layer.

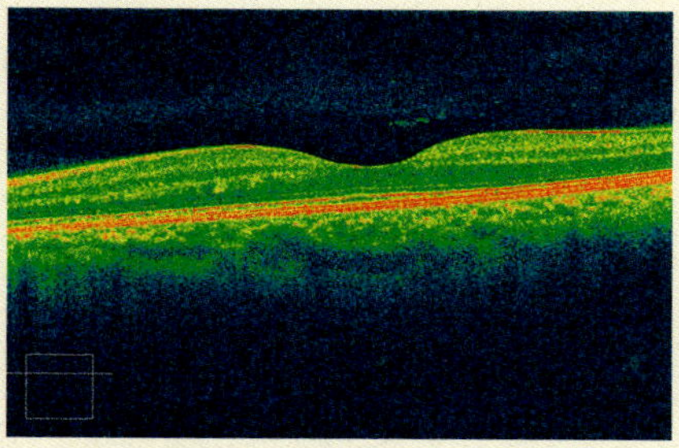

FIGURE 8-31. OCT OS, irregular shadows at external plexiform layer denoting macular edema, consistent with fluorescein findings and red-free photo.

Left eye: Cup-to-disc ratio is 0.7. Venous tortuosity is seen around the superior and inferior arcades. The superior vein at 12:00 veers nasally instead of its normal course in the direction of temporal retina. There is an abnormal light reflex at the nerve fiber layer of the superior arcade (Fig. 8-25). This can be prominently seen in the red-free photograph (Fig. 8-26).

Color photograph shows the blunting of the macular reflex (see Fig. 8-25). There are areas of retinal pigment epithelial depigmentation at 3:00 at the disc margin and the area at 9:00 from the fovea.

Red-free photograph shows the abnormal nerve fiber layer superiorly as a whitish area. This same phenomenon is seen in the inferotemporal nerve fiber layer as well. This may be a sign of nerve fiber layer loss as in chronic open angle glaucoma (see Fig. 8-26).

Fluorescein angiography OD: At 16 seconds, there is an abnormality of the foveal avascular zone. At 43 seconds, there is macular edema seen in the right eye, with an abnormal foveal avascular zone that is irregular (Figs. 8-27 and 8-28).
At 4 minutes of transit, during the late phase of the fluorescein angiogram, there is diffuse leakage around the fovea and macula. OCT scans show macular edema as well (Figs. 8-29 and 8-30).
Fluorescein angiography OS: At 4 minutes, 32 seconds, there are multiple microaneurysms in the foveal avascular zone and macula. There are more focal areas of macular edema (see Fig. 8-29). See the OCT scans (Fig. 8-31).

Comment

This patient has poor glycemic control, diabetic macular edema and needs to have laser treatment according to the ETDRS protocol. However, she has refused laser and wants to come back for monitoring. She was given an Amsler grid and a follow-up appointment in 1 month's time. We encouraged her to see a dietitian, to control her blood glucose, to follow the American Diabetes Association Diet, and to see her endocrinologist for better blood sugar control.

CLINICAL CORRELATIONS: Clinically Significant Macular Edema 20/50 to 20/80

Patient complaints: "I have trouble seeing for the past month."

Caveats: In young people who present with this complaint, be wary of poorly controlled diabetes, smoking, or alcoholism history. Consider that their diabetes is not really noninsulin dependent, or this type of patient may need insulin.

Case Study (Figs. 8-32–8-37)

6–1–2007: CTH is a 37-year-old Asian male engineer with decreased vision after laser treatment by another ophthalmologist. He is here for a second opinion.

V 20/60 PH 20/50
20/30 NIPH
Slit lamp examination
Cornea: Clear OU
Anterior chamber: Deep and quiet OU
Iris: Normal OU, no rubeosis OU
Lens: 1 + nuclear sclerosis OU
Applanation tonometry = 18/18 mm Hg (2:00 PM)
Gonioscopy: Open 360 degrees OU, no rubeosis OU

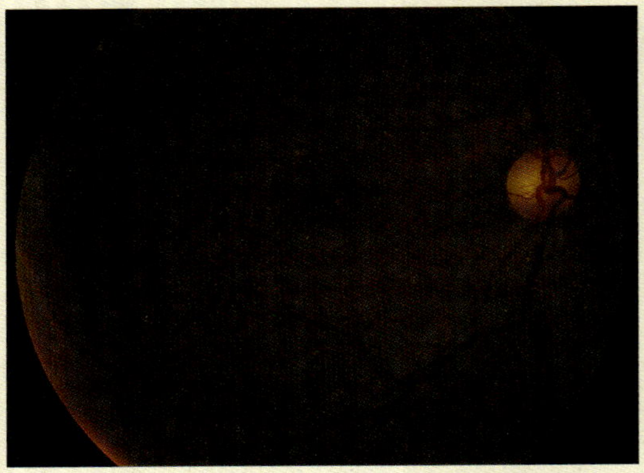

FIGURE 8-32. Photo OD, multiple hemorrhages and microaneurysms, venous loop.

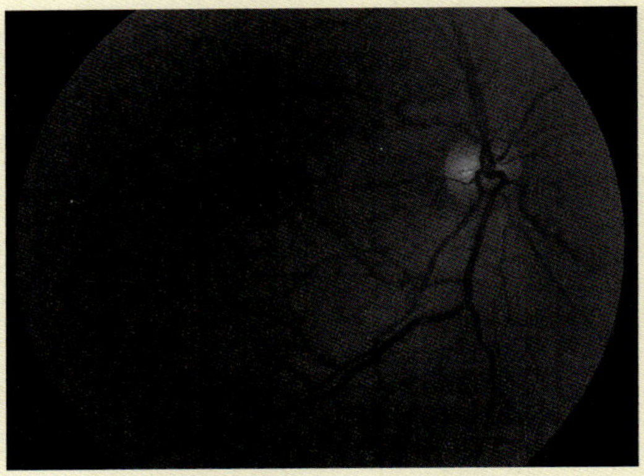

FIGURE 8-33. Red-free photograph OD, high contrast view of venous loop.

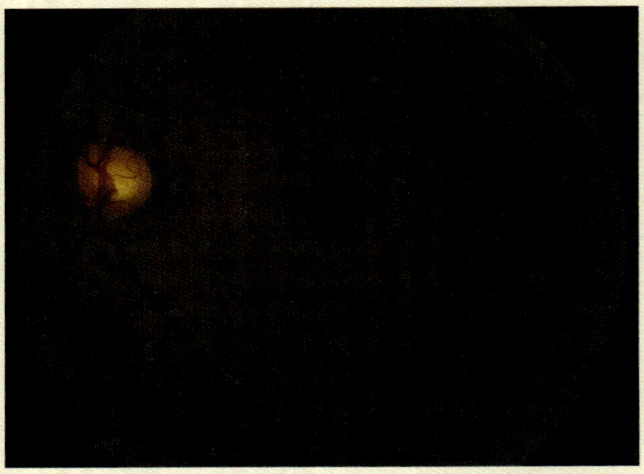

FIGURE 8-34. Photo OS, cotton-wool spot at 6:00, 7:00 near inferotemporal arcade.

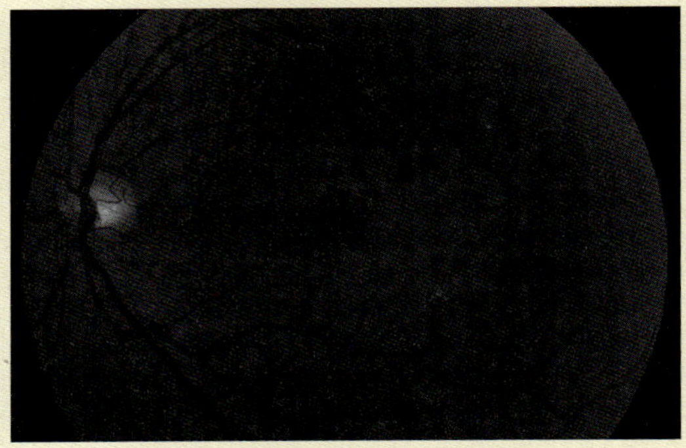

FIGURE 8-35. Red-free photograph OS, cotton-wool spots are seen more clearly with red free filter.

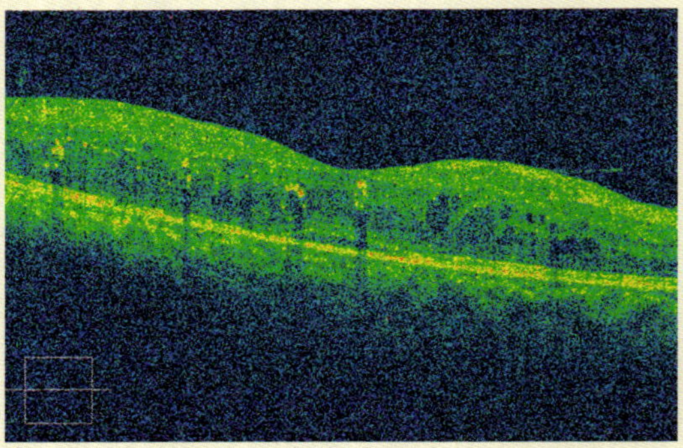

FIGURE 8-36. OCT OD, macular edema.

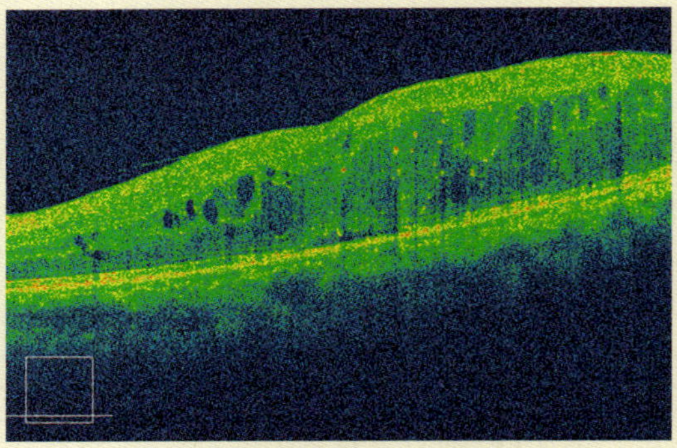

FIGURE 8-37. OCT OS, macular edema.

Dilated funduscopic examination:

Right eye: Dot blot hemorrhages, hard exudates in the macula, CSME. There is a cotton-wool spot in the inferotemporal aspect of the macula. There is a venous loop inferotemporally. This venous loop puts the patient in the nonproliferative diabetic retinopathy category.

Color fundus photography OD: Multiple hemorrhages and microaneurysms. Venous loop is seen. Hemorrhages are very clearly seen (Fig. 8-32).

Red-free photography OD: One can see nerve layer abnormality in the inferior arcade, suggesting some abnormalities. There is the high contrast view of the venous loop, inferotemporally, dot blot hemorrhages, and hard exudates in the macula (Fig. 8-33).
Left eye: More hard exudates are seen in the left eye than in the right eye, along the superior arcade and at 4:00 at edge of the macula. There are dot blot hemorrhages, and there is a cotton-wool spot at 6:00 and 7:00 near the inferotemporal arcade. There is CSME.
Color fundus photography OS: There is a dulled macular reflex with hard exudates superior to the fovea. Venous loop is seen. Cotton-wool spots along inferior arcade (Fig. 8-34).
Red-free photography OS: The hard exudates, microaneurysms, and hemorrhages are sharply defined with excellent contrast. The cotton-wool spots are seen at 6:00 and 7:00, well demarcated in the red-free photographs (Fig. 8-35).

Comment

This is a 37-year-old male with moderate nonproliferative diabetic retinopathy and CSME OU (Figs. 8-36 and 8-37).

He is a candidate for more focal macular laser photocoagulation. He needs a fluorescein angiogram to delineate the areas of treatment. He has had laser in the past. In 2009, as of this writing, this patient is also a candidate for bevacizumab or ranibizumab.

REFERENCES

1. http://diabetes.niddk.nih.gov/DM?PUBS/statistics/#allages. Accessed 1 January 2009.
2. Early Treatment Diabetic Retinopathy Study Research Group. Photocoagulation for diabetic macular edema. Early Treatment Diabetic Retinopathy Study report number 1. *Arch Ophthalmol.* 1985;103:1796–1806.
3. Mori F, Ishiko S, Kitaya N, et al. Use of scanning laser ophthalmoscope in clinically significant macular edema in type 2 diabetes mellitus. *Jpn J Ophthalmol.* 2002;46:650–655.
4. Hudson C, Flanagan JG, Turner GS, et al. Correlation of a scanning laser derived oedema index and visual function following grid laser treatment for diabetic macular oedema. *Br J Ophthalmol.* 2003;87:455–461.
5. Rohrschneider K, Bultmann S, Gluck R, et al. Scanning laser ophthalmoscope fundus perimetry before and after laser photocoagulation for clinically significant macular edema. *AMJ Ophthalmol.* 2003;87:455–461.
6. Williams MV, Baker DW, Parker RM, et al. Relationship of functional health literacy to patients' knowledge of their chronic disease. *Arch Int Med.* 1998;158:166–172.
7. Schillinger D, Grumbach K, Piette J, et al. Association of Health Literacy with Diabetes Outcomes. *JAMA.* 2002;288: 475–482.
8. Arevalo J, Fromow-Guerra J, Quiroz-Mercado H, et al. Primary Inravitreal Bevacizumab (Avastin) for Diabetic Macular Edema Results from the Pan-American Collaborative Retina Study Group at Month Follow-up. *Ophthalmology.* 2007;114(4):743–750.
9. Haritoglou C, Kook D, Neubauer A, et al. Intravitreal Bevacizumab (Avastin) Therapy for persistent diffuse diabetic macular edema. *Retina.* 2006;26(9):999–1005.
10. Williams P, Callanan D. Treating diabetic macular edema with ocular NSAIDs. http://www.retinalphysician.com/article.aspx?article = 101096. Accessed 12 February 2009.
11. Martidis A. Intravitreal triamcinolone for refractory diabetic macular edema. *Ophthalmol.* 2003;109:920–927.
12. Pendergast SD, Hassan TS, Williams GA, et al. Vitrectomy for diffuse macular edema associated with a taut premacular posterior hyaloid. *Am J Ophthalmol.* 2000;130:178–186.

SUGGESTED READINGS

1. Aiello LM, Wand M, Liang G. Neovascular glaucoma and vitreous hemorrhage following cataract surgery in patients with diabetes mellitus. *Am Acad Ophthalmol.* 1984;90:814–820.
2. American Academy of Ophthalmology. Preferred practice pattern. *Diabetic Retinopathy.* San Francisco, CA: American Academy of Ophthalmology; 1989.
3. Ashton N. The eye in malignant hypertension. *Trans Am Acad Ophthalmol Otolaryngol.* 1972;76:17–40.
4. Beetham WP. Diabetic retinopathy in pregnancy. *Trans Am Ophthalmol Soc.* 1950;48:205–219.
5. Blankenship GW. The lens influence on diabetic vitrectomy results. *Arch Ophthalmol.* 1980;98:2196–2198.
6. Blankenship GW. A clinical comparison of central and peripheral argon laser panretinal photocoagulation for proliferative diabetic retinopathy. *Ophthalmology.* 1988;95:170–177.
7. Blankenship GW, Flynn HW, Kokame GT. Posterior chamber intraocular lens insertion during pars plana lensectomy and vitrectomy for complications of proliferative diabetic retinopathy. *Am J Ophthalmol.* 1989;108:1–5.
8. Bresnick GH. Diabetic maculopathy: A critical review highlighting diffuse macular edema. *Ophthalmology.* 1983;90:1301–1317.

9. Bresnick GH. Background diabetic retinopathy. In: Ryan SJ, ed. *Retina*. St. Louis, MO: CV Mosby Co; 1989: 327–366.
10. Bresnick GH, Condit R, Syrjala S, et al. Abnormalities of the foveal avascular zone in diabetic retinopathy. *Arch Ophthalmol.* 1984;102:1286–1293.
11. Bresnick GH, Engerman R, Davis MD, et al. Patterns of ischemia in diabetic retinopathy. *Trans Am Acad Ophthalmol Otolaryngol.* 1976;81:694.
12. Diabetic Retinopathy Study Research Group. Photocoagulation treatment of proliferative diabetic retinopathy/vitrectomy study findings. *Am J Ophthalmol.* 1978;85:82–106.
13. Diabetic Retinopathy Study Research Group. Photocoagulation treatment of proliferative diabetic retinopathy; the second report of diabetic retinopathy/vitrectomy study findings. *Am J Ophthalmol.* 1978;85:82–106.
14. Diabetic Retinopathy Study Research Group. Report No 7. A modification on the Airlie House classification of diabetic retinopathy. *Invest Ophthalmol Vis Sci.* 1981;212:210–226.
15. Diabetic Retinopathy Study Research Group. Report no 14. Indication for photocoagulation treatment of diabetic retinopathy. *Int Ophthalmol Clin.* 1987;27:239.
16. Diabetic Retinopathy Study Research Group. Report no 14. Indication for photocoagulation treatment of diabetic retinopathy. *Int Ophthalmol Clin.* 1987;27:239–252.
17. Early Treatment Diabetic Study Research Group. Report No. 1. Photocoagulation for diabetic macular edema. *Arch Ophthalmol.* 1985;103:1796–1806.
18. Early Treatment Diabetic Retinopathy Study Research Group. Report no 2. Treatment techniques and clinical guidelines for photocoagulation of diabetic macular edema. *Ophthalmology.* 1987;947:761–774.
19. Early Treatment Diabetic Retinopathy Study Research Group. Report no 3. Techniques for scatter and local photocoagulation treatment of diabetic retinopathy. *Int Ophthalmol Clin.* 1987;274:254–264.
20. Early Treatment Diabetic Retinopathy Study Research Group. Report no 4. Photocoagulation for diabetic macular edema. *Int Ophthalmol Clin.* 1987;27:265–272.
21. Early Treatment Diabetic Retinopathy Study Research Group. Report no 9. Early photocoagulation for diabetic retinopathy. *Ophthalmology.* 1991;98:766–785.
22. Early Treatment Diabetic Retinopathy Study Research Group. Report no 12. Fundus photographic risk factors for progression of diabetic retinopathy. *Ophthalmology.* 1991;98:823–833.
23. Early Treatment Diabetic Retinopathy Study Research Group. Report no 13. Fluorescein angiographic risk factors for progression of diabetic retinopathy. *Ophthalmology.* 1991;98:834–840.
24. Ferris FL, Podgor MJ, Davis MD. The Diabetic Retinopathy Study Research Group. Report no 12. Macular edema in diabetic retinopathy study patients. *Ophthalmology.* 1987;94:754–760.
25. Frank RN. Etiology mechanisms in diabetic retinopathy. In: Ryan SJ, ed. *Retina*. St. Louis, MO: CV Mosby Co; 1989:30–326.
26. Frienkel N, Dooley SL, Metzger BE. Care of the pregnant woman with insulin-dependent diabetes. *N Engl J Med.* 1985;313:96–101.
27. Gass JDM. Retinal capillary disease. *Stereoscopic Atlas of Macular Diseases.* St Louis, MO: CV Mosby Co; 1987: 368–373.
28. Gass JDM, Norton EWD. Cystoid macular edema and papilledema following cataract extraction: A fluorescein funduscopic and angiographic study. *Arch Ophthalmol.* 1966;76:646–661.
29. Greenberg F, Lewis RA. Safety of fluorescein angiography during pregnancy [Letter] *Am J Ophthalmol.* 1990;110: 323–325.
30. Halperin LS, Olk RJ, Soubrane G, et al. Safety of fluorescein angiography during pregnancy. *Am J Ophthalmol.* 1990;109:563–566.
31. Hercules BL, Wozencroft M, Gayed II, Jeacock J. Peripheral retinal ablation in the treatment of proliferative diabetic retinopathy during pregnancy. *Br J Ophthalmol.* 1980;64:87–93.
32. Horvat M, Maclean H, Goldberg L, et al. Diabetic retinopathy in pregnancy: A 12-year prospective survey. *Br J Ophthalmol.* 1980;64:298–403.
33. Javitt J, Canner JK, Frank RG, et al. Detecting and treating retinopathy in patients with type I diabetes mellitus. *Ophthalmology.* 1990:483–495.
34. Javitt JC, Canner JK, Sommer A. Cost effectiveness of current approached to the control of retinopathy in type I diabetes. *Ophthalmology.* 1989:96–255.
35. Johnson GP. Pregnancy and diabetic retinopathy. *Am J Ophthalmol.* 1980;90:519–524.
36. Klein BEK, Davis MD, Segal P, et al. Diabetic retinopathy. Assessment of severity and progression. *Ophthalmology.* 1984;91:10–17.
37. Klein R, Klein BEK, Neider NW, et al. Diabetic retinopathy as detected using ophthalmoscopy, a non-mydriatic camera and standard fundus camera. *Ophthalmology.* 1985;92:485.
38. Kleiner RC, Elman MJ, Murphy RP, et al. Transient severe visual loss after panretinal photocoagulation. *Am J Ophthalmol.* 1988;106:298–306.
39. Kohner EM, Sleightholm M. Kroc Collaborative Study Group (appended). Does microaneurysm count reflect severity of early diabetic retinopathy? *Ophthalmology.* 1986;93:586–589.
40. Lee CM, Olk RJ. Modified grid laser photocoagulation for diffuse diabetic macular edema: Long term visual results. *Ophthalmology.* 1991;98:1594–1602.
41. McDonald HR, Schatz H. Macular edema following panretinal photocoagulation. *Retina.* 1985;5:5–10.
42. McDonald HR, Schatz H. Visual loss following panretinal photocoagulation for proliferative diabetic retinopathy. *Opthalmology.* 1985;92:388–393.
43. McEnery JK, Wong WP, Peyman GA. Evaluation of the teratogenicity of fluorescein sodium. *Am J Ophthalmol.* 1977;84:847–850.
44. Meyers SM. Macular edema after scatter laser photocoagulation for proliferative diabetic retinopathy. *Am J Ophthalmol.* 1980;90:210–216.
45. Moloney JB, Drury MI. The effect of pregnancy on the natural course of diabetic retinopathy. *Am J Ophthalmol.* 1982;93:745–756.
46. Moss SE, Klein R, Kessler SD, Richie KA. Comparison between ophthalmoscope and fundus photography in determining severity of diabetic retinopathy. *Ophthalmology.* 1985;92:62–67.

47. Niki T, Muraoka K, Shimizu K. Distribution of capillary nonperfusion in early-stage diabetic retinopathy. *Ophthalmology.* 1984;91:1431–1439.
48. Ohrt V. The influence of pregnancy on diabetic retinopathy with special regard to the reversible changes shown in 100 pregnancies. *Acta Ophthalmol.* 1984;62:603–616.
49. Olk RJ. Modified grid argon (blue-green) laser photocoagulation for diffuse diabetic macular edema. *Ophthalmology.* 1986;93:938–950.
50. Olk RJ. Argon green (514nm) versus krypton red (647 nm) modified grid laser photocoagulation for diffuse diabetic macular edema. *Ophthalmology.* 1990;97:1101–1113.
51. Phelps RL, Sakor P, Metzger BE, et al. Changes in diabetic retinopathy during pregnancy. *Arch Ophthalmol.* 1986;104:1806–1810.
52. Poliner LS, Christianson DJ, Escoffery RF, et al. Neovascular glaucoma after intracapsular and extracapsular cataract extraction in diabetic patients. *Am J Ophthalmol.* 1985;100:637–643.
53. Rice TA, Michels RG. Long term anatomic and functional results of vitrectomy for diabetic retinopathy. *Am J Ophthalmol.* 1980;90:297–303.
54. Rice TA, Michels RG, Maguire MG, et al. The effect of lensectomy on the incidence of iris neovascularization and neovascular glaucoma after vitrectomy for diabetic retinopathy. *Am J Ophthalmol.* 1983;95:1–11.
55. Salem H, Loux JJ, Smith S, et al. Evaluation of the toxicologic and teratogenic potentials of sodium fluorescein in the rat. *Toxicology.* 1979;12:143–150.
56. Shimizu K, Kobayaski Y, Muraoka K. Midperipheral fundus involvement in diabetic retinopathy. *Ophthalmology.* 1981;88:601–612.
57. Shirai S, Majima A. Effects of fluorescein-sodium injected to mother mice on the embryo. *Folia Ophthalmol Jpn.* 1975;26:132–137.
58. Sinclair SH, Nesler C, Foxman B, et al. Macular edema and pregnancy in insulin-dependent diabetes. *Am J Ophthalmol.* 1984;97:154–167.
59. Stark WJ Jr, Maumenee AE, Fagadau W, et al. Cystoid macular edema in pseudophakia. *Surv Ophthalmol.* 1984;28: 442–451.
60. Sunness JS. The pregnant woman's eye. *Surv Ophthalmol.* 1988;32:219–238.
61. Sussman EJ, Tsiaras WG, Soper KA. Diagnosis of diabetic eye disease. *JAMA.* 1982;247:3231–3234.
62. Ticho U, Patz A. The role of capillary perfusion in the management of diabetic macular edema. *Am J Ophthalmol.* 1973;76:880–886.
63. Tso MOM, Jampol LM. Pathophysiology of hypertensive retinopathy. *Ophthalmologica.* 1982;89:1132.
64. White P. Pregnancy and diabetes, medical aspects. *Med Clin North Am.* 1965;49:1015–1024.
65. Wilkinson CP. The clinical examination: Limitation and over utilization of angiographic services. *Ophthalmology.* 1986;93:401–404.
66. Yannuzzi LA, Roher KT, Tindel LJ, et al. Fluorescein angiography complication survey. *Ophthalmology.* 1986;93:611.

CHAPTER 9

Management of Proliferative Diabetic Retinopathy

When one third of the diabetic population does not appreciate that they have diabetes, it is common for retinal specialists to see patients who present with a vitreous hemorrhage.[1] The diagnosis of proliferative diabetic retinopathy (PDR) in such a clinical setting is made by examining the fellow eye. If the fellow eye has retina findings characterized by small hemorrhages, cotton-wool spots, macular edema and hard exudates rings, or other characteristics of diabetic retinopathy, then the patient is at risk for similar level of diabetic retinopathy in the eye with a vitreous hemorrhage. For a new patient who does not know his or her diabetes status, laboratory testing for HbA1c, fasting blood sugars (FBSs), lipid profiles, and creatinine must be done. Further testing with 3-hour glucose tolerance tests can be performed at the endocrinologist's office. The ophthalmologist may be the first physician to diagnose diabetes in this type of new patient with vision loss.

The risk of PDR is the greatest in those patients who have severe nonproliferative diabetic retinopathy (NPDR). Severe NPDR is described as having soft exudates (cotton-wool spots), intraretinal microvascular abnormalities (IRMAs), venous beading, extensive retinal hemorrhages, or microaneurysms (see Chapter 7). IRMAs can be new intraretinal vessels or dilated preexisting vessels. IRMAs are very difficult to see clinically and photographically. They are perhaps best seen with red-free photographs in the seven standard fields. Severe NPDR is defined as having three of the aforementioned four characteristics, each involving at least two quadrants of the fundus.[2] Once this occurs, the progression to PDR is within 15 months[2] (Figs. 9-1 to 9-4).

One of the reasons that IRMAs may be difficult to identify is that they can be transient. Cotton-wool spots usually disappear in 6 to 12 months. Blot hemorrhages and IRMAs disappear after extensive capillary closure. Capillary closure can be identified when the small vascular branches decrease in number and small arterioles become white threads, producing a picture described as "featureless retina." On fluorescein angiography, these areas are known to "capillary nonperfusion" (Figs. 9-5 and 9-6).

New vessels can arise anywhere but if they occur at the optic nerve (NVD), neovascular vessels are seen within 45 degrees from the optic nerve. They are commonly seen on the optic disc. Studies have documented 69% to 73% of neovascularization in PDR eyes is found on the optic disc.[3,4]

Neovascularization disc (NVD) can be seen as fine threadlike loops of vessels lying on the surface of the disc or bridging across the physiologic cup. They are usually easily identified but in their earliest stages, they may be overlooked with the low magnification of indirect ophthalmoscopy. They may be seen with a slit lamp examination using a 90 D or 60 D lens. They may be most easily identified with fundus photographs or fluorescein angiography. Fluorescein angiography can delineate new vessels at the optic disc because of their intense hyperfluorescence, which fills an increasingly larger area with each successive frame of the fluorescein angiogram (Figs. 9-7 and 9-8).

Techniques for finding the neovascularization elsewhere (NVE) and NVD and other characteristics in severe NPDR and PDR include the use of binocular indirect ophthalmoscopy, direct ophthalmoscopy, slit lamp biomicroscopy with a 90 or 60 D lens, and

FIGURE 9-1. Soft exudate or cotton-wool spot.

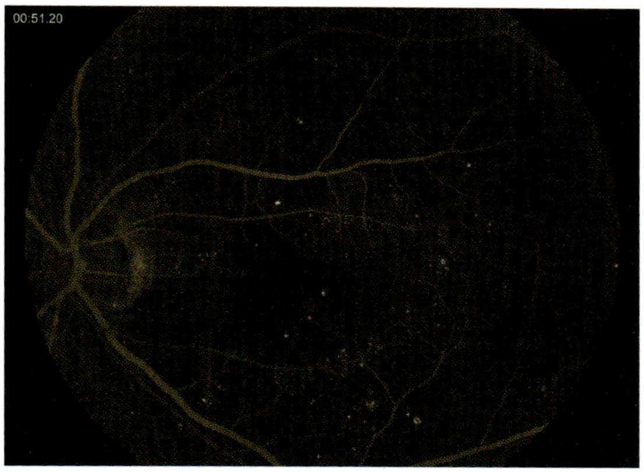

FIGURE 9-2. Intraretinal microvascular abnormality.

FIGURE 9-3. Venous beading.

FIGURE 9-4. Extensive retinal hemorrhages or microaneurysms.

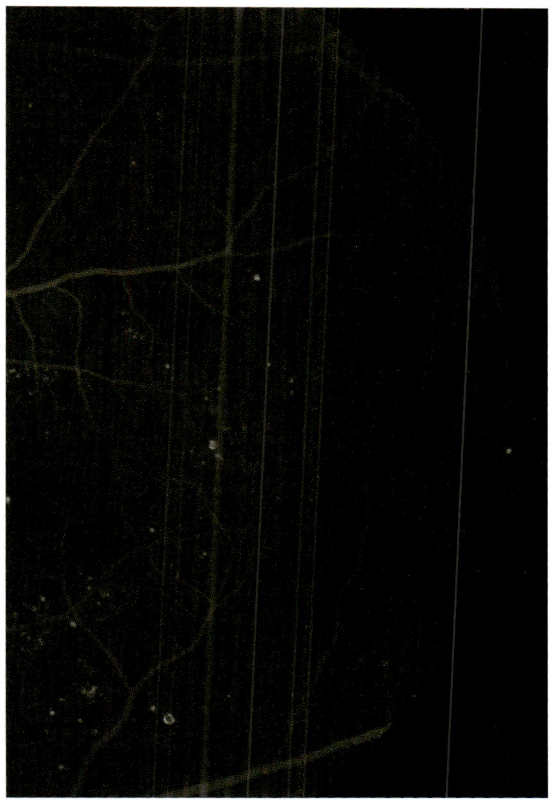

FIGURE 9-5. "Featureless retina."

FIGURE 9-6. "Featureless retina" and the fluorescein angiographic photo denoting capillary nonperfusion.

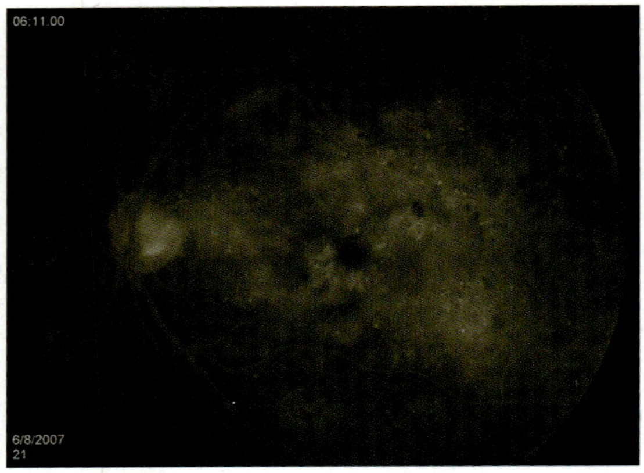

FIGURE 9-7. Fluorescein angiogram of disc neovascularization.

Goldmann contact lens. The goal is to find neovascular fronds 45 degrees from the optic nerve and examine the area 5 to 6 disc diameter (DD) from the optic nerve. It is essentially the area of the posterior pole to the equator, the area subtended by the seven standard photographic fields.

A fundus drawing with detailed notations in color is useful: red for new vessels elsewhere, noting if it is equatorial or anterior to the equator and the clock hour. The floating sheets of red blood cells imbedded in the vitreous gel can be color coded with shades of green, marking its location in space, with a diagram of the eye in cross section. NVE can be described in terms of the clock hour and the extent and the presence in the equator, in the posterior pole. Using light red to code the light vitreous hemorrhage enables the clinician to follow the progression of the hemorrhage at later follow-up appointments. In later examinations, the site of the original vitreous hemorrhage may reveal fronds of NVE, explaining the origin of the vitreous hemorrhage. In addition, this area may herald the site of future fibrovascular proliferation, also colored in green. Dense vitreous hemorrhage can be colored in dark green.

The Goldmann contact lens is excellent for examining the periphery if the clinician suspects NVE in the presence of a faint, diaphanous vitreous hemorrhage. The three

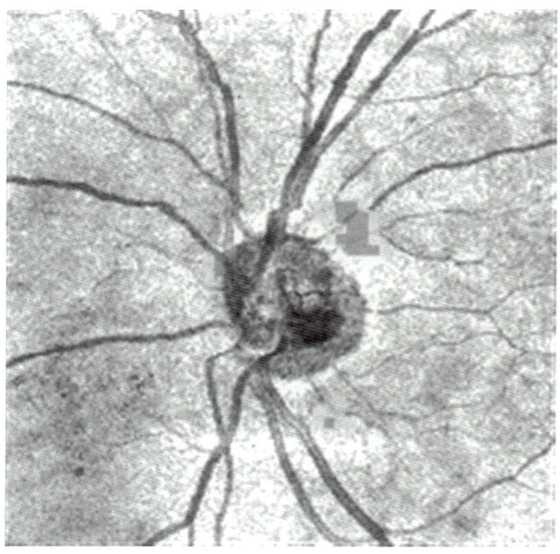

FIGURE 9-8. OCT, disc neovascularization, seen as a frond at the optic disc.

mirror lenses of the Goldmann contact lens allow navigation to the periphery and lucid areas where there is no vitreous blood.

In diabetic patients who are myopic, or who have had trauma to the orbit, the vitreous hemorrhage may be due to a retinal hole. Also in the setting of mild NPDR, short duration of diabetes, and good glycemic control, a vitreous hemorrhage may mean a retinal hole instead of PDR. Thus, examination of the periphery is important when the diabetic retinopathy does not equal the level of PDR and yet there is a vitreous hemorrhage. Always be suspicious that there is a retinal tear if the PDR or severe NPDR markers are not found on examination. Scleral depression and Goldmann contact lens examination of the retinal periphery in the eye with a vitreous hemorrhage lead to the discovery of a retinal hole.

When an eye has a vitreous hemorrhage, aim for a large pupillary dilation of 6 mm or 7 mm or more. Maximal pupillary dilation allows a view of the periphery which can give clues to the level of severe diabetic retinopathy with or without the presence of a retinal hole.

Stereoscopic fundus photographs using the 30 or 35 degree camera setting show early neovascularization of the optic disc and elsewhere. The seven standard fields are useful as well. Maximal pupillary dilation is important for a good fundus photograph. For follow-up visits, these photographs aid the clinician in pinpointing the progression of diabetic retinopathy.

Finding NVE and IRMAs may be difficult. In addition, differentiating between NVE and IRMA is a challenge. IRMAs may be extensive, and the NVE may not show classic frondlike patterns or wheel-spoke presentations. Frank NVE presents as extensions across arterial and venous systems in the equator and anterior to the equator. Older NVE is associated white fibrotic condensations adherent to the vitreous which are known as fibrovascular proliferations. These fibrovascular changes can occur as the NVE regresses or the fibrovascular changes occur after the resolution of a previous localized vitreous hemorrhage.

Using a Goldmann contact lens and the slit lamp biomicroscope, look at the equatorial mirror and then at the peripheral mirror for these areas of NVE. Start with low illumination but with a broad slit beam. This allows time for the examiner's eyes to be dark adapted. Then, use a very thin, bright slit beam to see more clearly if the area of neovascularization has an abnormal adherent relationship to the vitreous. Here, the three-dimensional quality of the NVE can be seen by using the slit beam at an angle to the viewing axis and in line with the viewing axis to see the characteristics about the NVE or IRMA and retinal surface.

Fluorescein angiography and fluorescein angioscopy can identify neovascularization versus IRMA. Neovascularization manifests as profound hyperfluorescence on fluorescein angiography. Fluorescein angioscopy is difficult to see in NVE in areas of equator and anterior to the equator because of the structural limitations of the fundus camera.

Lastly, if the clinician is suspicious of NVE and IRMAs, ask the patient to return in 1 month or sooner if his vision deteriorates. In careful follow-up in subsequent visits, the "suspicious" lesions become more pronounced and the level of diabetic retinopathy manifests.

New vessels may be barely visible at their inception. The caliber of the new vessels is 1/8 to 1/4 of that of a major vein at the optic disc margin. New vessels may be amorphous, without a pattern. Commonly, NVD are radiating spokes from the carriage wheel's center, with an associated circumferential vessel surrounding its periphery. NVD lie over vessels and seem to drain into veins. The superotemporal vein, seen in field 4, is the most common site of NVE, [3,4] occurring in about 27% of the 1,158 eyes under the DRS.[5] The inferotemporal field, field 5, has 17% of NVE seen out of 1,158 study eyes.[5] The inferonasal view of field 7 has 21% of the NVE seen out of 1,158 study eyes.[5]

The rate of growth of the NVE is variable. The change can vary between 1 week and several months. Early in the life of the patch of NVE, the vessels are bare. However, later, white fibrous tissue is adjacent to them. The fibrous proliferation contains fibrocytes and glial cells.[6,7] Their life cycle is that of proliferation followed by partial or complete regression.[3,8,9] Regression occurs when the wheel-shaped NVE has a decreasing number of vessels and caliber of the vessels in the center of the wheel. Next, there is a partial replacement of the NVE with fibrous tissue. Or paradoxically, the NVE patch enlarges but the peripheral vessels narrow. The regressing NVE can show sheathing of the vessels as well. The width of the sheath in the vessels of the NVE increases such that the NVE patch becomes a network of white lines without any red blood cells seen in the lumen. At this stage, there are new vessels forming at the edge of the patch of NVE. New vessels are seen at different stages of growth in different areas of the retina in the same eye.

The fibrovascular proliferation maybe translucent and are misinterpreted as inactive. Watch for any changes in the surrounding area. With more NVE, contraction of the fibrovascular proliferation can lead to separation from the retina, causing anterior-posterior traction. This type of traction retinal detachment is glistening white and concave. At this point, surgery is an option.

If contraction of the fibrovascular stalk does not occur but rather the NVE passes through all of its stages without affecting the patient's vision, the patient will be undergoing a quiescent stage of his or her PDR. The patient will have spontaneous regression of NVE leaving no adverse sequela for the patient.[10]

The posterior vitreous face touches the NVE patch and the NVE patch appears to be elevated. Adjacent to the patch of NVE adherent to the vitreous is a localized posterior vitreous detachment. The small localized vitreous detachment and the rest of the vitreous gel is close to the retina. As the posterior vitreous detachment becomes more extensive, the curved contour of the vitreous face is parallel to the surface of the retina and the NVE. The vitreous face is 0.5 to 2 DD from the surface of the retinal. Meanwhile, anatomically, the surface of the new vessels are adherent to the vitreous. As NVE networks get larger, the new vessels can be pulled away and can create a contraction and a traction retinal detachment.

The thickness of the posterior vitreous surface changes. At the site of NVE, the clinician can see the vitreous as a thick band using slit lamp biomicroscopy. This is probably due to fibrovascular proliferation along the posterior vitreous surface. There are alternating thicker and thinner adhesions to the vitreous, giving an undulating, textured, and irregular appearance to the vitreous and internal limiting membrane (ILM) interface. Lastly, the posterior vitreous surface is subtle and can be seen by using the binocular slit lamp's narrow slit beam to glide smoothly over the retina. The slit beam moves over the surface of the retina, while you are looking at the different types of light reflexes. Blood in the fluid vitreous, posterior to the detached vitreous gel, can languish on thew retina for weeks and months. However, blood inside the formed vitreous tends to lose color and becomes yellow or white before absorption is complete. This type of bleeding into the formed vitreous may require months to resorb. Unresolved vitreous hemorrhage ultimately needs surgery.

The contraction of the abnormal vitreous interface and fibrovascular proliferation may cause the macula to be dragged and distorted. Most commonly, the macula can be dragged nasally and vertically with overlying glistening white fibrous membranes.

Contraction of the extensive sheet of fibrovascular proliferation may lead to retinal detachment. The subsequent avulsion of a retinal vessel, usually a vein, can be accompanied by a vitreous hemorrhage. The retinal detachment may involve the entire macula causing a concave traction retinal detachment. Or in severe cases, sheets of fibrovascular proliferation are cross layered over the macula producing a traction retinal detachment. Associated holes can occur in the periphery as well, but this is rare.

Extensive NVE with large caliber new vessels accompany heavy fibroproliferation with tight vitreoretinal adhesions. Usually, these occur after a vitreous hemorrhage in the setting of an intact posterior hyaloid, adherent to the ILM. Contraction is followed by extensive retinal detachment. In those vitreous hemorrhages where there is little fibrovascular proliferation, NVE, and a posterior vitreous detachment, there is less risk for a traction retinal detachment. These vitreous hemorrhages when resolved, have a better visual prognosis than those vitreous hemorrhages with an intact hyaloid and severe fibrovascular proliferation.

CHIEF COMPLAINT

The patient may present with abrupt loss of vision or gradual loss of vision. The vision could be distorted reflecting the abnormality of the retinal surface and traction retinal detachment.

PAST MEDICAL HISTORY

In those instances of known diabetic patients who present with decreased vision, it is important to ask about their past history of fasting blood glucose, HbA1c, cholesterol levels, triglyceride levels, and creatinine levels.[11] In addition, ask about vision loss, past history of laser, macular laser, panretinal laser photocoagulation, and past vitrectomy surgery. In patients with moderate to severe diabetic retinopathy, it is important for the clinician to assess the risk of accelerating diabetic retinopathy. Does the patient have PDR, yet to be detected?

PHYSICAL EXAMINATION

PDR is the most severe type of retinal complication in a diabetic patient. As we are all aware, diabetic retinopathy is progressive. Thus, this patient presenting to the ophthalmologist's office has the most severe form of disease. He or she must have either had eye care in the distant past. Alternatively, he or she may never have received any eye care at all in his or her life.

If the patient has never received eye care from any eye care practitioner, the patient may be in denial. It is the responsibility of the ophthalmologist's office to provide patient education materials, all of which are available on the American Diabetes Association Web site.[1]

PATIENT HISTORY AND REVIEW OF SYSTEMS

In taking the patient history, one can assess if the patient is aware of his or her status of diabetes. By the time the PDR appears, the patient has impaired vision and there are other risk factors to ascertain.[11] Thus, the ophthalmologist and retinal specialist play an important role as an educator about diabetic retinopathy and diabetic eye disease. The ophthalmologist's office serves as a resource for community social services for diabetic patients with PDR. He or she may need to find a nutritionist, podiatrist, and psychologist. There is a high rate of depression among the chronically ill diabetic patients who have severe degrees of diabetic retinopathy.[12]

In one study, the combination of cognitive behavioral therapy and supportive diabetes education is an effective nonpharmacologic treatment for depression in Type 2 diabetic patients (Table 9-1). The behavioral therapy and education are associated with improved glycemic control.[13]

If the patient cannot remember the name of his or her medication or how long he or she has had the disease, he or she must have been newly diagnosed or unfamiliar with his or her diagnosis. In addition, the diagnosis of PDR could be new for him or her. Prior

TABLE 9.1 Education of Proliferative Diabetic Patient

1. Potential for severe vision loss if noncompliant with internal medicine physician.
2. Obesity and metabolic syndrome play a role in diabetic retinopathy
3. Lipid profiles
4. HbA1c and FBS
5. Kidney function

TABLE 9.2 Basic Health Literacy for the Diabetic Patient

1. Definition of Type 1 and Type 2 diabetes
2. The symptoms of hyperglycemia and hypoglycemia
3. Correlation of glycemic control and diabetic retinopathy
4. Correlation of glycemic control and systemic side effects: silent ischemia, diabetic retinopathy, renal insufficiency, hyperlipidemia, diabetic neuropathy, foot ulcers, and amputation
5. Diabetic diet: calorie counting, decreased portion size at meals, and ADA guidelines for diet
6. Oral medications and need for constant monitoring of diet
7. Insulin
8. See an ophthalmologist or retina specialist regularly if the patient has PDR.

to this visit, the patient may not have had any deterioration of vision affecting his or her activities of daily living. Or he or she could be in denial. In any case, we need to emphasize that the patient and the medical doctors are a "team." If the patient follows the instructions of his or her team of doctors, he or she will have a good treatment outcome. However, if the patient does not follow the treatment regimen for his or her diabetes, the treatment outcome may be disappointing.[11] Consequently, the patient may suffer accelerated, severe vision loss along with systemic complications involving the heart and kidneys.[11,14]

Similarly, in asking about the review of systems, the clinician gains an understanding of the patient's level of cardiovascular health, hypertension, and lipid metabolism.[5] All these factors play a role in taking care of the patient (Table 9-2). Weight issues and obesity play a role in diabetes and cardiovascular disease. According to the CDC, it is estimated that 33.3% of the men and 35.3% of the women in the United States are obese.[5] Smoking plays an adverse role in the development of diabetes.[14] Smoking has been associated with the development of NPDR.[14,15]

Lastly, excessive alcohol intake can hamper the compliance of an American Diabetes Association diet and is a risk factor in the development of diabetic retinopathy. Intake of a glass of wine is an additional 150 calories. These empty calories add nothing to the nutritional health of the diabetic patient.[15,16] Some patients will not give up their glass of wine. Therefore, they must learn to give up the 150 calories from their diet in other ways. Or they have to increase their exercise regimen to account for the 150 calories from alcohol (Table 9-3).

It is thought that the increase of obesity in the United States parallels the increase in the cases of diabetes. Roughly, one third of adults in the United States are obese. In patients with diabetes, cardiovascular disease is a comorbid risk factor: the diagnosis of cardiovascular disease has been reported by 38.1% of adults with diabetes.[11] Obesity is a particular problem in patients who have PDR. Since adipocytes are thought to play a role in insulin resistance, the obese diabetic will have a hard time controlling his or her blood sugar and therefore, the natural progression of the diabetic retinopathy will continue unabated. The United Kingdom Prospective Diabetes Study (UKPDS) data shows that for every decrease of 1% of the HbA1c, the risk of diabetic retinopathy is lowered by 37%.[17]

For PDR patients, the metabolic syndrome is a concern. The metabolic syndrome is a set of interrelated risk factors of metabolic origins which promote the development of atherosclerotic cardiovascular disease and increase the risk of developing Type 2 diabetes

TABLE 9.3 Web Sites for Patient Education

www.diabetes.org (American Diabetes Association)
www.aace.com (American Association of Clinical Endocrinologists)
www.mayoclinic.com (Mayo Clinic's web site for the diabetic diet)
http://diabetes.niddk.nih.gov/dm/pubs/eating_ez/ (The NIH's web site for diabetic diet)

mellitus. The metabolic risk factors are atherogenic dyslipidemia, elevated blood pressure, and elevated plasma glucose. Thus, patients with the metabolic syndrome are at increased risk of developing diabetes.

These metabolic syndrome risk factors affect cardiovascular and vascular status, thereby affecting blood flow and perfusion. In turn, the low blood flow and resultant ischemia would cause abnormal endothelial cell and pericyte function in the diabetic patient. Thus, the additive effects of vascular disease and diabetes worsen the visual function.

FAMILY HISTORY

Patients with family members with blindness from diabetic retinopathy are a red flag for the ophthalmologist. Family history of death related to diabetes implies that the patient may have genetic predisposition to severe diabetes and its complications.

EXAMINATION

Patients with Visual Acuity of 20/20 to 20/40

Visual acuity, slit lamp examination, and retinal examination are the standard examination techniques. Patients with PDR may present with visual acuity of 20/20 to 20/40 range. These patients may have NVE or NVD but are asymptomatic. Asymptomatic patients who have no visual complaints will find it difficult to accept the diagnosis of PDR. Thus, the office staff or office nurse may need to educate these patients about their disease.

Other Findings

Macular edema can occur in the setting of any level of diabetic retinopathy. While these macular edema and PDR patients may not need fluorescein angiography for their diagnosis of macular edema, the fluorescein angiography will delineate areas of NVE and areas of capillary nonperfusion. The extent of neovascularization of the retina will determine high-risk characteristics as recorded by the DRS.[18]

Patients will need panretinal photocoagulation if they have both optic NVD and other areas of retinal neovascularization (NVE). If they have only one of the risk factors of the high-risk characteristics, they could wait for their photocoagulation but they must be monitored. In addition, their labs must be updated for the evaluation of FBS, HbA1c, and hyperlipidemia (Table 9-4).

Patients with Visual Acuity of 20/50 to 20/80

Mild vitreous hemorrhage and/or macular edema can occur with NVE or NVD can lead to this level of visual acuity. The patient may present with 20/50 to 20/80 visual acuity because of previously treated panretinal photocoagulation and new or residual macular edema. These patients need fluorescein angiography to delineate the etiology of their visual loss especially if there is no media opacity to explain the visual loss.

TABLE 9.4 High-Risk Characteristics for PDR

1. NVE + NVD (<standard photograph 10A)
2. NVE + NVD (<standard photograph 10A) + VH or preretinal hemorrhage
3. NVE + NVD (≥standard photograph 10A)
4. NVE + NVD (≥ standard photograph 10A) + vitreous hemorrhage/preretinal hemorrhage

NVD, neovascularization at the disc, new vessels located at or within 1 DD of the disc;
NVE, neovascularization elsewhere; VH, vitreous hemorrhage.

Patients with Visual Acuity of 20/100 to 20/400

As the vision worsens, the patient usually has a vitreous hemorrhage. In dense vitreous hemorrhages, there may be a traction retinal detachment or severe macular edema. Fluorescein angiography and optical coherence tomography (OCT) can characterize the retina only if the fundus view is clear. If a vitreous hemorrhage is present, ultrasound studies should be performed.

PHYSICAL EXAMINATION

Visual Acuity Measurement

Assuming that the patient's previous medical records are available, the ophthalmologist can check the deterioration or improvement of his visual acuity. Watch the patient's pattern of ambulation to assess his or her peripheral vision. In examining him for visual acuity measurement, look to see if he misses the central letter of each visual acuity line or if he has to "search" to find the letters on the eye chart. Searching eye movements indicate poor vision or abnormal visual field changes.

Slit Lamp Examination

Slit lamp examination can diagnose iris rubeosis. Examine closely the iris margin for small red tufts or dots of neovascularization. Use gonioscopy to inspect the angle. Once there is rubeosis iridis and or angle neovascularization, the patient will have neovascularization of the retina in the periphery known as NVE. Neovascularization of the optic disc is easy to find if it is florid. It is difficult to see early disc neovascularization but the red-free photographs will be helpful at the 20 degree angle. NVD is seen easily with fluorescein angiography. Similarly, NVE is seen easily with fluorescein angiography.

Neovascularization of the fundus, from the equator of the retina to the anterior aspects of the retina, is hard to examine by indirect ophthalmoscope. For small fronds of neovascularization at the posterior pole, slit lamp biomicroscopy with the 90 D lens or the Goldmann contact lens can detect these changes. The fundus camera can facilitate detection of these neovascular fronds in fields 1 and 2, using the seven standard diabetic fields. For the area of the equator to the periphery, the fundus camera can be used in the red-free setting.

Optical Coherence Tomography

In vitreous hemorrhage patients, the OCT scan will not be helpful because of optical aberrations. Neovascular fronds cannot be visualized with OCT scans. However, macular edema will be delineated clearly with OCT.

Ultrasonography

Ultrasonic evaluation is used to ascertain the integrity of the retina in patients with media opacity. If there is a retinal detachment, surgery should be performed immediately. If there is no retinal detachment, waiting can be as short as 1 month before performing vitrectomy. If vision deteriorates in the 1-month waiting period, or if the patient cannot perform activities of daily living or perform work-related functions, the retina surgeon can suggest earlier vitrectomy.

Vitrectomy

The recommended timing of vitrectomy for severe PDR and vitreous hemorrhage is 3 months for Type 1 diabetes and 6 months for Type 2 diabetes.[19] Surgical goals include removal of vitreous hemorrhage to create a clear medium for vision, excision of posterior hyaloid face, epiretinal fibrovascular membranes or its attachments to relieve vitreoretinal traction, and application of endolaser photocoagulation to achieve regression of neovascularization and proliferation.

The basic pathophysiology of a vitreous hemorrhage occurring in PDR involves vitreoretinal adhesions centered around vascular epicenters. Abrams has studied 100 consecutive eyes undergoing their first vitrectomy for diabetic retinopathy.[20] He finds that 22% have minimal or no posterior vitreous detachment, but present with preretinal hemorrhage, dragged macula, or tractional diabetic macular edema. Thirty-one percent of the eyes have only a partial vitreous detachment, with vitreous attached at the posterior pole and mid periphery, and 39% the vitreous is attached at the posterior pole only and not at the periphery. Eight percent of the eyes have a total posterior vitreous detachment.[20]

Evaluating vitreoretinal adhesions, Abrams finds that 86% of the eyes had one point of focal vitreoretinal adhesion.[20] Multiple focal adhesions are more common. Thirty-three percent of the eyes had more than one focal adhesion but no traction retinal detachment. Forty-one percent had more than one adhesion with a traction retinal detachment. The vitreous may separate partially from the retinal around some adhesions. Additional vitreoretinal proliferation may occur around epiretinal membranes around an adhesion and therefore forms a broader attachment. The retina around the adhesions may remain attached or may develop into purely tractional or a combined traction/rhegmatogenous retinal detachment.

Vitreoretinal adhesions can be separated into those with and without infolding of the underlying retina. This may be caused by a large patch of neovascularization. These are difficult to peel since the underlying retina can seem alternately stiff and avascular or atrophic and avascular. The underlying retina is almost always detached.

If the vitreous hemorrhage is dense, no fundus details are visible and ultrasonagraphy shows retinal detachment involving the macula, combined traction/rhegmatogenous retinal detachment, severe fibrovascular proliferation, and vitrectomy is indicated.

In severe PDR and vitreous hemorrhage cases, the favorable prognosis eyes are those with a traction retinal detachment of short duration, limited extent of the macular detachment, presence of preoperative panretinal photocoagulation, and the absence of vitreous hemorrhage and severe neovascularization.[21–30]

When surgeons have broadened the indication to include traction detachment threatening the macula, early vitrectomy can cause macular distortion, metamorphopsia, loss of central visual field, and a reduction in visual acuity.[31–33]

Macular detachments whose duration is greater than 6 months to a year do not yield useful vision. Surgery is not commonly performed in these cases.

Vitrectomy indications have been expanded to include macular edema with a taut posterior hyaloid,[34] without a taut posterior hyaloid face,[35] vitreopapillary traction.[36,37] As such, postoperative complications can arise in the eyes after vitrectomy such as recurrent vitreous hemorrhage, anterior hyaloidal fibrovascular proliferation, and fibrinoid syndrome.

TREATMENT

Nonsurgical Treatment

Some patients want a nonsurgical option. The clinician must document this with the patient's signature on the medical chart. The risks and benefits of waiting for a spontaneous clearing of a vitreous hemorrhage must be explained to the patient and his or her family.

If there is only a vitreous hemorrhage without a retinal detachment, the patient can wait for 3 to 6 months. However, waiting for the vitreous hemorrhage to clear spontaneously when there is a retinal detachment is not the standard of care and this must be explained to the patient. A second opinion can be suggested. Again, an informed decision statement must be given to the patient and the patient must sign the statement that he or she is fully aware that he or she is taking his or her eyesight to a dangerous level of risk because he or she refuses surgery.

Laser

Laser in the eye with a vitreous hemorrhage can be done if there is a view of the retina with the Rodenstock lens or laser lens. If there is a quadrant of retina that can be identified, laser photocoagulation can be done in that quadrant. It would not be surprising that a quadrant of laser can improve vision in the next few days. Much, of course, depends on the degree of diabetic control as well. Intravitreal bevacizumab may be used in conjunction with laser, as well.

Laser Techniques

Scatter treatment is done with burns spaced about one half to one burn width apart, extending from the posterior pole to the equator and often completed in a single sitting. The argon treatment technique noted in the DRS states 800 to 1,600 burns, 500 μm spot size, of 0.1 second duration. The DRS specifies that the treatment be applied directly to new vessels elsewhere (NVE).[38–40]

Intravitreal Bevacizumab (Avastin)

Bevacizumab may be injected in an eye with a vitreous hemorrhage but without a retinal detachment. Intravitreal bevacizumab may be a compromise that the patient can agree to undertake if he or she refuses vitrectomy.[41–47]

Regression of retinal neovascularization has been noted in two patients with diabetic vitreous hemorrhage at 1 month follow-up visit. Each of the patients has had two injections of bevacizumab.[41–47]

Intravitreal bevacizumab is used prior to the vitrectomy surgery to change the vascular endothelial growth factor state of the eye. Some surgeons have noted marked improvement in the neovascularized fronds on the retina with the use of intravitreal injections of bevacizumab 5 to 7 days prior to the surgery.[41–48] There have been reported complications of traction retinal detachment after bevacizumab intravitreal injections. Arevalo et al.[46] reported 11 eyes out of 211 intravitreal injections of bevacizumab have had refractory PDR despite panretinal photocoagulation. The traction retinal detachments occur between 3 and 31 days, at an average of 13 days. The 11 eyes of the 11 patients have had a history of poor glycemic control.[46]

The complication rate of intravitreal bevacizumab is low, reported to be <0.21% among 7,113 injections given to 5,228 patients, in an Internet survey given to physicians worldwide.[47] The physician reported that complications were corneal abrasion, lens injury, endophthalmitis, retinal detachment, inflammation or uveitis, cataract progression, acute vision loss, central retinal artery occlusion, subretinal hemorrhage, retinal pigment epithelium tears, blood pressure elevation, transient ischemic attack, and cerebrovascular accident and death.

Intravitreal Triamcinolone

Intravitreal injections prior to vitrectomy surgery have been popular prior to the advent of the bevacizumab. Intravitreal triamcinolone has been used during vitrectomy surgery before the advent of bevacizumab.[48] In one European study, the use of intravitreal triamcinolone at the time of vitrectomy compared to controls showed no significant difference in postoperative visual acuity.[48] More surgeons have switched to the use of bevacizumab intravitreally prior to vitrectomy surgery. Retina surgeons have noted marked improvement in the PDR with triamcinolone in the days prior to bevacizumab.

CLINICAL CORRELATIONS: Proliferative Diabetic Retinopathy

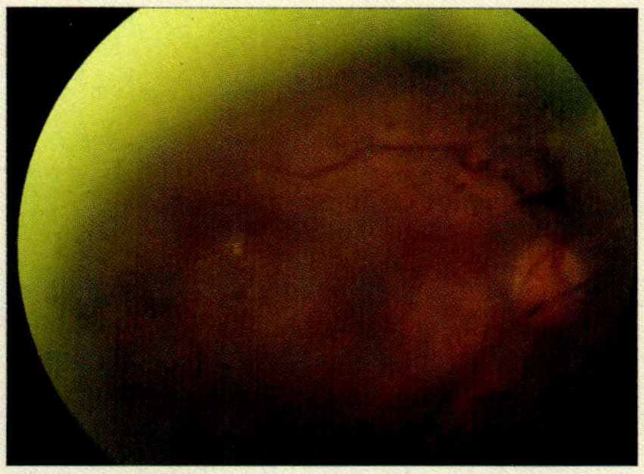

FIGURE 9-9. 52-year-old Caucasian male, banker with loss of vision Photo OD, vitreous hemorrhage.

FIGURE 9-10. Fluorescein angiogram OD, 1 minute, 14 seconds transit, fibrovascular stalk at superior disc.

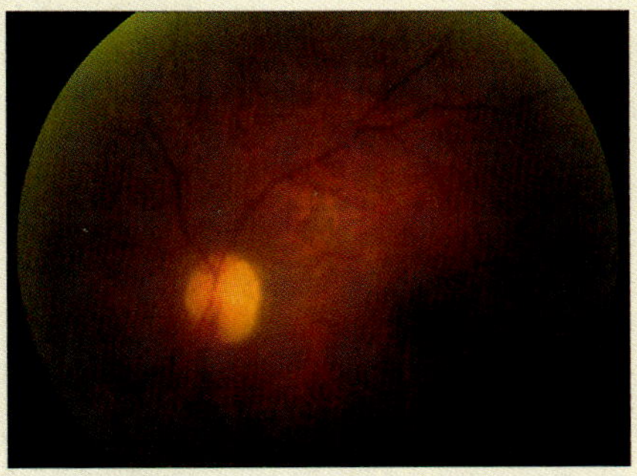

FIGURE 9-11. Photo OS, vitreous hemorrhage.

FIGURE 9-12. Fluorescein angiogram OS, 48 seconds transit, superior to disc, there is neovascularization.

Patient complaints: "I have trouble seeing for the past month but it has gotten worse this past week."

Caveats: For diabetic patients, this is a nonspecific complaint. They could have macular edema or PDR. Other considerations are retinal vascular occlusions and transient ischemic attacks.

Case Study (Figs. 9-9–9-12)

10–29–2007: 52-year-old Caucasian male, banker, who notes loss of vision. He has had an 8-year history of using insulin with a total duration of diabetes of 15 years. He has a sedentary lifestyle. He remembers lifting heavy luggage at the airport 1 month ago.

V Hand motion
20/80 NIPH
Slit lamp examination
Cornea: Clear OU
Anterior chamber: Deep and quiet OU
Iris: Normal OU, no rubeosis OU
Lens: 1 + nuclear sclerosis OU
Applanation tonometry = 14/14 mm Hg (10:00 AM)
Gonioscopy: Open 360 degrees OU, no rubeosis OU

Dilated funduscopic examination:

Right eye: Vitreous hemorrhage is seen, the optic nerve can be identified. Superiorly, there is a fibrovascular stalk OD. The blood is densest at this area, superior optic disc. This is PDR. By tilting the eye and by ductional movement, the entire area of the retina can be seen. There is no retinal detachment. Scleral depression identifies the ora serrata and the peripheral retina is attached.

Color fundus photography OD: Vitreous hemorrhage with the area of hemorrhage arising from the superior optic disc.

Red-free photography OD: Hemorrhage appears black and is more clearly delineated.

Left eye: Vitreous hemorrhage is seen and the superior and inferior arcades can be identified. There is no retinal detachment.

Color fundus photography OS: Less dense vitreous hemorrhage.

Red-free photography OS: More of the retina vessels can be identified in the red-free photograph.

Comment

PDR in a 52-year-old male, 15-year duration of diabetes, and insulin usage for the past 8 years. He needs to see an endocrinologist for better glycemic control. For every 1% decline of HbA1c, there is a 35% decline in diabetic retinopathy according to the UKPDS study. In addition, normal HbA1c = 6% and he is far from the target goal. Panretinal laser photocoagulation is recommended for both eyes. However, treatment may not be completed due to poor visualization.

CLINICAL CORRELATIONS: Proliferative Diabetic Retinopathy

Patient complaints: "I cannot see the computer."

Caveats: Poor compliance and inadequate glycemic control.

Case Study I (Figs. 9-13–9-16)

54-year-old Caucasian female with loss of vision. She has been ignoring her diabetes because she was taking care of a sister dying of breast cancer. She is a comptroller for a major corporation. She has had previous retinal laser in both eyes in another city several years ago.
Fasting blood glucose = 145 mg/dL, HbA1c = 6.9%, Cholesterol = 163 mg/dL, triglycerides 108 mg/dL, HDL = 60 mg/dL, LDL = 81 mg/dL, BUN = 31 mg/dL (normal 7–25 mg/dL), BUN/creatinine ratio = 31 (normal 10 to 20)

V Hand motion
20/80 PH 20/40
Slit lamp examination
Cornea: Clear OU
Anterior chamber: Deep and quiet OU
Iris: Normal OU, no rubeosis OD but iris rubeosis at 1:00 to 3:00 at edge of iris. The iris neovascularization is seen under an intense slit beam under a dark room setting (overhead lights out and clinician's own eyes are dark adapted).Gonioscopy: Neovascularization seen in the left eye at 3:00.
Lens: 1 + nuclear sclerosis OU
Applanation tonometry = 14/14 mm Hg (10:00 AM)
Gonioscopy: Open 360 degrees OU, rubeosis OS at 3:00

Dilated funduscopic examination:

Right eye: Vitreous hemorrhage is seen, with a preretinal hemorrhage seen in the inferior arcade. There is disc neovascularization greater than standard 10A photograph. This fulfills the high risk criteria for PDR.
Color fundus photography OD: Vitreous hemorrhage with previous laser seen inferiorly.
Red-free photography OD: Venous loops seen more clearly, temporal to the macula, in the red-free photograph. The disc neovascularization is better seen in the red-free photographs as well.
Left eye: Mild, less dense vitreous hemorrhage is seen. Smaller preretinal hemorrhage is seen inferotemporally.
Color fundus photography OS: Less dense vitreous hemorrhage. Laser seen inferiorly.
Red-free photography OS: Hemorrhages are more clearly delineated in red-free photographs than in the color photographs.

Comment

PDR in a patient with poor glycemic control. Patient has early renal dysfunction. Poor renal function can lead to later macular edema and retention of fluid. The elevated HbA1c demonstrates poor glycemic control over the past 6 months.

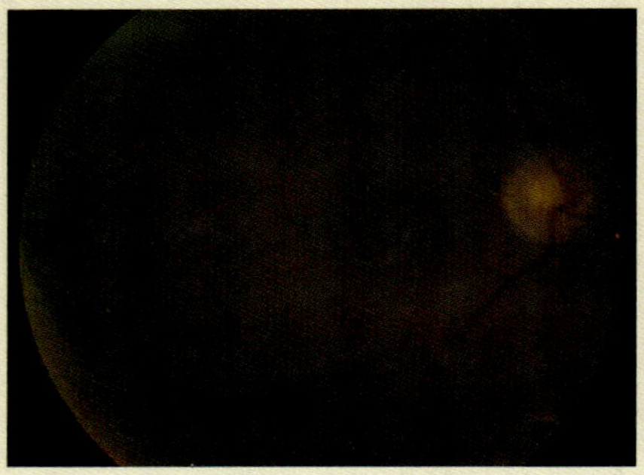

FIGURE 9-13. 54-year old-Caucasian female with loss of vision. Photo OD, vitreous hemorrhage, disc neovascularization.

FIGURE 9-14. Red free photograph OD, venous loops are prominent.

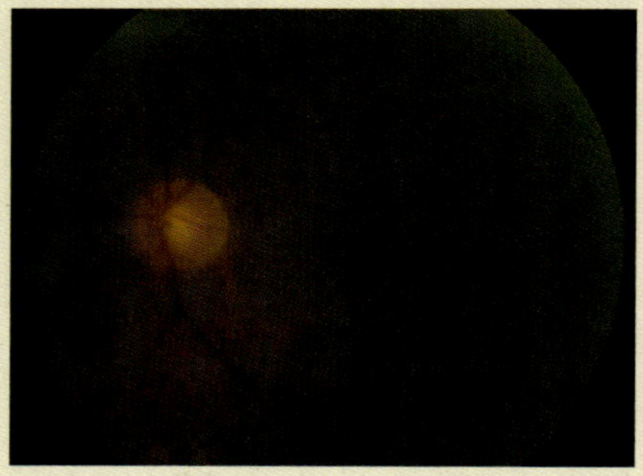

FIGURE 9-15. Photo OS, vitreous hemorrhages, preretinal hemorrhage.rhages, preretinal hemorrhage.

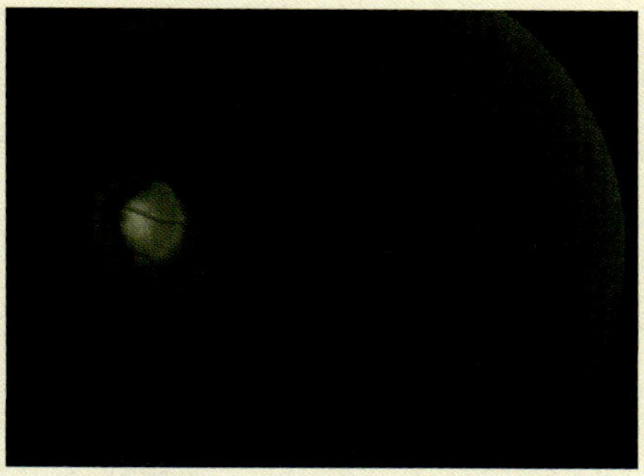

FIGURE 9-16. Red-free photograph OS, hard exudates are prominent.

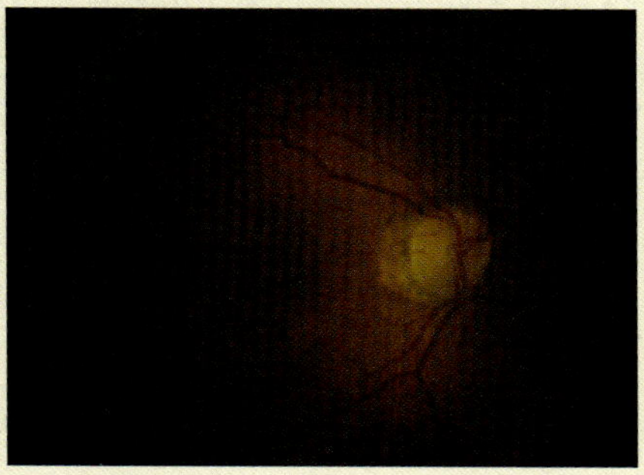

FIGURE 9-17. 80-year-old Caucasian female with bilateral loss of vision, gradually over 6 months. Photo OD, mild vitreous hemorrhage.

FIGURE 9-18. Photo OS, vitreous hemorrhage.

Case Study II (Figs. 9-17 and 9-18)

11–21–2006: 80-year-old Caucasian female with bilateral loss of vision, gradually over 6 months. She has just relocated to this area. She has had 20 years of hypertension, 15 years of Type 2 diabetes, and she has intermittent eye pain.

V Hand motion
Hand motion
Slit lamp examination
Cornea: Clear OU
Anterior chamber: Deep and trace flare noted OU
Iris: Very small areas of iris atrophy noted in her blue irides OU, at the iris crypts at 12:00 OD and 1:00 OS.
Lens: 2 + nuclear sclerosis OU
Applanation tonometry = 26/26 mm Hg (10:00 AM)
Gonioscopy: Open 360 degrees OU, trace rubeosis OU
OD: Fine arborization, rubeosis is 12:00
OS: Fine arborization, rubeosis is 1:00 to 3:00

Dilated funduscopic examination:

Right eye: Light vitreous hemorrhage is seen, the optic nerve can be identified. This is PDR. Presumably, there is NVE rather than at the optic disc. The view is obscured because of the fine vitreous hemorrhage. She must have chronic poor glycemic control.
Color fundus photography OD: Vitreous hemorrhage without a site of neovascularization.
Left eye: Vitreous hemorrhage is seen and the superior and inferior arcades can be identified. There is no retinal detachment.
Color fundus photography OS: Less dense vitreous hemorrhage, poor delineation of retinal details.

Comment

PDR in an 80-year-old female with 15-year duration of diabetes. She needs to see an endocrinologist for better glycemic control. Her HbA1c is 7.0% which is elevated but her FBS is 130 meaning that she has some issues with glycemic control. Perhaps diet modification can help this elderly Type 1 diabetic patient. Panretinal laser photocoagulation is recommended for both eyes. In addition, she may be a candidate for gonioscopic laser at the new vessels in her angle. She needs antiglaucoma treatment such as a beta-blocker (timolol maleate 1/2% BID OU) and a glaucoma consultation. Laser treatment should be initiated for the PDR immediately in the office or as soon as possible.

REFERENCES

1. www.diabetes.org/home.jsp. Accessed 1 March 2009.
2. Diabetic Retinopathy Study Research Group. Photocoagulation treatment of proliferative diabetic retinopathy: The second report of the Diabetic Retinopathy Study findings. *Ophthalmology*. 1978;85:82–106.
3. Davis M. Vitreous contraction in proliferative diabetic retinopathy. *Arch Ophthalmol.* 1965;74:741–751.
4. Taylor E, Dobree J. Proliferative diabetic retinopathy: Site and size of initial lesions. *Br J Ophthalmol.* 1970;54:11–18.
5. Prudhomme G, Rand L. The Diabetic Retinopathy Research Group: Distribution of maximum grade of lesions in proliferative diabetic retinopathy. *Invest Ophthalmol Vis Sci.* 1981;21:210–226.
6. Kampik A, Kenyon K, Michels R, et al. Epiretinal and vitreous membranes: Comparative study of 56 cases. *Arch Ophthalmol.* 1981;99:1445–1454.
7. Nork T, Wallow I, Sramek S, et al. Mueller's cell involvement in diabetic retinopathy. *Arch Ophthalmol.* 1987;105: 1424–1429.
8. Davis M. Natural history of diabetic retinopathy. In: Kimura S, Caygill W, eds. *Vascular Complications of Diabetes Mellitus.* St Louis, MO: Mosby; 1967.
9. Dobree J. Proliferative diabetic retinopathy: Evolution of retinal lesions. *Br J Ophthalmol.* 1964;48:637–649.
10. Bandello F, Gass J, Lattanzio R, et al. Spontaneous regression of neovascularization at the disc and elsewhere in diabetic retinopathy. *Am J Ophthalmol.* 1996;122:494–501.
11. Buse JB, Ginsburg HN, Bakris GL, et al. Primary prevention of cardiovascular disease in people with diabetes mellitus: A scientific statement for the American Heart Association and American Diabetes Association. *Diabetes Care.* 2007;30:162–172.
12. De Groot M, Anderson R, Freedland KE, et al. Association of depression and diabetes complications: A meta-analysis. *Psychosomatic Med.* 2001;63:619–630.
13. Lustman PJ, Griffith LS, Freedland KE, et al. Cognitive behavior therapy for depression in Type 2 diabetes mellitus. *Ann Int Med.* 1998;129:613–621.
14. Coffey JT, Brandle M, Zhou H, et al. Valuing health-related quality of life in diabetes. *Diabetes Care.* 2002;25: 2238–2243.
15. Rimm EB, Chan J, Stampfer MJ, et al. Prospective study of cigarette smoking, alcohol use, and the risk of diabetes in men. *BMJ.* 1995:310:555–559.
16. Young RJ, McCulloch DK, Prescott RJ, et al. Alcohol: Another risk factor for diabetic retinopathy? *BMJ.* 1984;288: 1035–1037.
17. Stratton IM, Adler AI, Neil HAW, et al. Association of glycaemia with macrovascular and microvascular complications of type 2 diabetes (UKPDS 35): Prospective observational study. *BMJ.* 2000;321:405–412.
18. Diabetic Retinopathy Study Research Group. DRS Report No. 3: Four risk factors for severe visual loss in diabetic retinopathy. *Arch Ophthalmol.* 1979;97:654–655.
19. Ho T, Smiddy WE, Flynn HW. Vitrectomy in the management of diabetic eye disease. *Surv Ophthalmol.* 1992;37: 190–202.
20. Eliott D, Lee MS, Abrams GW. Proliferative Diabetic Retinopathy: Principles and techniques of surgical treatment, page 2414 in www.retinatext.com. Accessed 15 March 2009.
21. Peyman GA, Huamonte FU, Goldberg MF, et al. Four hundred consecutive pars plana vitrectomies with the vitreophage. *Arch Ophthalmol.* 1978;96:45–50.
22. Thompson JT, de Bustros S, Michels RG, et al. Results and prognostic factors in vitrectomy for diabetic vitreous hemorrhage. *Arch Ophthalmol.* 1987;105:191–199.
23. Blankenship GW. Preoperative prognostic factors in diabetic pars plana vitrectomy. *Ophthalmology.* 1982;89: 1246–1254.
24. Ho T, Smiddy WE, Flynn HW. Vitrectomy in the management of diabetic eye disease. *Surv Ophthalmol.* 1992;37: 190–202.
25. Aaberg TM. Pars plana vitrectomy for diabetic traction retinal detachment. *Ophthalmology.* 1981;88:639–642.
26. Charles S. Vitrectomy for retinal detachment. *Trans Ophthalmol Soc UK.* 1980; 100:542–552.
27. Michels RG. Vitrectomy for complications of diabetic retinopathy. *Arch Ophthalmol.* 1978;96:237.
28. Thompson JT, De Bustros S, Michels RG, et al. Results and prognostic factors in vitrectomy for diabetic traction retinal detachment of the macula. *Arch Ophthalmol.* 1987;105:497–502.
29. Tolentino FI, Freeman HM, Tolentino FL. Closed vitrectomy in the management of diabetic traction retinal detachment. *Ophthalmology.* 1980;87:1078–1089.
30. Rice TA, Michels RG, Rice EF. Vitrectomy for diabetic traction retinla detachment involving the macula. *Am J Ophthalmol.* 1983;95:22–33.
31. Bresnick GH, Haight B, de Venecia G. Retinal wrinkling and macular heterotopia in diabetic retinopathy. *Arch Ophthalmol.* 1979;97:1890–1895.
32. Bresnick GH, Smith V, Pokorny J. Visual function abnormalities inmacular heterotopia caused by proliferative diabetic retinopathy. *Am J Ophthalmol.* 1981;92:85–102.
33. Michael JC, De Venecia G, Bresnick GH. Macular heterotopia in proliferative diabetic retinopathy. *Arch Ophthalmol.* 1994;112:1455–1459.
34. Lewis H, Abrams GW, Blumenkranz MS, et al. Vitrectomy for diabetic macular traction and edema associated with posterior hyaloid traction. *Ophthalmology.* 1992;99:753–759.
35. Rosenblatt BJ, Shah GK, Sharma S, et al. Pars plana vitrectomy with internal limiting membranectomy for refractory diabetic macular edema without a taut posterior hyaloid. *Graefes Arch Clin Exp Ophthalmol.* 2005;253:20–25.
36. Kroll P, Wiegand W, Schmidt J. Vitreopapillary traction in proliferative diabetic vitreoretinopathy. *Br J Ophthalmol.* 1999;83:261–264.
37. McLeod D. Diabetic tractional papillopathy: A new (and true) nosological entity? *Br J Ophthalmol.* 1999;83:257–258.
38. Aiello LM, Berocal J, Davis M, et al. The Diabetic Retinopathy Study. *Arch Ophthalmol.* 1973;90:347–348.
39. The Diabetic Retinopathy Study Research Group. Preliminary report on effects of photocoagulation therapy. *Am J Ophthalmol.* 1976;81:83–396.
40. The Diabetic Retinopathy Study Research Group. Indications for photocoagulation treatment of diabetic retinopathy. DRS report no. 14. *Int Ophthalmol Clin.* 1987;27:239–253.

41. Spaide RF, Fisher YL. Intravitreal bevacizumab (Avastin) treatment of proliferative diabetic retinopathy complicated by vitreous hemorrhage. *Retina*. 2006;26:275–278.
42. Avery RL, Pearlman J, Pieramici DJ, et al. Intravitreal bevacizumab (Avastin) in the treatment of proliferative diabetic retinopathy. *Ophthalmology*. 2006;113:1695–1715.
43. Oshima Y, Sakaguchi H, Gomi F, et al. Regression of iris neovascularization after intravitreal bevacizumab (Avastin) in patients with proliferative diabetic retinopathy. *Am J Ophthalmol*. 2006;142:155–158.
44. Bakri SJ, Donaldson MJ, Link TP. Rapid regression of disc neovascularization in a patient with proliferative diabetic retinopathy. *Eye*. 2006;20:1474–1475.
45. Mason JO, Albert MA Jr, Mays A, et al. Regression of iris neovascular iris vessels by intravitreal bevacizumab. *Retina*. 2006;26:839–841.
46. Arevalo JF, Maia M, Flynn HW Jr, et al. Tractional retinal detachment following intravitreal bevacizumab (Avastin) in patients with severe proliferative diabetic retinopathy. *Br J Ophthalmol*. 2008;92:213–216.
47. Fung AE, Rosenfield PJ, Reichel E. The International Intravitreal Bevacizumab Safety Survey: Using the internet to assess drug safety worldwide. *Br J Ophthalmol*. 2006;90:1344–1349.
48. Jonas JB, Sofker A, Degenring R. Intravitreal triamcinolone acetonide as an additional tool in pars plana vitrectomy for proliferative diabetic retinopathy. *Eur J Ophthalmol*. 2003;13:468–473.

CHAPTER 10

Indications for Vitrectomy

VITREOUS ANATOMY

The vitreous is a translucent gel when it is in its normal state. The vitreous is a three-dimensional interactive matrix of collagen fibers with contractile properties and hyaluronic acid gel. The vitreous is in contact with the macula, pars plana, ciliary body, and retina in a sphere with a concavity for the lens. As aging occurs, the gellike structure becomes liquefied. In disease states such as diabetes, blood cells can be interspersed in the three-dimensional matrix, and the patient sees floaters. Or, in a dense vitreous hemorrhage, the patient experiences a loss of vision.

In visualizing the vitreous, the surgeon should start at the preoperative examination with dynamic ultrasound. Watch the movement of the vitreous with the epiretinal and periretinal membranes. Place the ultrasound probe at each clock hour of the retina to see the movement of the vitreous gel as the eye moves to the right, left, up, and down.

If there is a view of the vitreous and retina, the surgeon can use the Goldmann three-mirror lens to observe the peripheral vitreous, equator, midvitreous, and anterior vitreous. Consider the vitreous anatomy as one would enter the eye from anterior to posterior, using the Goldmann three-mirror lens. Take notes of various vitreous adhesions to retinal surfaces.

When examining the clear media in a patient with a traction retinal detachment from diabetic retinopathy, consider the anatomy of the vitreous and retina interface. Epiretinal membranes are white with a dull matte finish. The retina has a shiny, reflective sheen and is a slightly different shade of beige color than a white epiretinal membrane.

In cases of an incomplete posterior vitreous detachment, the epiretinal membrane will be attached at some places to the posterior hyaloid face. There will be areas where the tension of the vitreous gel pulls on the epiretinal membrane. This is an area of vitreous traction. It is at these "tension" points that microdissection and delamination can be initiated. These geometric forces can be seen by the preoperative examination.

The differences in the anterior-posterior direction of tension cause different types of epiretinal membrane formation. Tangential traction will cause starfolds and puckerlike folds. The most common type of epiretinal membrane in diabetic patients is anterior-posterior traction at sites of neovascularization and inflammation. The result is a plateau type of membrane structure.

In diabetic membranes, the epiretinal membrane may be pulling on the atrophic retina which has been thinned from lack of oxygen or chronic ischemia. These membranes look to be fully integrated with the retina. For these membranes, removing the anterior-posterior traction near the membrane or en bloc resection can be performed safely.

MEMBRANE PEELING

The posterior hyaloid can be identified with a soft-tipped silicone suction cannula. When suction is lightly applied, the cannula becomes occluded by the vitreous gel as the cannula is brought close to the retinal surface. The cortical vitreous can be seen with the staining techniques of intravitreal injection of the dye such as fluorescein, indocyanine green, or trypan blue. Triamcinolone with its particulate matter may also be injected following core vitrectomy. The particles become entangled in the cortical vitreous, thus "labeling" the vitreous and its interface with epiretinal membranes. Residual triamcinolone appears to be well tolerated but can be associated with ocular hypertension, cataract, and sterile uveitis. The cortical vitreous is then peeled from the inner retinal surface, creating a posterior vitreous detachment. This can be done with the suction cutting instrument or cannula using active suction (100 to 200 mm Hg) at the area next to the optic nerve where the retina is thick and strong, able to tolerate some tissue manipulation in the posterior-anterior direction. Alternatively, the use of a bent myringotomy blade in the dominant hand, or of a light pick in the nondominant hand, may be useful in this maneuver. With the creation of a posterior vitreous detachment, the surgeon can visualize a floating Weiss' ring. The vitrectomy is then completed, and removal of the posterior cortical vitreous is confirmed by the reaction of the brushing motion of the soft-tipped cannula.

Epiretinal membranes may be removed at this point using a bent myringotomy blade and intraocular forceps. Indirect ophthalmoscopy of the entire retina is performed to examine for iatrogenic retinal breaks and retinal detachments. Air-fluid exchange is then performed. Rapid accumulation of intravitreal fluid on the retinal surface usually occurs quickly, within the first 10 minutes after the air-fluid exchange. Therefore, many retinal surgeons allow at least 10 minutes to elapse before aspirating the accumulated intravitreal fluid. This technique would prepare for a maximal intravitreal gas bubble postoperatively. Face-down positioning is required postoperatively to provide retinal tamponade and repair of the diabetic traction retinal detachment.

A nonclearing vitreous hemorrhage in a diabetic patient is an indication for surgery. The timing of surgery is urgent if there is a traction retinal detachment threatening the macula. In the Diabetic Retinopathy Vitrectomy Study, vitreous hemorrhages were monitored for 6 months, however, that was in the era before optical coherence tomography (OCT) and before small incision vitrectomy surgery.

In many situations, vitrectomy for a diabetic patient is done within a few weeks of presentation to the ophthalmologist's office. In these cases, the patient is a poor historian and is unable to say how long he has had the loss of vision. In other cases, the patient already has rubeosis of the iris and/or neovascular glaucoma or that his activities of daily living are severely hampered.

The surgical intervention begins with the preoperative consent. The team of physicians, consulting internist, endocrinologist, cardiologist, and nephrologist need to be consulted. In the cases of severe proliferative diabetic retinopathy, it is important to have medical clearance

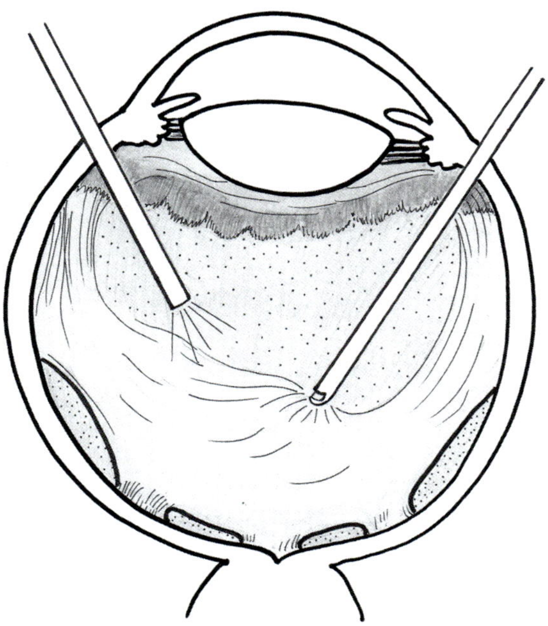

FIGURE 10-1. Core vitrectomy.

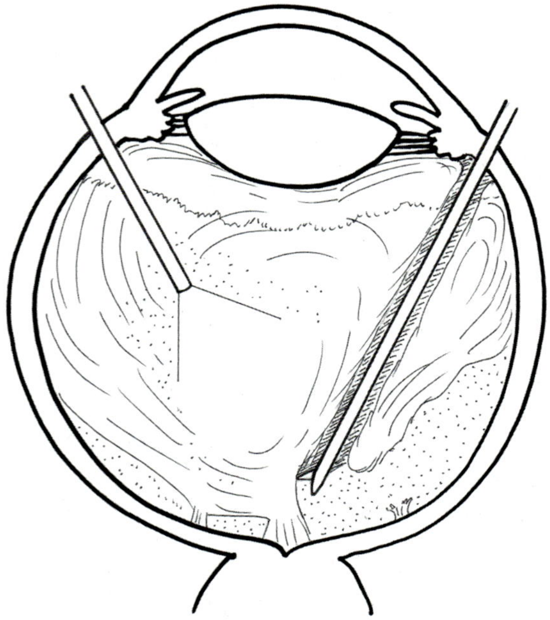

FIGURE 10-2. En bloc resection, step 1.

since the patient usually has other signs of systemic complications of diabetes. The most important risk factor for this patient is the cardiovascular risk factors. In fact, the need for diabetic vitrectomy surgery correlates with poor survival within 5 years of the surgery.[1]

In a core pars plana vitrectomy, where there is bright red, vitreous blood with ultrasonic evidence of attached retina, the light pipe can be used in the first part of the surgery to delineate the type of vitreous gel present. The vitreous can be dense clots or vitreous gel suffused with red blood cells. The light reflex shows the surgeon the texture of the vitreous (Fig. 10-1).

As the light pipe advances deeper into the posterior pole, the light reflections can help with the visualization of the vitreous gel and allow the surgeon to do en bloc dissection (Fig. 10-2). Using en bloc dissection, the vitreous gel, which is only partially detached, and the accompanying vitreoretinal membranes are removed as a single unit (see Fig. 10-2). Similarly, for new traction retinal detachment, membrane peeling and en bloc dissection techniques can be utilized (Fig. 10-3). While for some surgeons, the en bloc dissection

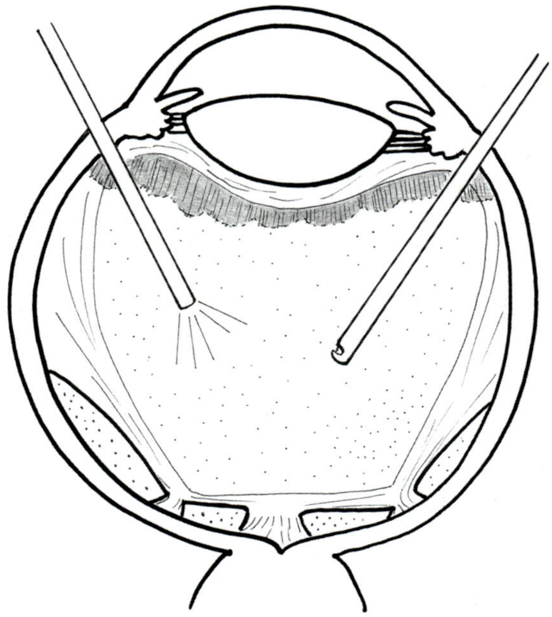

FIGURE 10-3. New traction retinal detachment, step 2.

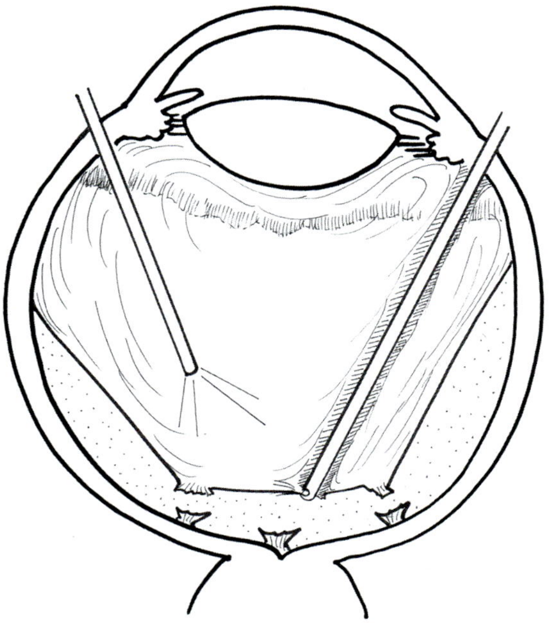

FIGURE 10-4. En bloc resection of traction retinal detachment.

technique serves to perform surgery with the minimal risk to the underlying retina (Fig. 10-4) because the countertraction of the vitreous gel enables the release of the adhesions of the membranes to the vitreous. All techniques utilize the fluidics of the vitrectomy probe, suction forces, and the response of the retina to the dissection techniques of the surgeon.

Other techniques include delamination and methods of releasing the focal vitreoretinal adhesion with localized truncation of the anterior vitreoretinal forces of membranes. If there are tangential adhesions, membrane peeling is a challenge: care must be taken to create a space between the underlying retina and the overlying membrane. In that space, safe removal of the membrane can be performed.

In summary, all safe membrane peeling revolves around the creation of a space between the underlying retina and the membrane. If possible, the membrane can be removed by the vitrectomy probe with its cutting and suction action, thereby removing traction. For diabetic traction retinal detachments, membrane peeling techniques are based on the least trauma to the underlying atrophic or abnormally vascularized retina. In diabetic traction retinal detachments, the surgeon is concerned about bleeding from the fibrovascular membranes as well.

Using the smaller gauge instrumentation for pars plana vitrectomy, a 23- or 25-gauge system makes the vitrectomy very simple and accessible. Postoperatively, the patient has an excellent cosmetic result. The 23-gauge system has many compatible forceps and tools that can be used with the 23-gauge port of entry.

Of note, if the vitreous hemorrhage is dense, full of red clots of blood or old discolored heme, the 23-gauge system and 25-gauge system will take longer to remove the blood than the 20-gauge system. However, with practice and patience, the surgery results will be the same. There is precise control of the cutting action and the suction with the use of the small caliber instrumentation, thus, most retinal surgeons have converted to the smaller gauge systems.

MEMBRANE PEELING FOR TRACTION RETINAL DETACHMENT

Once there is a traction retinal detachment of the macula, the clinician can measure the amount of traction with the OCT, fundus camera, and fluorescein angiography. There is usually a glial membrane that initiates the process of fibrovascular formation and consequent traction retinal detachment.

Traction retinal detachments occur after a vitreous hemorrhage or recurrent vitreous hemorrhage despite panretinal photocoagulation. These detachments are common and are common indications for pars plana vitrectomy with membrane peeling. Typically, the detachment is between the optic nerve and the macula.

There are two types of traction retinal detachment, (i) in the setting of active proliferative diabetic retinopathy, never having had panretinal laser photocoagulation and (ii) in the setting of multiple panretinal photocoagulation sessions. The first type is an active process where the fibrous bands have juicy red blood vessels and the retina that is being pulled upward and is encased in fresh, glistening glial tissue. This type of traction retinal detachment bleeds easily intraoperatively. Preoperatively, the retina surgeon could consider using intravitreal bevacizumab. The injection makes the activity of the blood vessels become less pronounced and hence less of an intraoperative bleeding hazard at the time of surgery.

The second type of traction retinal detachment, in the setting of old panretinal photocoagulation, is challenging because the surrounding tissue of the traction retinal detachment is thin and atrophic. Careful delamination is necessary rather than tissue manipulation of the atrophic retina. This type of thinned retina can lead to iatrogenic tears. Indirect membrane peeling using viscoelastic substances or silicon-tipped instruments are indicated for this type of traction retinal detachment repair.

At the time of vitrectomy surgery, while removing the blood, attention is paid to the anterior vitreous and then going more deeply into the posterior vitreous. At this point, the thickened vitreous at the periphery can be removed. For the peeling of the membrane, the process can start at the optic disc where the membrane is the thickest and then peeled across the papillomacular bundle, toward the fovea. Some surgeons like to start temporal to the macula and peel toward the fovea. The judgment of where to begin peeling depends on where the membrane is the thickest and where the surgeon can get the best control with the intraocular forceps to initiate the peeling. Bent 20-gauge needle is still a simple instrument to raise a membrane edge. There are diamond-tipped spatula needles as well.[2]

Delaminating scissors are useful for relieving the anterior-posterior traction. Various soft-tipped needles are useful in raising the edge in the membrane peeling process and continuing the peeling motion (Fig. 10-5).

If there are tangential adhesions, membrane peeling is a challenge: care must be taken to create a space between the underlying retina and the overlying membrane. In that space, safe removal of the membrane can be performed.

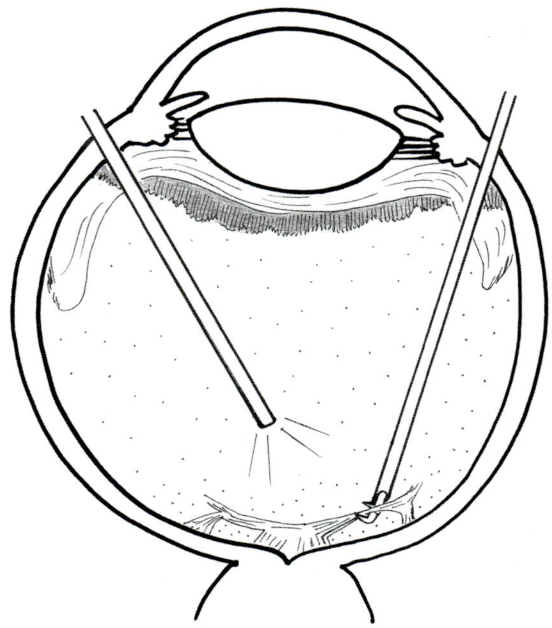

FIGURE 10-5. Membrane peeling with scissors.

In summary, all safe membrane peeling revolves around the creation of a space between the underlying retina and the membrane. If possible, the membrane can be removed by the vitrectomy probe with its cutting and suction action, thereby removing traction. For diabetic traction retinal detachments, membrane peeling techniques are based on the least trauma to the underlying atrophic or abnormally vascularized retina. In diabetic traction retinal detachments, the surgeon is concerned about bleeding from the fibrovascular membranes as well.

GENERAL INDICATIONS FOR VITRECTOMY

The obvious indication for vitrectomy is the presence of a nonclearing vitreous hemorrhage and/or the appearance of the traction retinal detachment as noted by the Diabetic Retinopathy Vitrectomy Study Research Group.[3] However, 30 years later, the indications have included refractory macular edema.[4] The diagnostic instrumentation, such as OCT and ultrasonography, has enabled earlier diagnosis of the vitreous-internal limiting membrane interface changes heralding traction retinal detachments. Thus, early surgical interventions are possible and are being met with great success (Table 10-1).

The Future

23- and 25-gauge Vitrectomy for Complex Vitreoretinal Disease

Machemer introduced pars plana vitrectomy with a 17-gauge vitrector, and in 1974, O'Malley created a 20-gauge vitreous cutter. In 1990, De Juan and Hickingbotham developed 25-gauge instruments for vitrectomy. These instruments allow for the creation of sclerotomy sites that are self-sealing and are sutureless.

The 25-gauge microcannular system includes a microcannula, an insertion trocar, an infusion cannula, a plug forceps, and a cannula plug. The microcannula consists of a thin-walled tube 3 to 4 mm in length with an outer diameter of approximately 0.55 to 0.60 mm. The insertion trocar has a sharp tip that has a continuous collar attached to the microcannula. This allows easy entry into the conjunctiva and sclera. The 25-gauge infusion cannula can be inserted into its microcannula. No sutures are needed.

The plugs are designed to fit into the microcannulas for temporary closure. The 25-gauge infusion cannula can be inserted into the microcannula system. No suture is needed.

A variety of instruments are designed for the 25-gauge system: a vitreous cutter, illumination probe, intraocular microforceps, rigid retinal pick, flexible and extendable retinal pick, microvitreoretinal blade, tissue manipulator, soft-tip cannula, and intraocular laser probe.

As of this writing, 23-gauge vitrectomy is commonplace among operating rooms of all vitreoretinal surgeons. Now, the 25-gauge vitrectomy procedure is becoming more common.[5–8]

Both the 23- and 25-gauge systems share advantages: sutureless vitrectomy surgery, less induced astigmatism, early recovery of visual acuity, and less postoperative pain.

There are new innovations in 25-gauge instruments. There is a 25-gauge vitreous forceps with a short length, only 28 mm. This forceps is three times as stiff as the standard

TABLE 10.1 Indications for Vitrectomy in Diabetic Eyes

Nonclearing vitreous hemorrhage
Nonclearing vitreous hemorrhage with a traction retinal detachment
Severe diffuse DME, refractory to laser photocoagulation
Severe diffuse DME with rapid loss of central vision

one used in 23-gauge instrumentation. A high-performance vitreous cutter is available, with the Accurus system.[9] The cutting rate, flow rate, and duty cycle of the vitrectomy probe are 2,500 cycles/minute, 7.30 mL/minute (cutter on) and 42% (full open time/total one cycle time). A 15-degree curved vitreous cutter is also useful for peripheral vitreous removal and delamination of the membranes that are located around the macular area. A 25-gauge diamond dusted membrane scraper and backflush instruments are available as well.

VITRECTOMY FOR DIABETIC MACULAR EDEMA

The vitreous is thought to play a role in the development of diabetic macular edema (DME).[10,11] DME causes vascular permeability via two proposed mechanisms: mechanical or physiologic. For years, surgical procedure is performed because of macular traction and abnormality of the posterior hyaloid. Literature has cited two possible reasons why vitrectomy is effective for the treatment of DME.[12–16] One reason is the physical release of the tractional forces that the vitreous gel exerts on the macula.[4] The other reason is that the vitrectomy improves the oxygenation of the macula, thereby decreasing its vascular permeability and subsequent resolution of DME.[15,16]

Stefansson et al. used oxygen sensors at the retinal surface, and they have found that retinal oxygen tension increases after the removal of vitreous gel, and the posterior pole becomes perfused by the oxygen rich aqueous humor.[15,16] The more rapid clearing of the growth factors in the vitrectomized eye has been postulated as a potential mechanism for this purpose. Supporting the hypothesis of Stefansson et al., the vascular endothelial growth factor (VEGF) is known to be up-regulated by hypoxia and down-regulated by increased oxygenation.[17] Thus, many authors speculate that vitrectomy improves oxygenation of the posterior segment, leading to down-regulation of VEGF, decreased vasopermeability, and decreased macular thickness.[18,19]

The Diabetic Retinopathy Clinical Research Network (DRCR.net) designed a prospective cohort study. As of December 2007, there were 241 eyes enrolled with DME. Eighty-five eyes met the criteria for primary cohort group with Snellen visual acuity of 20/63 to 20/400, OCT center subfield greater than 300 μm, and not undergoing cataract surgery at the time of vitrectomy. Median preoperative acuity for the 85 eyes was 20/80 with median OCT central subfield thickness of 413 μm. Indications for surgery include 49% unresponsive to DME therapies and 70% vitreomacular interface abnormalities. Fifty percent of the eyes had a surgery with a 25-gauge vitrectomy system. Epiretinal membranes were peeled in 61% of the cases. ILM was removed in 64% of the cases. Sixty-six percent of the cases had pharmacologic agents to visualize the membranes. Intraoperative laser was used in 54% of cases, and corticosteroids were injected into 68%.

Pars plana vitrectomy for refractory macular edema has been changed with the advent of bevacizumab. The use of bevacizumab has made it possible to treat severe macular edema as an adjunct to vitrectomy or as a "stand-alone" treatment. In Pendergast's article, the technique focused on the removal of the anterior-posterior traction caused by the ILM and vitreous interface.[4] With the use of bevacizumab in the treatment of diffuse DME, OCT central subfield thickness has been shown to decrease in some studies. As more DRCR.net results are published about vitrectomy for DME, more will be elucidated about the "taut premacular posterior hyaloid"[4] which plays a role in diffuse DME. The "taut premacular hyaloid" is usually attached to the ILM. Pendergast's original paper has reported 55 eyes of 50 diabetic patients with diffuse, clinically significant macular edema.[4] They had an average preoperative visual acuity of 20/160, and the final corrected visual acuity was 20/80. Eyes with 20/200 or worse preoperative vision responded less favorably to vitrectomy in the Pendergast study, thus suggesting further studies are needed for severe DME eyes. In the future, we may see additional multicentered, clinical, prospective trials which demonstrate the usefulness of bevacizumab for the severe macular edema eyes.

REFERENCES

1. Vote, BJ, Gamble GD, Polkinghorne, PJ. Auckland Proliferative Diabetic Vitrectomy Fellow Eye Study. *Clin Exp Ophthalmol.* 2004;32(4) 397–403.
2. Tolentino FA, Wu G. Diamond-dusted microspatula tips for vitreoretinal surgery. *Arch Ophthalmol.* 1987;105:1732–1733.
3. Diabetic Retinopathy vitrectomy Study Research Group. Early vitrectomy for severe vitreous hemorrhage in diabetic retinopathy; four year results of a randomized trial. *Arch Ophthalmol.* 1990;108:958–964.
4. Pendergast SD, Hassan TS, Williams GA, et al. Vitrectomy for diffuse diabetic macular edema associated with a taut premacular posterior hyaloid. *Am J Ophthalmol.* 2003;130:178–186.
5. Fujii GY, De Juan E Jr, Humayun MS, et al. Initial experience using the transconjunctival sutureless vitrectomy system for vitreoretinal surgery. *Ophthalmology.* 2002;109:1814–1820.
6. Ibarra MS, Hermel M, Prenner JL, et al. Long-term outcomes of transconjunctival sutureless 25 gauge vitrectomy. *Am J Ophthalmol.* 2005;139:831–839.
7. Oshima Y, Ohji M, Tano Y. Surgical outcomes of 25-gauge transconjunctival vitrectomy combined with cataract surgery for vitreoretinal disease. *Ann Acad Med Singapore.* 2006;35:175–180.
8. Okamoto F, Okamoto C, Sakata K, et al. Changes in corneal topography after 25-gauge transconjunctival sutureless vitrectomy versus after 20-gauge standard vitrectomy. *Ophthalmology.* 2007;114:2138–2141.
9. Fang SY, Humayun MS. Performance analysis of new generation vitreous cutters. *Graefes Arch Clin Exp Ophthalmol.* 2008;246:61–67.
10. Nasrallah FP, Van De Velde F, Jalkh AE, et al. Importance of the vitreous in young diabetics with macular edema. *Ophthalmology.* 1989;96:1511–1516.
11. Nasrallah FP, Jalkh AE, Van Coppenolle F, et al. The role of the vitreous in diabetic macular edema. *Ophthalmology.* 1988;95:1335–1339.
12. Lewis H, Abrams GW, Blumenkranz MS, et al. Vitrectomy for diabetic macular traction and edema associated with posterior hyaloidal traction. *Ophthalmology.* 1992;99:753–759.
13. Christoforidis JB, D'Amico DJ. Surgical and other treatments of diabetic macular edema: An update. *Int Ophthalmol Clin.* 2004;44:139–160.
14. Harbour JW, Smiddy WE, Flynn HW Jr, et al. Vitrectomy for diabetic macular edema associated with a thickened and taut posterior hyaloid membrane. *Am J Ophthalmol.* 1996;121:405–413.
15. Micelli Ferari T, Cardascia N, Durante G, et al. Pars plana vitrectomy in diabetic macular edema. *Doc Ophthalmol.* 1999;97:471–474.
16. Stefansson E, Novack RI, Hatchell D. Vitrectomy prevents retinal hypoxia in branch retinal vein occlusion. *Invest Ophthalmol Vis Sci.* 1990;31:284–289.
17. Stefansson E, Landers MBI, Wolbarsht ML. Increased retinal oxygen supply following pan-retinal photocoagulation and vitrectomy and lensectomy. *Trans Am Ophthalmol Soc.* 1981;79:307–334.
18. Aiello LP. Vascular endothelial growth factor and the eye: Biochemical mechanisms of action and implications for novel therapies. *Ophthalmic Res.* 1997;29:354–362.
19. Aiello LP, Avery R, Arrigg P, et al. Vascular endothelial growth factor in ocular fluid of patients with diabetic retinopathy and other retinal disorders. *N Engl J Med.* 1994;331:1480–1487.

SUGGESTED READINGS

1. Aiello LM, Wand M, Liang G. Neovascular glaucoma and vitreous hemorrhage following cataract surgery in patients with diabetes mellitus. *Am Acad Ophthalmol.* 1984;90:814–820.
2. American Academy of Ophthalmology. Preferred practice pattern. *Diabetic Retinopathy.* San Francisco, CA: American Academy of Ophthalmology; 1989.
3. Arevalo JF, Fromnow-Guerra J, Quiroz-Mercado H, et al. Pan American Collaborative Retina Study Group. Primary intravitreal bevacizumab (Avastin) for diabetic macular edema: Results from the Pan-American Collaborative Retina Study Group at 6-month follow-up. *Ophthalmology.* 2007;114:743–750.
4. Ashton N. The eye in malignant hypertension. *Trans Am Acad Ophthalmol Otolaryngol.* 1972;76:17–40.
5. Beethan WP. Diabetic retinopathy in pregnancy. *Trans Am Ophthalmol Soc.* 1950;48:205–219.
6. Blankenship GW. The lens influence on diabetic vitrectomy results. *Arch Ophthalmol.* 1980;98:2196–2198.
7. Blankenship GW. A clinical comparison of central and peripheral argon laser panretinal photocoagulation for proliferative diabetic retinopathy. *Ophthalmology.* 1988;95:170–177.
8. Blankenship GW, Flynn HW, Kokame GT. Posterior chamber intraocular lens insertion during pars plana lensectomy and vitrectomy for complications of proliferative diabetic retinopathy. *Am J Ophthalmol.* 1989;108:1–5.
9. Bresnick GH, Condit R, Syrjala S, et al. Abnormalities of the foveal avascular zone in diabetic retinopathy. *Arch Ophthalmol.* 1984;102:1286–1293.
10. Bresnick GH, Engerman R, Davis MD, et al. Patterns of ischemia in diabetic retinopathy. *Trans Am Acad Ophthalmol Otolaryngol.* 1976;81:694.
11. Diabetic Retinopathy Study Research Group. Photocoagulation treatment of proliferative diabetic retinopathy; the second report of diabetic retinopathy/vitrectomy study findings. *Am J Ophthalmol.* 1978;85:82–106.
12. Diabetic Retinopahty Study Research Group. Report no 14. Indication for photocoagulation treatment of diabetic retinopathy. *Int Ophthalmol Clin.* 1987;27:239–252.
13. Early Treatment Diabetic Retinopathy Study Research Group. Report no 9. Early photocoagulation for diabetic retinopathy. *Ophthalmology.* 1991;98:766–785.
14. Early Treatment Diabetic Retinopathy Study Research Group. Report no 12. Fundus photographic risk factors for progression of diabetic retinopathy. *Ophthalmology.* 1991;98:823–833.
15. Ferris FL, Podgor MJ, Davis MD. The Diabetic Retinopathy Study Research Group. Report no 12. Macular edema in diabetic retinopathy study patients. *Ophthalmology.* 1987;94:754–760.
16. Frienkel N, Dooley SL, Metzger BE. Care of the pregnant woman with insulin-dependent diabetes. *N Engl J Med.* 1985;313:96–101.

17. Gass JDM. Retinal capillary disease. In: *Stereoscopic Atlas of Macular Diseases*. St. Louis, MO: CV Mosby Co; 1987: 368–373.
18. Gass JDM, Norton EWD. Cystoid macular edema and papilledema following cataract extraction: A fluorescein funduscopic and angiographic study. *Arch Ophthalmol.* 1966;76:646–661.
19. Greenberg F, Lewis RA. Safety of fluorescein angiography during pregnancy [Letter]. *Am J Ophthalmol.* 1990;110:323–325.
20. Halperin LS, Olk RJ, Soubrane G, et al. Safety of fluorescein angiography during pregnancy. *Am J Ophthalmol.* 1990;109:563–566.
21. Hercules BL, Wozencroft M, Gayed II, Jeacock J. Peripheral retinal ablation in the treatment of proliferative diabetic retinopathy during pregnancy. *Br J Ophthalmol.* 1980;64:87–93.
22. Horvat M, Maclean H, Goldberg L, et al. Diabetic retinopathy in pregnancy: A 12-year prospective survey. *Br J Ophthalmol.* 1980;64:298–403.
23. Javitt JC, Aiello LP, Bassi LJ, et al. Detecting and treating retinopathy in patients with type I diabetes mellitus. *Ophthalmology.* 1991;98:1565–1574.
24. Johnson GP. Pregnancy and diabetic retinopathy. *Am J Ophthalmol.* 1980;90:519–524.
25. Klein, R. The epidemiology of diabetic retinopathy: Findings from the Wisconsin Epidemiologic Study of Diabetic Retinopathy. *Int Ophthalmol Clin.* 1987;27:230–238.
26. Klein R, Klein BEK, Moss SE, et al. The Wisconsin Epidemiologic Study of Diabetes Retinopathy. II. Prevalence and risk of diabetic retinopathy when age at diagnosis is less than 30 years. *Arch Ophthalmol.* 1984;102:520–526.
27. Klein R, Klein BEK, Moss SE, et al. The Wisconsin Epidemiologic Study of Diabetic Retinopathy. III. Prevalence and risk of diabetic retinopathy when age at diagnosis is 30 or more years. *Arch Ophthalmol.* 1984;102:527–532.
28. Klein R, Klein BEK, Moss SE, et al. The Wisconsin Epidemiologic Study of Diabetic Retinopathy. IV. Diabetic macular edema. *Ophthalmology.* 1984;91:1464–1474.
29. Klein R, Klein BEK, Moss SE, et al. The Wisconsin Epidemiologic Study of Diabetic Retinopathy. IX. Four-year incidence and progression of diabetic retinopathy when age at diagnosis is less than 30 years. *Arch Ophthalmol.* 1989;107: 237–242.
30. Klein R, Klein BEK, Moss SE, et al. The Wisconsin Epidemiologic Study of Diabetic Retinopathy. X. Four-year incidence and progression of diabetic retinopathy when age at diagnosis is 30 years or more. *Arch Ophthalmol.* 1989;107: 244–249.
31. Klein R, Klein BEK, Moss SE, et al. The Wisconsin Epidemiologic Study of Diabetic Retinopathy. XI. The incidence of macular edema. *Ophthalmology.* 1989;96:1501–1510.
32. Kleiner RC, Elman MJ, Murphy RP, et al. Transient severe visual loss after panretinal photocoagulation. *Am J Ophthalmol.* 1988;106:298–306.
33. Lee CM, Olk RJ. Modified grid laser photocoagulation for diffuse diabetic macular edema: Long-term visual results. *Ophthalmology.* 1991;98:1594–1602.
34. McDonald HR, Schatz H. Macular edema following panretinal photocoagulation. *Retina.* 1985;5:5–10.
35. McDonald HR, Schatz H. Visual loss following panretinal photocoagulation for proliferative diabetic retinopathy. *Ophthalmology.* 1985;92:388–393.
36. McEnery JK, Wong WP, Peyman GA. Evaluation of the teratogenicity of fluorescein sodium. *Am J Ophthalmol.* 1977;84:847–850.
37. Meyers SM. Macular edema after scatter laser photocoagulation for proliferative diabetic retinopathy. *Am J Ophthalmol.* 1980;90:210–216.
38. Moloney JB, Drury MI. The effect of pregnancy on the natural course of diabetic retinopathy. *Am J Ophthalmol.* 1982;93:745–756.
39. National Society to Prevent Blindness, Operational Research Department. *Vision Problems in the US: A Statistical Analysis.* New York: National Society to Prevent Blindness; 1980:1–46.
40. Ohrt V. The influence of pregnancy on diabetic retinopathy with special regard to the reversible changes shown in 100 pregnancies. *Acta Ophthalmol.* 1984;62:603–616.
41. Olk RJ. Modified grid argon (blue-green) laser photocoagulation for diffuse macular edema. *Ophthalmology.* 1986;93:938–950.
42. Olk RJ. Argon green (514 nm) versus krypton red (647 nm) modified grid laser photocoagulation for diffuse diabetic macular edema. *Ophthalmology.* 1990;97:1101–1113.
43. Phelps RL, Sakor P, Metzger BE, et al. Changes in diabetic retinopathy during pregnancy. *Arch Ophthalmol.* 1986;104:1806–1810.
44. Poliner LS, Christianson DJ, Escoffery RF, et al. Neovascular glaucoma after intracapsular and extracapsular cataract extraction in diabetic patients. *Am J Ophthalmol.* 1985;100:637–643.
45. Rice TA, Michels RG. Long term anatomic and functional results of vitrectomy for diabetic retinopathy. *Am J Ophthalmol.* 1980;90:297–303.
46. Rice TA, Michels RG, Maguire MG, et al. The effect of lensectomy on the incidence of iris neovascularization and neovascular glaucoma after vitrectomy for diabetic retinopathy. *Am J Ophthalmol.* 1983;95:1–11.
47. Salem H, Loux JJ, Smith S, et al. Evaluation of the toxicologic and teratogenic potentials of sodium fluorescein in the rat. *Toxicology.* 1979;12:143–150.
48. Shirai S, Majima A. Effects of fluorescein-sodium injected to mother mice on the embryo. *Folia Ophthalmol Jpn.* 1975;26:132–137.
49. Sinclair SH, Nesler C, Foxman B, et al. Macular edema and pregnancy in insulin-dependent diabetes. *Am J Ophthalmol.* 1984;97:154–167.
50. Stark WJ Jr, Maumenee AE, Fagadau W, et al. Cystoid macular edema in pseudophakia. *Surv Ophthalmol.* 1984;28: 442–451.
51. Sunness JS. The pregnant woman's eye. *Surv Ophthalmol.* 1988;32:219–238.
52. Ticho U, Patz A. The role of capillary perfusion in the management of diabetic macular edema. *Am J Ophthalmol.* 1973;76:880–886.
53. Tso MOM, Jampol LM. Pathophysiology of hypertensive retinopathy. *Ophthalmologica.* 1982;89:1132.
54. White P. Pregnancy and diabetes, medical aspects. *Med Clin North Am.* 1965;49:1015–1024.
55. Yannuzzi LA, Roher KT, Tindel LJ, et al. Fluorescein angiography complication survey. *Ophthalmology.* 1986;93:611.

CHAPTER 11

Diabetes in Pregnancy

Hyperglycemia affects 8% of all pregnancies in America.[1] Preexisting diabetes affects 1% of all pregnancies. The hyperglycemia exists with Type 1 diabetes or gestational Type 2 diabetes. During the first trimester of pregnancy, hyperglycemia is associated with higher risk of spontaneous abortion and fetal malformations. In the third trimester, hyperglycemia increases the risk of macrosomia and metabolic complications at birth, increased incidence of caesarean section, and increased admission rates to newborn intensive care units. Risk of these birth complications is proportional to the degree of maternal hyperglycemia (Table 11-1).

PATHOPHYSIOLOGY

Maternal Fetal Metabolism in Normal Pregnancy

With each meal, the pregnant woman experiences a complex set of maternal hormonal actions: rise in blood glucose, followed by secondary secretion of pancreatic insulin, glucagons, somatomedins, and adrenal catecholamines. Pregnant women develop hypoglycemia between meals and during sleep because the fetus continues to draw glucose across the placenta from the maternal bloodstream even during periods of fasting. Interprandial hypoglycemia increases as the pregnancy progresses and the glucose demand of the fetus increases.

Placental steroid and peptide hormones (estrogens, progesterone, and chorionic somatomammotropin) rise throughout the second and third trimesters. In the later stages of pregnancy, the levels of these hormones rise, creating increasing tissue insulin resistance despite increased insulin secretion, a response to the increased feeding. The mean insulin levels are 50% higher in the third trimester compared to the nonpregnant state[2] (Tables 11-2 and 11-3).

The Diabetic Pregnancy

If the maternal pancreatic insulin response cannot meet the needs of the increased feeding, then maternal and fetal hyperglycemia is the end result. The recurrent postprandial hyperglycemia is a cause for the increased growth of the fetus, leading to macrosomia. The episodes of maternal and fetal hyperglycemia are accompanied by fetal hyperinsulinemia. Fetal hyperinsulinemia promotes excessive nutrient storage, resulting in macrosomia. The fetal conversion of excess glucose into fat causes a depletion of fetal oxygen levels. The relative fetal hypoxia causes surges in adrenal catecholamines which in turn causes hypertension, cardiac hypertrophy, erythropoietin stimulation, red cell hyperplasia, and increased hematocrit. Polycythemia with a hematocrit over 65% occurs in 5% to 10% of newborns with diabetic mothers. This finding appears to be related to the level of glycemic control and level of fetal hypoxia. Elevated hematocrit in the neonate leads to poor circulation and hyperbilirubinemia.[3]

TABLE 11.1 Risk Factors for Type 1 Pregnant Diabetic Patients

Acceleration of diabetic retinopathy
1. Elevated HbA1c
2. Longer duration of diabetes
3. Higher systolic blood pressure

In the United States, 23.6 million people or approximately 7% of the population have diabetes. Another 6 to 7 million may be undiagnosed. An additional 57 million Americans are prediabetic and will become diabetic.[4] While 3% to 10% of all pregnancies are complicated by diabetes, 90% of the diabetic pregnancies are due to gestational diabetes. The remaining 8% of the diabetic pregnancies are due to preexisting, insulin resistant or Type 2 diabetes.[3]

Diabetic Retinopathy in Pregnancy

The National Eye Institute (NEI), a division of the National Institutes of Health, states that "…during pregnancy, diabetic retinopathy may be a problem for women with diabetes. To protect vision, every pregnant woman with diabetes should have a comprehensive dilated eye exam as soon as possible." In addition, the NEI also recommends that "your doctor may recommend additional exams during your pregnancy."[5] Thus, the official recommendations of National Institute of Health, an agency of the U.S. Department of Health and Human Services, suggest that diabetic pregnant women have dilated retinal exams. Studies involving diabetic retinopathy and pregnancy have shown that in Type 1 diabetic patients, elevated HbA1c, longer duration of diabetes, and higher systolic blood pressure were correlated with the progression of retinopathy[5–7] (Table 11-4).

Gestational Diabetes Mellitus

Epidemiology

Gestational Diabetes Mellitus (GDM) is a condition in which women without previously diagnosed diabetes exhibit high blood glucose levels during pregnancy. Gestational diabetes has few symptoms, and is commonly diagnosed by fasting blood sugar (FBS) screening during pregnancy. Gestational diabetes affects 3% to 10% of pregnancies.

Factors in the apparent increase in GDM are varied. Prevalence of obesity in youth is thought to be due to low levels of physical activity and high levels of caloric intake. There is improved survival of female infants whose birth weights are at the extremes of the normal range. As adults, these infants will have altered insulin action and/or insulin secretory

TABLE 11.2 The Risk Factors for GDM

1. Previous history of GDM, prediabetes, impaired glucose tolerance, and impaired fasting glycemia.
2. Family history with first-degree relative with Type 2 diabetes
3. Maternal age (women over age 35)
4. Ethnic background: African Americans, Afro-Caribbeans, Native Americans, Hispanics, Asians, Pacific Islanders, and South Asian Indians of the India subcontinent
5. Overweight and obesity
6. Previous pregnancy which resulted in a child with high birth weight ≥4,000 g
7. Smokers
8. Polycystic ovarian syndrome

TABLE 11.3 Risk Factors for Pregnant Diabetic Patients

Acceleration of diabetic retinopathy
Lipid profiles (cholesterol and triglycerides)
Glycemic control over the course of her 9-month gestation
Level of diabetic retinopathy in the first trimester will progress into the third trimester. Hypertension status
Kidney status.

capacity that may predispose them to the development of GDM. Birth weight history may be helpful in the risk assessment of GDM.[8]

No specific cause has been identified, but it is believed that the hormones produced during pregnancy increase insulin resistance resulting in impaired glucose tolerance. The action of insulin as it binds to the insulin receptor is thought to be affected by pregnancy hormones.[2] The interference of insulin receptor binding probably occurs at the level of the cells signaling pathway at the insulin receptor. Since insulin promotes the entry of glucose into the cell, insulin resistance prevents glucose from entering the cell and as a result, glucose remains in the blood stream. Plasma glucose levels rise and more insulin is needed to overcome this resistance. In a normal pregnancy, insulin is produced at 1.5 to 2.5 times the normal nonpregnant state.

Insulin resistance is a normal occurrence in the second trimester of pregnancy, which then progresses to levels seen in nonpregnant patients with Type 2 diabetes in the third trimester. Women with GDM have an insulin resistance that is not compensated with increased production of insulin in the beta cells of the pancreas.[2] Placental hormones and to a lesser extent, increased fat deposits during pregnancy seem to mediate insulin resistance during pregnancy. Cortisol and progesterone are the main culprits, but human placental lactogen, prolactin, and estradiol are contributing factors to insulin resistance during pregnancy.[2]

It is postulated that there is a chronic beta-cell defect that is present in the prepregnancy and postpregnancy states and is accompanied by increasing blood glucose concentration. Thus, at the time of the diagnosis of GDM, some of the women may have had preexisting glucose intolerance that is demonstrated by glucose tolerance screening in pregnancy.

While it is unclear why some patients are unable to balance insulin needs and develop GDM, a number of explanations have been given, similar to those with Type 2 diabetes: obesity, autoimmunity, and gene mutations. In one study evaluating Pima Indian women with diabetes during pregnancy, the authors find that the 68 children of 49 mothers who had diabetes during pregnancy have a higher prevalence of obesity than the 541 control children born of 134 women who were prediabetic or than the 1,326 children of 446 mothers who remained nondiabetic. At 15 to 19 years of age, 58% of the offspring of diabetics weigh 140% or more of their desirable weight as compared with 25% of the of the prediabetics and 17% of the offspring of nondiabetics. Obesity in the children is directly related to maternal diabetes. The findings suggest that prenatal environment

TABLE 11.4 Diabetic Pregnancy Guidelines

American association of clinical endocrinologists
HbA1c < 6%
FBS range: 60 and 90 mg/dL
1 hr postprandial plasma glucose ≤120 mg/dL.

Source: Moloney JB, Drury MI. The effect of pregnancy on the natural course of diabetic retinopathy. *Am J Ophthalmol.* 1982;93:745–756.

of the offspring of diabetic women results in the development of obesity in childhood and adolescence.[9] Several humoral autoimmune markers have been found in GDM, islet cell antibodies (ICA) and ICA+ patients have poor glucose tolerance. Antibodies against glutamic acid decarboxylase (GAD) are detected in sera of Type 1 diabetics before and at the onset of the disease. In the study by Falluca et al.,[10] GAD positivity was found in 3.6% of 83 GDM patients and 3.8% of 79 Type 2 diabetic pregnant women and none of the 64 pregnant nondiabetic women. These results suggest that the two diabetic pregnant populations have the same disposition to develop Type 1 diabetes and are likely to share the same disease.[10]

Genetic predisposition to GDM has been suggested since GDM clusters in families. Women with mutations in MODY (maturity onset diabetes of the young) genes often present with GDM. Common variants in several candidate genes (potassium inwardly rectifying channel subfamily J, member 11 (KCNJ11) glucokinase (GCK), hepatocyte nuclear factor-1 alpha (HNFIA) have been demonstrated to increase the risk of GDM.[11]

Risk Factors for Gestational Diabetes Mellitus

Prevalence of gestational diabetes is related to the patient's race and culture. Prevalence rates are higher in African, Hispanic, Native American, and Asian women than in white women. Only 1.5% to 2% of Caucasian women develop GDM, whereas Native Americans from the Southwestern region of the United States have rates as high as 15%. In Hispanic, African American and Asian populations, the incidence is 5% to 8%. In these high-risk populations, the recurrence risk with future pregnancies has been reported as high as 68%. In patients with gestational diabetes, their risk of developing diabetes later in life is approximately 20% to 50%.[5] In a study of Navajo women, the risk of diabetes after GDM was estimated to be 50% to 70% after 11 years.[5,12,13]

All patients with gestational Type 2 diabetes should be advised to have medical nutritional therapy at the time of diagnosis. Medical nutrition therapy should focus on food choices that allow for adequate energy intake to provide appropriate weight gain, normoglycemia, and the absence of ketones.

While weight loss during pregnancy is not recommended, obese or overweight women with gestational Type 2 diabetes may benefit from modest exercise and carbohydrate restriction. Given the stringent glycemic targets suggested during pregnancy, the patient should monitor blood glucose frequently and maintain a dietary log. The record of the patient's meals will provide useful information about the patient's dietary compliance to the obstetrician, endocrinologist, and nutritionist.

In the first trimester, the gestational diabetic patient may be sent to the ophthalmologist or retinal specialist for an evaluation. Baseline examination and fundus photographs are useful for documentation. While gestational diabetic patients usually do not have diabetic retinopathy in the first trimester, they can develop loss of vision as their diabetes worsens. At that point, additional ophthalmic follow-up is needed. Specifically, if the patient has symptoms such as decreased vision while reading or transient visual loss, increasing levels of HbA1c or worsening glycemic control, or elevated systolic blood pressure, she may be at risk for retinal changes. Thus, she may need more frequent follow-up with an ophthalmologist.

In a pregnant patient with existing diabetic retinopathy, her retinopathy frequently worsens during pregnancy.[14] Even in prepregnancy planning, these women patients with known diabetic retinopathy should be seen by a retinal specialist. They should be counseled on their risk of developing diabetic retinopathy. They should also be told that their diabetic retinopathy can worsen during pregnancy unless they aim for glycemic control and good nutritional habits.

In a pregnant patient with a duration of diabetes of 15 years or more, they will need to see a retinal specialist.[14] At the minimum, this type of patient will have mild nonproliferative diabetic retinopathy (NPDR) that will progress by the third trimester. For this group of patients, watch for clinically significant macular edema that may necessitate laser. By the time of delivery, these groups of patients require follow-up care until they stop breast feeding. Encourage them to do Amsler grid testing at home. They should be instructed to return to the retinal specialist's office if there is deterioration of vision on Amsler grid testing in the postpartum period.

Women with diabetes who become pregnant should have a dilated fundus examination in the first trimester and followed as closely as needed. They should be seen in every trimester by a retinal specialist.

Ask the patient to send her HbA1c and FBSs to the ophthalmologist as well.[14] If the HbA1c rises over 7.0 and then to 7.5, then with every 0.5% climb with each trimester, the patient will be at risk for acceleration of her diabetic retinopathy.[14] It is important to be wary of new changes of her retinal status. She may be developing background diabetic retinopathy or mild NPDR with macular edema if her FBSs rise along with HbA1c.

During the first trimester of pregnancy, hyperglycemia increases the risk of spontaneous abortion and fetal malformation. Later in pregnancy, hyperglycemia increases the risk of macrosomia and metabolic complications at birth. According to the guidelines from the American Academy of Clinical Endocrinologists, the pregnant diabetic patient should ideally have a HbA1c ≤6%, fasting blood glucose <125 mg/dL, and nonfasting plasma glucose <200 mg/dL.[15]

The American Diabetes Association guidelines suggest FBS < 95 mg/dL, 1 hour postprandial <140 mg/dL, 2 hour postprandial glucose of <120 mg/dL. Blood pressure should be maintained <130/80 mm Hg.[15,16]

In addition, ask the patient for a copy of her lipid profiles. This information would allow the ophthalmologist to watch for any large increases in cholesterol and triglycerides between the first and third trimester. If the patient has diabetic retinopathy, the rise in lipid profiles will add to the hard exudates formation that can occur in the retina.

For the pregnant diabetic patient, the severity of her retinopathy will be dependent on her glycemic control over the course of her 9-month gestation. Whatever the level of diabetic retinopathy in the first trimester, there will be a progression into the third trimester. The progression can be mild or moderate or severe depending on the patient's level of glycemic control and her overall health. Contributing factors are her hypertension status and kidney status.

Macular Edema

Macular edema can present at any stage of the diabetic pregnancy. The edema can be quite severe and can require laser in the first, second, and third trimesters (Figs. 11-1–11-7).

Progression of Diabetes can be Rapid between First and Second Trimester

Rapid progression of diabetic retinopathy can occur in patients who have had juvenile onset diabetes and are now pregnant. Patients can progress from quiescent proliferative diabetic retinopathy (PDR) to newly aggressive PDR during the pregnancies.[17,18]

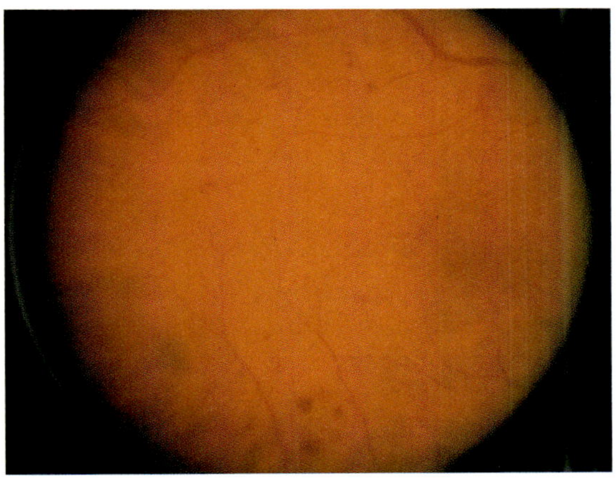

FIGURE 11-1. Pregnant Type 1 diabetic patient, 37-year-old female G0P1 for evaluation, Type 1 diabetes 10 years, first trimester vision 20/40 OU, Photo OD, dot blot hemorrhages, macular edema.

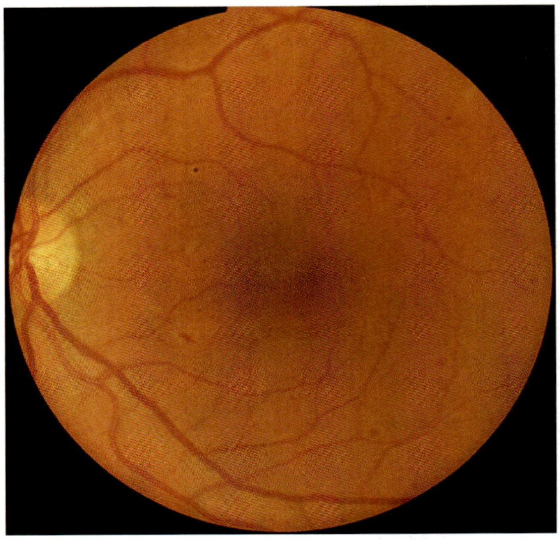

FIGURE 11-2. First trimester, V 20/80 OS, Photo OS, dot blot hemorrhages, macular edema, flame-shaped hemorrhage along inferotemporal arcade.

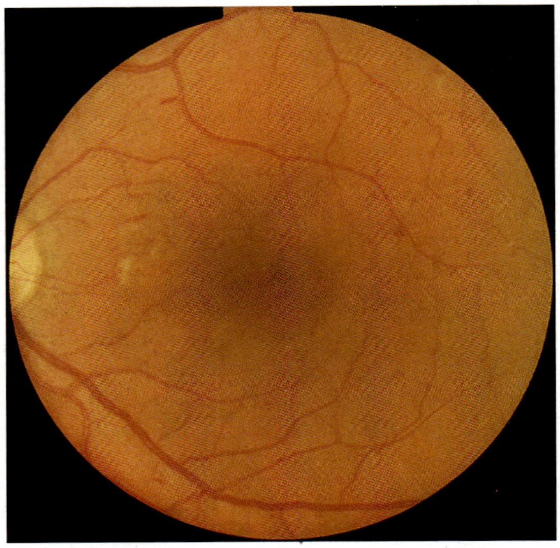

FIGURE 11-3. Second trimester, Photo OS, new cotton-wool spot is noted in addition to the hemorrhages.

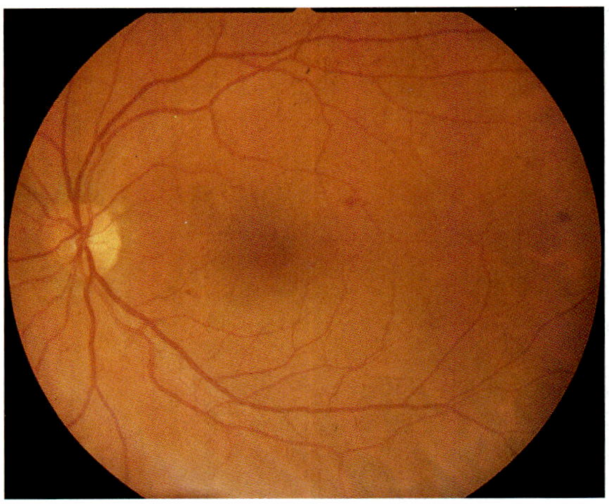

FIGURE 11-4. Six months postpartum, V 20/20 OS, Photo OS, note the resolution of the hemorrhages and cotton-wool spot.

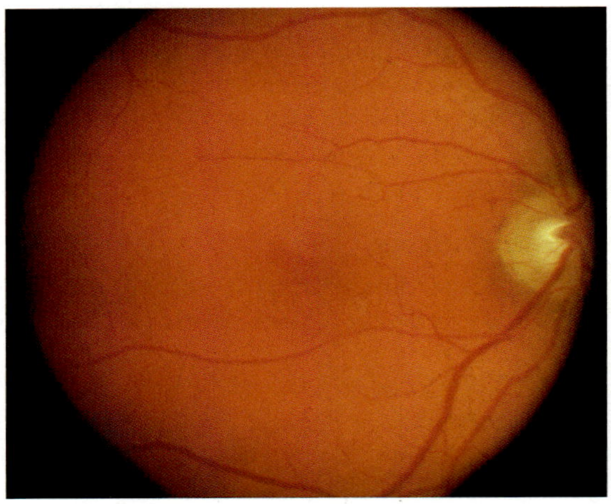

FIGURE 11-5. A 40-year-old female, G1P0 with Type 1 diabetes for 15 years, first trimester, V 20/40 OD, Photo OD, clinically significant macular edema noted. She refused laser.

Additional panretinal photocoagulation may be necessary for these patients. There can be sites of bleeding from areas of neovascularization which develop as the pregnancy progresses.

Proliferative Diabetic Retinopathy in a Pregnant Diabetic Patient

For the pregnant patient with PDR, consider immediate laser panretinal photocoagulation. Suggest monthly follow-up visits to monitor her progress. It is not unusual to see vitreous hemorrhage during the second trimester of pregnancy when the pregnancy hormones are maximal and there is maximal insulin resistance. In the Diabetes and Early Pregnancy Study, Chew et al.[19] studied 155 diabetic women from the preconception period to early postpartum period of 1 month. They found that 6.3% developed PDR when they initially

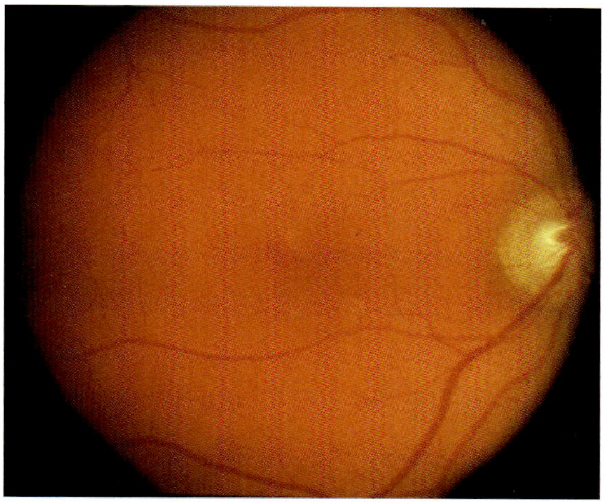

FIGURE 11-6. One month later, V 20/60, clinically significant macular edema seen.

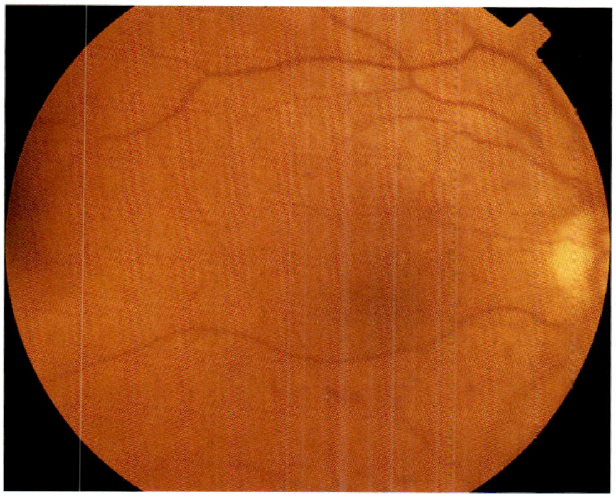

FIGURE 11-7. A 39-year-old female, Type 1 diabetes for 20 years, G1P0, V 20/40 OD, first trimester, Photos OD, dot blot hemorrhages, cotton-wool spots, clinically significant macular edema seen.

presented at preconception baseline with mild NPDR. However, 29% of the pregnant women developed diabetic retinopathy if their preconception examination showed moderate to severe NPDR.[19] Thus, diabetic patients planning their pregnancies should aim for optimal control of their diabetes before pregnancy.

Traction Retinal Detachment in a Pregnant Diabetic Patient

Traction retinal detachment in a pregnant diabetic patient is a rare complication. Approximately 6.25% of eyes in one study manifest the complication of PDR associated with a traction retinal detachment.[17] These patients are usually Type 1 diabetic patients who have had poor prenatal care. These patients will have a severe and accelerated course of diabetic retinopathy during gestation.

Predictors of Progression of Retinopathy

In the literature, pregnant diabetic patients who present with no or mild background diabetic retinopathy at the onset of pregnancy can progress to a worse state of disease. The rate of progression ranges from 8%[18] to 21%.[19] Some authors cite a progression rate of 25%.[20] In the Diabetes in Early Pregnancy Study, 140 patients without PDR were studied at preconception.[19] Fundus photographs were taken within 5 weeks of conception. Of these 140 patients, 10.3% progressed to retinopathy even if at baseline examination they had no diabetic retinopathy. In the group of pregnant patients with mild NPDR showing microaneurysms only, progression occurred in 21.1%. If the baseline was mild NPDR, 18.8% showed progression.

However, in patients with moderate to severe nonproliferative diabetic retinopathy at baseline, they had a 54% risk of progressive changes.[19] Glycemic control is an important predictor of progression of diabetic retinopathy.[21]

In addition, for pregnant diabetic patients, a rapid near normalization of glycemic control by continuous subcutaneous insulin infusion can accelerate progress of retinopathy in poorly controlled diabetic patients.[22] In Laatikainen's study, the diabetic pregnant patients who progressed were characterized by long duration of Type 1 diabetes (>15 years) and poor HbA1c at presentation (HbA1c >7%). The study shows that 65% of patients with frank retinopathy at onset of pregnancy continued to progress to worse retinopathy. Also there was a degree of symmetry both in the development of diabetic retinopathy and the final outcome. Thus, changes in the first eye serve as a predictor for the progression of retinopathy in the second eye.

POST PARTUM

Regression of diabetic retinopathy is thought to occur in the postpartum period (see Figs. 11-1–11-5). Thus in some instances, greater than 80% progress occurs during the postpartum period all within the first 8 weeks of the postpartum period.[17] Some patients fail to receive prior photocoagulation during their pregnancy for their proliferative disease because the treating ophthalmologist believes that regression would normally occur postpartum. Unfortunately, those patients go on to have aggressive PDR that develop into vitreous hemorrhage, traction retinal detachment, and neovascular glaucoma.[20]

SURGICAL MANAGEMENT DURING PREGNANCY

The most common indications for surgery are nonclearing vitreous hemorrhage, traction retinal detachment, combined rhegmatogenous retinal detachment and traction retinal detachment, and neovascular glaucoma. There are technical challenges in managing the pregnant patient for surgery. She may need local anesthesia. In addition, the pregnant woman has to be lying down on her back, pressing on her vena cava, during the surgery. This position may be uncomfortable for the pregnant patient. In addition, repeated surgery may be required and then there is the question of repeated anesthesia for the pregnant patient and the unborn fetus. General anesthesia is recommended for the patient in the latter part of the second trimester or third trimester of pregnancy. Anesthetic agents are to be avoided during the organogenesis of the first trimester of pregnancy.

REFERENCES

1. ACOG technical bulletin. Diabetes and pregnancy. Number 200. Committee on Technical Bulletins of the American College of Obstetricians and Gynecologists. *Int J Gynaecol Obstet.* 1995;48:331–339.
2. Goldstein BJ. *The Patient with Type 2 Diabetes.* Newtown: Handbooks in Health Care Co.; 2008.
3. Moore TR, Warshak C. *Diabetes Mellitus and Pregnancy.* http://emedicine.medscape.com/article/127547-overview. Accessed 1 March 2009.
4. http://www.diabetes.org/diabetes-statistics/cost-of-diabetes-in-us.jsp. Accessed 1 March 2009.
5. http://www.nei.nih.gov/health/diabetic/retinopathy.asp. Accessed 24 January 2009.
6. Axer-Siegel R, Hod M, Fink-Cohen S, et al. Diabetic retinopathy during pregnancy. *Ophthalmology.* 1996;103:1815–1819.
7. Moloney JB, Drury MI. The effect of pregnancy on the natural course of diabetic retinopathy. *Am J Ophthalmol.* 1982;93:745–756.
8. Metzger BE, Buchanan TA, Coustan DR, et al. Summary and recommendations of the fifth international workshop-conference of gestational diabetes mellitus. *Diabetes Care.* 2007;30:S251–S260.
9. Pettitt DJ, Baird HR, Aleck KA, et al. Excessive obesity in offspring of Pima Indian women with diabetes during pregnancy. *N Engl J Med.* 1983;308:242–245.
10. Falluca F, Tibert C, Torresi P, et al. Autoimmune markers of diabetes in diabetic pregnancy. *Ann Ist Super Sanita.* 1997;33:425–428.
11. Shaat N, Group L. Genetics of gestational diabetes mellitus. *Curr Med Chem.* 2007;14:569–583.
12. Kim C, Newton KM, Knopp RH. Gestational diabetes and the incidence of Type 2 diabetes: A systematic review. *Diabetes Care.* 2002;25(10):1862–1868.
13. Steinhart JR, Sugarman JR, Connell FA. Gestational diabetes is a herald of NIDDM in Navajo women. High rate of abnormal glucose tolerance after GDM. *Diabetes Care.* 1997;20(6):943–947.
14. Klein BE, Moss SE, Klein R. Effect of pregnancy on progression of diabetic retinopathy. *Diabetes Care.* 1990;13:34–40.
15. AACE Diabetes Mellitus Clinical Practice Guidelines Task Force. American Association of Clinical Endocrinologists medical guidelines for clinical practice for the management of diabetes mellitus. *Endocr Pract.* 2007;13(suppl 1):S3–S68.
16. American Diabetes Association. Standards of medical care in diabetes—2007. *Diabetes Care.* 2007;30(suppl 1):S4–S41.
17. Chan WC, Lim LT, Quinn M J, et al. Management and outcome of sight-threatening diabetic retinopathy in pregnancy. *Eye.* 2004;18:826–832.
18. Rodman H, Singerman LJ, Aiello L, et al. Diabetic retinopathy and its relationship to pregnancy. In: Merkaty T, Adams P, eds. *The Diabetic Pregnancy: A Perinatal Perspective.* New York: Grune & Stratton; 1979.
19. Chew EY, Mills JL, Metzger BE, et al. Metabolic control and the progression of retinopathy: The diabetes in early pregnancy study. *Diabetes Care.* 1995;18:631–637.
20. Chan WC, Lim LT, Quinn MJ, et al. Management and outcome of sight-threatening diabetic retinopathy in pregnancy. *Eye.* 2004;18:826–832.

21. Finnlauszus J, Klebe G. Diabetic retinopathy in pregnancy during tight metabolic control. *Acta Obstet Gynecol Scand.* 2001;79:367–370.
22. Laatikainen L, Teramo K, Hieta-Heikurainen H, Koivisto V, Pelkonen R. A controlled study of the influence of continuous subcutaneous insulin infusion treatment on diabetic retinopathy during pregnancy. *Acta Med Scand.* 1987;221:367–376.

SUGGESTED READINGS

1. Beethan WP. Diabetic retinopathy in pregnancy. *Trans Am Ophthalmol Soc.* 1950;48:205–219.
2. Best RM, Chakravarthy U. Diabetic retinopathy in pregnancy. *Br J Ophthalmol.* 1997;81:249–251.
3. Dibble CM, Kochenour NK, Worley RJ, et al. Effect of pregnancy on diabetic retinopathy. *Obstet Gynecol.* 1982;59:699–704.
4. Frienkel N, Dooley SL, Metzger BE. Care of the pregnant woman with insulin- dependent diabetes. *N Engl J Med.* 1985;313:96–101.
5. Greenberg F, Lewis RA. Safety of fluorescein angiography during pregnancy [Letter]. *Am J Ophthalmol.* 1990;110:323–325.
6. Halperin LS, Olk RJ, Soubrane G, et al. Safety of fluorescein angiography during pregnancy. *Am J Ophthalmol.* 1990;109:563–566.
7. Horvat M, Maclean H, Goldberg L, et al. Diabetic retinopathy in pregnancy: A 12-year prospective survey. *Br J Ophthalmol.* 1980;64:298–403.
8. Johnson GP. Pregnancy and diabetic retinopathy. *Am J Ophthalmol.* 1980;90:519–524.
9. Laatikainen L, Larinkari J, Teramo K. Occurrence and prognostic significance of retinopathy in diabetic pregnancy. *Metab Paediatr Ophthalmol.* 1980;4:191–195.
10. Maloney JB, Drury MI. The effect of pregnancy on the natural course of diabetic retinopathy. *Am J Ophthalmol.* 1982;93:745–756.
11. McEnery JK, Wong WP, Peyman GA. Evaluation of the teratogenicity of fluorescein sodium. *Am J Ophthalmol.* 1977;84:847–850.
12. Ohrt V. The influence of pregnancy on diabetic retinopathy with special regard to the reversible changes shown in 100 pregnancies. *Acta Ophthalmol.* 1984;62:603–616.
13. Phelps RL, Sakol P, Metzger BE, et al. Changes in diabetic retinopathy during pregnancy. Correlations with regulation of hyperglycaemia. *Arch Ophthalmol.* 1986;104:1806–1810.
14. Price JH, Hadden DR, Archer DB, Harley JM. Diabetic retinopathy in pregnancy. *Br J Obstet Gynaecol.* 1984;91:11–17.
15. Rosenn B, Miodovnik M, Kranias G, et al. Progression of diabetic retinopathy in pregnancy: Association with hypertension in pregnancy. *Am J Obstet Gynecol.* 1992;166:1214–1218.
16. Salem H, Loux JJ, Smith S, et al. Evaluation of the toxicologic and teratogenic potentials of sodium fluorescein in the rat. *Toxicology.* 1979;12:143–150.
17. Serup L. Influence of pregnancy on diabetic retinopathy. *Acta Endocrinol (Copenh).* 1986;22(Suppl):122–124.
18. Shirai S, Majima A. Effects of fluorescein-sodium injected to mother mice on the embryo. *Folia Ophthalmol Jpn.* 1975;26:132–137.
19. Sinclair SH, Nesler C, Foxman B, et al. Macular edema and pregnancy in insulin-dependent diabetes. *Am J Ophthalmol.* 1984;97:154–167.
20. Sunness JS. The pregnant woman's eye. *Surv Ophthalmol.* 1988;32:219–238.
21. The Diabetes Control, Complications Trial Research Group. Effect of pregnancy on microvascular complications in the diabetes control and complications trial. *Diabetes Care.* 2000;23:1084–1091.
22. White P. Pregnancy and diabetes, medical aspects. *Med Clin North Am.* 1965;49:1015–1024.
23. Yannuzzi LA, Roher KT, Tindel LJ, et al. Fluorescein angiography complication survey. *Ophthalmology.* 1986;93:611.

CHAPTER 12

Complications

PATIENT EXPECTATIONS AND PATIENT EDUCATION

Patients with severe visual loss despite successful surgery can be depressed and despondent because of their postoperative recovery period. In addition, these patients may have to change their activities of daily living and rearrange their work schedules to accommodate their visual rehabilitation schedule.[1] During this time, it is important to address the patients' short-term and long-term expectations. At this time, if the clinician senses that the patient feels morose or pensive about his long-term prognosis of visual recovery, the clinician can suggest a consultation with a social worker, psychologist, or psychiatrist. It is important that postoperative patients have support systems or else their sense of despair can turn into anger. The anger then turns into litigious behavior.[2]

Health Literacy

Functional literacy or the ability to understand the complex maneuvers in traction retinal detachment and vitrectomy surgery is important. In a study with 402 patients with diabetes and hypertension, 92% of the patients understood that blood pressure of 160/100 mm Hg is "high" compared to 55% of patients with poor literacy skills. Functional illiteracy is a problem in educating patients about chronic diseases and their health outcomes.[3]

In another study involving 408 patients with Type 2 diabetes, the authors found that those patients who have poor health literacy will have poor glycemic control and higher rates of retinopathy. Thus, inadequate health education may account for diabetes-related problems in disadvantaged populations.[4] Thus, in patients who are poorly educated or who have marginal understanding of the complexity of the surgery and surgical expectations, the retinal surgeon and staff must be constantly vigilant in educating and reeducating the patient and family members in order to manage postoperative expectations.

To improve management of patient expectations for surgery and postoperative visual loss, referral to behavioral therapists may be helpful. In a study with 51 patients with Type 2 diabetes and major depression, the researchers found that after cognitive behavioral therapy, the mean hemoglobin A1c levels were lower than those of the control group.[5]

Poor Visual Outcome but Great Anatomical Results

In diabetic patients, there is a risk of poor postoperative visual acuity despite excellent anatomic surgical results. The most important point to stress to the diabetic patient is that the recovery period is slow and is to be expected. Emphasize that it is "normal" to have a prolonged visual recuperation. The rods and cones must be anatomically aligned without edema for the visual recovery to occur. We have instances where the patient sees 20/25 after detachment surgery but the optical coherence tomography (OCT) scan shows edematous fluid. Or conversely, there is a small amount of macular edema or central subfield thickness on the OCT, yet the vision is 20/100.

In cases of prolonged, poor postoperative visual outcome, persisting 6 months or more, one would consider ERG testing to evaluate the health of the rods and cones. Interestingly, the ERG will improve by 6 to 8 weeks postoperatively mirroring the improvement in visual acuity.

Vitrectomy

Vitrectomies for vitreous hemorrhage may seem uncomplicated to the patient however, there are complications associated with unexpected findings intraoperatively. A dense vitreous hemorrhage may reveal a combined traction and rhegmatogenous retinal detachment in a proliferative diabetic retinopathy (PDR) eye. Combined traction and rhegmatogenous retinal detachment are serious adverse side effects of the disease and may have a poor visual prognosis. Favorable preoperative prognostic factors include a visual acuity of 5/200 or better, absence of rubeosis, and absence of macula retinal detachment.[6,7] Thus, it is important to communicate the favorable and unfavorable prognostic factors to the patient and family prior to surgery. As a consequence, the patient can manage his or her expectations of the surgery.

Laser Burns and Consequent Laser-Induced Atrophy of the Retina

Laser complications can occur with diode laser and panretinal photocoagulation. The deeper tissue penetration that occurs with diode laser may then damage the short ciliary nerves. When the eye is anesthetized, the laser surgeon may not be aware of the damage to the nerves. After the procedure tonic pupils can be noted in the patients.[8]

Panretinal photocoagulation can cause macular edema if a heavy treatment of more than 1,000 to 1,200 burns is performed in one setting. This can occur because the retina is already ischemic and releases vascular endothelial growth factors (VEGFs) as well as inflammatory cells.[9]

Postoperatively after panretinal laser photocoagulation, there can be macular gliosis as well. This is most likely due to the contracting of the posterior hyaloid membrane as it stretches over the arcades in the equatorial aspect of the vitreous interface with the internal limiting membrane Thus, macular edema can occur as the blood supply is distorted after laser. Postoperatively, the physician can use nonsteroidal anti-inflammatory drug (NSAID) eyedrops or steroid eyedrops. There is also a role for anti-VEGF injections such as bevacizumab to treat residual macular edema.[9]

TREATMENT OF COMPLICATIONS AFTER PANRETINAL PHOTOCOAGULATION FOR PROLIFERATIVE DIABETIC RETINOPATHY

In refractory cases of poor visual acuity after panretinal photocoagulation in the presence of macular edema, one can initiate a trial of NSAIDs and/or carbonic anhydrase inhibitors. They may aid in the resolution of residual postoperative macular edema after panretinal photocoagulation. These agents are sometimes used as long as 3 months after surgery for postoperative macular edema after vitrectomy and membrane peeling.

Vascular Endothelial Growth Factor

VEGF has been shown to be an angiogenic inducer in various in vivo and in vitro models.[9,10] VEGF has been known to increase retinal vascular permeability by increasing the phosphorylation of tight junction proteins.[10] Hypoxia has been shown to induce VEGF gene transcription.[10] It has been shown that there are elevated levels of VEGF in ocular fluids in patients with PDR.[10,11] Thus, with that type of background, anti-VEGF drugs such as bevacizumab have been used for PDR and persistent proliferative diabetic rertinopathy despite laser treatment.[10–15] In some surgical cases with severe PDR and associated traction retinal detachment, bevacizumab may be injected preoperatively. Postoperative injections of bevacizumab may be used as well.

MRI IMAGING AND UNEXPLAINED VISUAL LOSS AFTER TREATMENT

In some instances when a patient presents for a second opinion after having had previous retinal detachment and diabetic vitreous hemorrhage surgery with poor visual acuity results, one might consider optic nerve imaging of the retina and the visual pathways in the brain.

PDR or quiescent PDR can have associated loss of vision from anterior ischemic optic neuropathy (AION). It can present with disc edema in the setting of quiescent PDR and eventually, the disc edema becomes AION or it can spontaneously resolve without any visual symptoms. In patients with diabetes and asymptomatic optic disc edema, 31% of these patients will go onto AION.[8]

MACULAR LASER COMPLICATIONS

Macular laser in diabetic patients can lead to scar enlargement over time. The grid pattern treatment for clinically significant macular edema may lead to later enlargement of the laser burns.[8] The scars can be in the form of retinal pigment epithelial hypertrophy and retinal pigment epithelial hyperplastic scar formation. Schatz et al.[16] evaluated 203 eyes and found that there was a 5% incidence of scar formation. The pre-scar formation and post-op laser visual acuity was 20/40. After scar enlargement in the fovea, the visual acuity deteriorated to 20/100 to 20/200.

Macular laser in patients with posterior hyaloidal traction can lead to macular edema. Kaiser's study evaluated nine eyes of nine patients with diabetic macular edema and posterior hyaloidal traction on clinical examination.[17] Eight of the nine eyes had grid or focal macular laser for diabetic macular edema. All nine eyes had a thickened, taut, glistening posterior hyaloid on clinical slit lamp biomicroscopic examination, with no posterior vitreous separation. Kaiser et al.[17] defined the taut glistening posterior hyaloid interface with macular edema as a tractional component in diabetic macular edema. Fluorescein angiography showed all nine eyes as having early hyperfluorescence with deep, diffuse, late leakage in the macular area consistent with the theory of the tractional forces exerted on the macular edema, associated with the posterior hyaloid. OCT revealed retinal thickening in all nine eyes with a mean retinal thickness of 556.9 μm. In addition, eight of the nine eyes had a shallow macular traction detachment associated with the posterior hyaloid traction. Thus, eyes with diabetic macular edema associated with posterior hyaloid traction may have a shallow, subclinical, macular detachment.[8] These changes in the retinal architecture may be observed if the patient does not note any improvement of vision. Serial OCT testing can be performed to document any changes in the macula in the postlaser period.

Treatment of Diabetic Macular Edema

Nonsteroidal Anti-Inflammatory Drugs

Residual diabetic macular edema may be addressed with NSAID topical eyedrops. The use of NSAID eyedrops have been commonplace for the treatment of cystoid macular edema after cataract surgery. Now with the advent of OCT scans where postlaser diabetic macular edema can present with cystic spaces and edema at Henle layer, similar to the cystoid macular edema setting in cataract surgery, NSAID eyedrops can be part of the retinal specialist's armamentarium. The NSAID eyedrops work on the alternate complement pathway and may have an effect in improving the patient's vision.[18–21]

Acetazolamide

Acetazolamide, a carbonic anhydrase inhibitor, has been used to treat macular edema in uveitis and it has been found to be useful in treating diabetic macular edema.[22–26] Giusti et al.[23] evaluated the use of acetazolamide for macular edema and found that macular edema improves the fluorescein angiographic findings in diabetic macular edema patients. With Heidelberg retina angiography and computerized perimetry (Octopus 2000 R), there was documented improvement in Giusti's study in his sample of 12 diabetic patients, five with Type 1 and seven with Type 2 diabetes. Visual acuity outcome varies only slightly.[23]

It is thought that the diffuse leakage from the RPE responds to carbonic anhydrase treatment due to the modulation of membrane-bound carbonic anhydrase receptors in the retinal pigment epithelium. These receptors have lost its polarized distribution in the presence of macular edema. It is also thought that carbonic anhydrase inhibitors work on the alternate complement pathway which is involved in the release of VEGF factors in inflammation in age-related macular degeneration and diabetic retinopathy.[22–26]

While some retinal specialists suggest a starting dose of CAI 500 mg per day for a month, we use a starting dose of 250 mg per day especially for our elderly patients who take diuretics. The elderly may be sensitive to hypovolemia and require hospitalization if the dose is not titrated. If in doubt, ask the family practitioner or internal medicine physician who cares for the patient.[26]

Intravitreal Triamcinolone Acetonide

Intravitreal injection of 4 mg triamcinolone acetonide subconjunctivally can be used to treat macular edema unresponsive to macular laser photocoagulation.[27] Massin et al.[27] evaluated 12 patients with diabetic macular edema for a follow-up of 3 months. Seven of the 12 patients had 6 months of follow-up. The average macular thickness was 509.6 μm in the injected eyes, versus 474.4 μm in the control eyes. Four weeks postinjection, the average macular thickness by OCT was 207.3 μm in injected eyes and 506.7 μm in the control eyes. After 12 weeks, the average macular thickness was 207 and 469.3 μm, respectively ($p = 0.005$). However, the difference between the macular thickness of the injected and control eyes was no longer significant at 24 weeks because of the recurrence of macular edema in 5 of 12 injected eyes. Before triamcinolone injection, the ETDRS visual acuity score was found to be an average of 47.8 letters in the treated eyes, versus 51.9 letters in the control eyes. Twelve and twenty-four weeks later, the ETDRS visual acuity was approximately the same in the treated and untreated eyes. Neither group improved visual acuity, and there was improvement only in the pathological thickness of the macula as measured by OCT. In 6 of the 12 triamcinolone treated eyes, intraocular pressure measurement was greater than 25 mm Hg, and was controlled by topical, antiglaucoma medication.[27]

Intravitreal Bevacizumab

A 2006 study evaluating intravitreal bevacizumab enrolled 51 consecutive patients with diffuse diabetic macular edema. All patients had one injection of 1.25 mg of bevacizumab and had 6 weeks of follow-up. Twenty-three patients (45%) had 12 weeks of follow-up. OCT thickness decreased from baseline average of 501 μm to 425 μm postinjection.[28]

In 2007, Arevalo and the PanAmerican Collaborative Retina Study Group evaluated 110 eyes with diabetic macular edema.[29] Seventy-eight eyes of 64 consecutive patients had a minimum follow-up of 6 months and mean age of 59.7 years. The patients were treated with at least one intravitreal injection of 1.25 mg or 2.5 mg of bevacizumab and underwent ETDRS visual acuity testing, OCT, and fluorescein angiography. The main measures of outcome were OCT and fluorescein angiography. Sixteen of the 78 eyes (20.5%) needed a second injection and 6 eyes (7.7%) needed a third injection. Mean central macular thickness at baseline by OCT was 387 μm and decreased to a mean central macular thickness of 275.7 μm at the end of follow-up. Both doses of 1.25 mg or 2.5 mg of bevacizumab were found to be effective.[29]

Intravitreal Bevacizumab and Intravitreal Triamcinolone

In a 2006 study, 28 patients were assigned to receive a single intravitreal injection of 4 mg/0.1 mL triamcinolone acetonide versus 1.5 mg/0.06 mL of bevacizumab. The OCT and ETDRS visual acuity were the main outcome measures. The authors conclude that a single injection of triamcinolone may be advantageous over bevacizumab based on OCT measurements of central macular thickness and visual acuity.[30]

Intravitreal bevacizumab and intravitreal triamcinolone have been used together in clinical practice. In a study involving 115 eyes of 101 patients with refractory diabetic macular edema, enrolled in a prospective, controlled randomized pilot study, three consecutive intravitreal injections of bevacizumab have a beneficial effect on refractory diabetic macular edema in terms of central macular thickness as measured by OCT and visual acuity. The adjunctive use of intravitreal triamcinolone in the first injection induced earlier visual acuity improvement but there were no long-term significant adverse side effects.[31]

REFERENCES

1. Jacobson AM. The psychological care of patients with insulin dependent diabetes mellitus. *N Engl J Med.* 1996;334: 1249–1253.
2. Kraushar MR. Medical malpractice experiences of vitreoretinal specialists: Risk prevention strategies. *Retina.* 2003;23:523–529.
3. Williams MV, Baker DW, Parker RM, et al. Relationship of functional health literacy to patients' knowledge of their chronic disease. *Arch Int Med.* 1998;158:166–172.
4. Schillinger D, Grumbach K, Piette J, et al. Association of health literacy with diabetes outcomes. *JAMA.* 2002;288: 475–482.
5. Lustman PJ, Griffith LS, Freedland KE, et al. Cognitive behavior therapy for depression in Type 2 diabetes mellitus. *Ann Int Med.* 1998;129:613–621.
6. Rice TA, Michels RG, Rice EF. Vitrectomy for diabetic rhegmatogenous retinal detachment. *Am J Ophthalmol.* 1983;95:34–41.
7. Thompson JT, De Bustros S, Michels RG, et al. Results and prognostic factors in vitrectomy for diabetic traction–rhegmatogenous retinal detachment. *Arch Ophthalmol.* 1987;105:503–511.
8. Patel JI, Jenkins L, Benjamin L, Webber S. Dilated pupils and loss of accommodation following diode panretinal photocoagulation with sub-tenon local anaesthetic in four cases. *Eye.* 2002;16:628–632.
9. McDonald HR, Schatz H. Macular edema following panretinal photocoagulation. *Retina.* 1985;5:5–10.
10. Ferrara N. Vascular endothelial endothelial growth factor-induced retinopathy in the nonhuman primate. *Am J Ophthalmol.* 2002;133:373–385.
11. Tolentino MJ, McLeod DS, Taomoto M, et al. Pathologic features of vascular growth factor: Basic science and clinical progress. *Endocr Rev.* 2004;25:581–611.
12. Adamis AP, Miller JW, Bernal MT, et al. Increased vascular endothelial growth factor levels in the vitreous of eyes with proliferative diabetic retinopathy. *Am J Ophthalmol.* 1994;118:45–450.
13. Aiello LP, Avery RL, Arrigg PG, et al. Vascular endothelial growth factor in ocular fluid of patients with diabetic retinopathy and other retinal disorders. *N Engl J Med.* 1994;331:1480–1487.
14. Spaide RF, Fisher YL. Intravitreal bevacizumab (avastin) treatment of proliferative diabetic retinopathy complicated by vitreous hemorrhage. *Retina.* 2006;26:275–278.
15. Avery Rl, Pearlman J, Pieramici DJ, et al. Intravitreal bevacizumab (Avastin) in the treatment of proliferative diabetic retinopathy.*Ophthalmology.* 2006;113:1695–1705.
16. Schatz H, Madeira D, McDonald HR, et al. Progressive enlargement of laser scars following grid laser photocoagulation for diffuse diabetic macular edema. *Arch Ophthalmol.* 1991;109:1549–1551.
17. Kaiser P, Riemann C, Sears J, Lewis H. Macular traction detachment and diabetic macular edema associated with posterior hyaloidal traction. *Am J Ophthalmol.* 2001;131:44–49.
18. Guex-Crosier Y. The pathogenesis and clinical presentation of macular edema in inflammatory disease. *Doc Ophthalmologica.* 1999;97:297–309.
19. Williams P, Callanan D. Treating diabetic macular edema with ocular NSAIDS. http://www.retinalphysician.com/article.aspx?article = 101096. Accessed 28 February 2009.
20. Sivaprasad S, Bunce C, Wormald R. Non-steroidal anti-inflammatory agents for cystoid macular edema following cataract surgery: A systematic review. *Br J Ophthalmol.* 2005;89:1420–1422.
21. Kern TS, Miller CM, Du Y, et al. Topical administration of nepafenac inhibits diabetes-induced retinal microvascular disease and underlying abnormalities of retinal metabolism and physiology. *Diabetes.* 2007;56:373–379.
22. Whitcup SM, Csaky KG, Podgor MJ, Chew EY, Perry CH. A randomized, masked, cross-over trial of acetazolamide for cystoid macular edema in patients with uveitis. *Ophthalmology.* 1996;103:1054–1062.
23. Giusti C, Forte R, Vingolo EM, et al. Is acetazolamide effective in the treatment of diabetic macular edema? *A Pilot Study Int Ophthalmol.* 2001;24:79–88.
24. Purushottam J, Bora PS, Bor NS. The role of complement system in ocular diseases including uveitis and macular degeneration. *Mol Immunol.* 2007;44:3901–3908.
25. Meleth AD, Agron E, Chan CC, et al. Serum inflammatory markers in diabetic retinopathy. *Invest Ophthalmol Vis Sci.* 2005;46:4295–4301.
26. Wolfensberger TJ. The role of carbonic anhydrase inhibitors in the management of macular edema. *Doc Ophthalmol.* 1999;97:387–397.

27. Massin P, Audren F, Haouchine B, et al. Intravitreal triamcinolone acetonide for diabetic diffuse macular edema. *Ophthalmology.* 2004;111:218–224.
28. Haritoglou C, Kook D, Neubauer A, et al. Intravitreal bevacizumab (Avastin) therapy for persistent diffuse diabetic macular edema. *Retina.* 2006;26:999–1005.
29. Arevalo JF, Fromow-Guerra J, Quiroz Mercado H, et al. Pan-American Collaborative Retina Study Group. Primary intravitreal bevacizumab (Avastin) for diabetic macular edema: Results from the Pan-American Collaborative Retina Study Group at 6-month follow-up. *Ophthalmology.* 2007;114:743–750.
30. Paccola L, Costa RA, Folgosa MS, et al. Intravitreal triamcinolone versus bevacizumab (Avastin) for treatment of refractory diabetic macular edema. *Br J Ophthalmol.* 2008;92:76–80.
31. Ahmadieh H, Ramezani A, Shoeibi N, et al. Intravitreal bevacizumab with or without triamcinolone for refractory diabetic macular edema; a placebo-controlled, randomized clinical trial. *Graefe's Arch Clin Exp Ophthalmol.* 2008;246: 483–489.

SUGGESTED READINGS

1. Almoq Y, Goldstein M. Visual outcome in eyes with asymptomatic optic disc edema. *J Neurophthalmol.* 2003;23: 204–207.
2. Antcliff RJ, Marshall J. The pathogenesis of edema in diabetic maculopathy. *Semin Ophthalmol.* 1999;14:223–232.
3. Bakri SJ, Donaldson MJ, Link TP. Rapid regression of disc neovascularization in a patient with proliferative diabetic retinopathy following adjunctive intravitreal bevacizumab. *Eye.* 2006;20:1474–1475.
4. Funatsu H, Yamashita H, Ikeda T, et al. Vitreous levels of interleukin-6 and vascular endothelial growth factor are related to diabetic macular edema. *Ophthalmology.* 2003;110:1690–1696.
5. Funatsu H, Yamashita H, Sakata K, et al. Vitreous levels of interleukin-6 and vascular endothelial growth factor and intercellular adhesion molecule I are related to macular edema. *Ophthalmology.* 2005;112:806–816.
6. Gillies MC, Sutter FK, Simpson JM, et al. Intravitreal triamcinolone for refractory diabetic macular edema: Two-year results of a double-masked, placebo-controlled, randomized clinical trial. *Ophthalmology.* 2006;113:1533–1538.
7. Malacaze F, Clamens S, Simorre-Pinatel V, et al. Detection of vascular endothelial growth factor messenger RNA and vascular endothelial growth factor-like activity in proliferative diabetic retinopathy. *Arch Ophthalmol.* 1994;112: 1476–1482.
8. Maturi RK, Bleau LA, Wilson DL. Electrophysiologic findings after intravitreal bevacizumab (Avastin) treatment. *Retina.* 2006;26:270–274.
9. Oshima Y, Sakaguchi H, Gomi F, Tano Y. Regression of iris neovascularization after intravitreal injection of bevacizumab in patients with proliferative diabetic retinopathy. *Am J Ophthalmol.* 2006;142:155–158.
10. Shahar J, Avery RL, Heilweil G, et al. Electrophysiologic and retinalpenetration studies following intravitreal injection of bevacizumab (Avastin). *Retina.* 2006;26:262–269.

CHAPTER 13

Diabetes and Glaucoma

NEOVASCULAR GLAUCOMA

"If an adult presents with bilateral rubeosis iridis, diabetes mellitus should be considered the most likely cause." This statement was made by glaucoma surgeons Higginbotham and Yang.[1] Thus, the clinician must have a high index of suspicion for diabetic patients with severe nonproliferative diabetic retinopathy or proliferative diabetic retinopathy (PDR). Ischemia is thought to play an important role in this disease. The bilaterality of the rubeosis iridis suggests a systemic disease.

Historically, in the medical literature, neovascular glaucoma is associated most strongly with retinal venous obstructive diseases (36.1%), diabetic retinopathy (32.2%), and carotid obstructive disease (12.9%). Other less common causes are central retinal artery obstruction (3.8%), combined retinal arterial and venous obstruction (3.8%), and rhegmatogenous retinal detachment (1.5%). The rest of the 3.5% is comprised of vitreous wick syndrome, radiation retinopathy, syphilitic vasculitis, nonrhegmatogenous retinal detachment associated with malignant melanoma and angiomatosis retinae, squamous cell carcinoma of the conjunctiva, and carotid sinus fistula.[2]

Gartner and Henkind[3] elucidated the causes of neovascularization of the iris and that neovascular glaucoma causes 20% of all eye enucleations (Table 13-1).

However, when one looks at the causes of neovascularization of the iris and neovascular glaucoma, central retinal vein occlusion usually is associated with a systemic vascular disorder such as hypertension or diabetes. In that context, diabetes plays a large role in the incidence of neovascular glaucoma.

In one study by Klein et al.,[4] a cohort of people with diabetes self-reported glaucoma. Data were taken from an 11-county area of southern Wisconsin. Two thousand three hundred and sixty-six diabetics were part of the evaluation over a 10-year period. The authors found that the 10-year incidence of glaucoma was 3.7% in the younger onset people. It was 6.9% in the older onset people not using insulin and 11.8% in the older onset people using insulin. Univariate analyses showed that in the younger onset people, there was a greater body mass index. In the older age group of noninsulin users, there was a longer duration of diabetes, history of cataract surgery, and increased severity of diabetic retinopathy at baseline.

Older onset diabetics who were using insulin had longer duration of diabetes, higher intraocular pressure (IOP), history of cataract surgery at baseline, and an increased risk of glaucoma.[4] In multivariate analyses, only age was significantly related to increased incidence of glaucoma in younger onset people. Age, IOP, and insulin use were significantly associated with increased risk in the older onset group.[4]

The incidence of neovascular glaucoma and vitreous hemorrhage after cataract surgery in diabetic patients has been studied by Aiello et al.[5] in 154 patients. After intracapsular cataract extraction in patients with active PDR, the incidence was 40% for the development of rubeosis iridis/neovascular glaucoma.[5] In patients with active PDR, there was a 20% incidence of vitreous hemorrhage. However, in eyes with no diabetic retinopathy or background diabetic retinopathy, the incidence was 6.5% for the development of vitreous hemorrhage. In eyes without regard to preoperative diabetic retinopathy, the incidence of rubeosis iridis/neovascular glaucoma was 7.8%.[5] From the glaucoma surgeon's perspective,

TABLE 13.1 Causes of Neovascularization of the Iris

Vascular disorders
Central retinal vein occlusion
Central retinal artery occlusion
Branch vein occlusion
Carotid occlusive disease
Takayasu disease
Giant cell arteritis
Carotid artery ligation
Carotid-cavernous fistula
Leber military aneurysms
Retrolental fibroplasias
Sturge-Weber disease with choroidal hemangioma
Ocular disease
Uveitis
Endophthalmitis
Sympathetic ophthalmia
Vogt-Koyanagi syndrome
Retinal detachment
Coats disease
Eales disease
Pseudoexfoliation of the lens capsule
Essential iris atrophy
Glaucoma
Open-angle glaucoma
Closed-angle glaucoma
Secondary glaucoma
Surgery and radiation therapy
Retinal detachment surgery
Vitrectomy
Laser coreoplasty
Cataract extraction
Radiation
Trauma
Systemic diseases
Diabetes
Norrie disease
Sickle Cell disease
Neurofibromatosis
Lupus erythematosus
Marfan syndrome
Neoplastic disease
Retinoblastoma
Choroidal melanoma
Iris melanoma
Metastatic carcinoma
Reticulum cell sarcoma of the ciliary body

Source: Data from Gartner S, Henkind P. Neovascularization of the iris (rubeosis iridis). *Surv Ophthalmol.* 1978;22:291–312.

the teaching was that 20% of the eyes enucleated were due to neovascular glaucoma.[3] Of eyes not enucleated, after cyclocryotherapy, more than half suffered severe vision loss.[3]

Sivak-Callcott et al.[6] performed a meta-analysis of the literature from 1966 to the present. The current literature reaffirms the need for a full ocular examination when there is a high index of suspicion, undilated gonioscopy and pupil examination. The recommendations for treatment include treatment of the underlying disease, complete panretinal photocoagulation (PRP) in retinal ischemia is a factor. Medical control of the elevated IOP and medical treatment of the accompanying inflammation are needed. If medical treatment is inadequate for the control of the IOP, then glaucoma surgery is necessary. While the ideal glaucoma surgery is still controversial, trabeculectomy with antimetabolite therapy, aqueous shunt implants, diode laser cyclophotocoagulation, or cycloablation with cryopexy are the preferred treatment modalities.[6]

In a diabetic patient who presents with unilateral rubeosis iridis, loss of vision, and central retinal vein occlusion, the IOP will be low, and the patient will be in the fifth decade slightly younger than a nondiabetic patient with a CRVO.[2] The patient will most likely have an ischemic CRVO. Forty percent of the patients in this group develop neovascular glaucoma within 7 months, and 50% develop neovascular glaucoma after 3 years.[7]

In cases of marked asymmetry of diabetic retinopathy and unilateral rubeosis iridis, where upon PRP does not eliminate anterior segment neovascularization, think about carotid occlusive disease. Carotid artery obstruction produces bilateral rubeosis iridis only in 8% of the cases.[8] IOP can be normal despite 360 degrees of peripheral anterior synechiae (PAS). In fact, only one third of the patients have elevated IOP with PAS.[9] These diabetic patients with carotid artery disease may present with a painful red eye, periorbital pain, engorged episcleral and conjunctival vessels, a cloudy cornea, ischemic uveitis with cells and flare in the anterior chamber, rubeoisis iridis, venous stasis retinopathy, and a decreased central retinal arterial pressure as measured by ophthalmodynamometry. Cataracts are seen as a late finding. When there is severe eye and periorbital pain, send the patient for an emergency sedimentation rate to evaluate for temporal arteritis. In cases with severe pain, the majority of patients may have normal IOP or low IOP because of hypoperfusion of the ciliary body and thus a decreased rate of aqueous production.[8]

Once carotid occlusive disease is suspected, fluorescein angiography will show delayed filling of the arteriovenous phase, areas of choroidal hypoperfusion, or areas of capillary nonperfusion. Systemic workup would involve carotid artery ultrasonography; magnetic resonance angiography of the carotid artery, echocardiography of the heart, Holter monitoring can be performed.

The presence of any neovascularization is an indication for PRP. The PRP will cause a regression of the iris neovascularization. This can be done in patients who are awaiting surgical treatment of their carotid occlusive disease.

The postoperative IOP should be followed closely because glaucoma can develop after reperfusion of the ischemic ciliary body. It is important to control IOP in order to prevent further optic nerve damage. Medical therapy, trabeculectomy, and cyclocryotherapy have been ineffective, and some glaucoma surgeons recommend the use of a seton implant such as a Molteno implant or other implants. Anticoagulation with aspirin is suggested as well, while awaiting the definitive procedure of carotid artery surgery.

Pathophysiology

The common factor of neovascular glaucoma and diabetes is retinal ischemia. Vasoproliferative factors such as VEGF are thought to play a role in rubeosis iridis. There are some case reports on the use of intravitreal bevacizumab (Avastin) for the treatment of neovascular glaucoma among glaucoma surgeons.[10,11]

Neovascularization of the iris begins as endothelial budding from capillaries or venules in the iris. New vessels form at the pupillary zone or iris periphery where there are many capillaries. However, new vessels can arise in the iris stroma as well. The new vessels tend to grow in the anterior surface of the iris and are thin walled. These new vessels leak fluorescein because their endothelium has gaps and fenestrations as recorded in electron microscopy studies.[12]

Accompanying the new vessels is the proliferation of myofibroblasts, resulting in the formation of a fibrovascular membrane.[13] The myofibroblasts contract, causing the fibrovascular membrane to shrink, flatten the iris, and lose their surface architecture. As the membrane shrinks, the posterior pigment layer of the iris may be pulled anteriorly onto the anterior iris surface, creating ectropion uveae. If the sphincter muscle becomes distorted, the condition is called ectropion of the sphincter muscle. In late iris

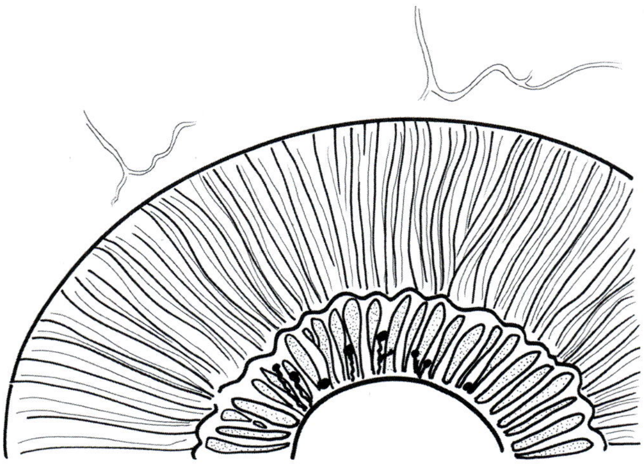

FIGURE 13-1. Iris neovascularization.

neovascularization, the progressive fibrosis causes loss of the dilator muscle function and partial atrophy of the sphincter muscle. This explains the fixed dilated pupil and unresponsive iris seen in advanced cases of neovascular glaucoma.

As iris neovascularization moves to the angle, the fibroavascular membrane adheres to the cornea, iris, and causes PAS. Furthermore, if the fibrovascular membrane progresses further, secondary angle closure can occur.

Diagnosis

The key in the diagnosis of neovascularization of the iris is a high index of suspicion and early diagnosis. The diagnosis of neovascular glaucoma begins with the slit lamp examination, under high magnification (Fig. 13-1). Look for the new iris vessels at the papillary margin, the usual site of origin. This is especially difficult in darkly pigmented irides.

As the iris neovascularization progresses over time, the iris new vessels extend from the papillary margin to the periphery of the iris. A reddish coloration may be visible, but this is advanced rubeosis iridis. These iris new vessels with their abnormal fenestrations of endothelial cells will tend to leak and cause the formation of a hyphema in some patients. At this stage, the patient is still asymptomatic, without pain, and can have only minor changes in visual acuity, and the IOP can still be normal.

As neovascularization of the iris progresses, the new vessels are visible over the peripheral iris and in the angle. The new vessels may form anastomoses with the circumferential ciliary body artery, which is another site of neovascularization.

In the later stages of rubeosis iridis, the PAS and ectropion uveae become visible. If PAS occlude enough of the angle, then elevated IOP will occur and angle-closure glaucoma will occur (Table 13-2).

TABLE 13.2 Diagnosis of Rubeosis Iridis

1. High index of suspicion
2. Highest magnification on slit beam with highest intensity of light
3. Look at pupillary margin
4. Look at iris periphery
5. Look for reddish hue at pupillary margin
6. Gonioscopy with highest magnification and highest intensity of light at slit lamp
7. Light pressure with contact gonioscopic lens may make neovascularization collapse and look "invisible" to the eye
8. Fluorescein angiography of iris
9. Late rubeosis iridis is ectropion uveae

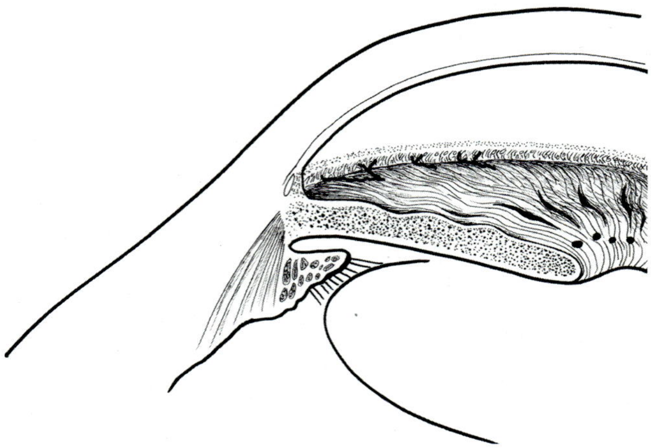

FIGURE 13-2. Iris neovascularization at the angle.

Gonioscopy

New vessels in the angle will only appear if iris neovascularization is already present in the iris (Fig. 13-2). Wand recommends highest magnification with the slit beam and the highest light intensity offered by the slit lamp with the Goldmann goniolens.[14] Another caveat is that if a contact goniolens is used, even the slightest pressure will collapse the new vessels thus making visualization impossible. Invisible to the examiner is the clear fibrovascular membrane found with the new vessels. Another last caveat: the angle may be completely closed by PAS, but the examiner mistakes this for a normal angle.

Fluorescein Angiography

Fluorescein angiography can identify new vessels at least 1 month prior to being seen on the iris surface.[15] The iris vessels are tortuous and leak fluorescein. The vessels travel radially without creating little branches. The leakage can appear as luminous dots at the papillary margin.

Not all iris vessels are iris neovascularization. Normal iris vessels can be seen in the elderly who have atrophic irides and light-colored irides. These normal vessels are radially

TABLE 13.3 Medical Treatment of Neovascular Glaucoma

1. Atropine 1% eyedrops
2. Aqueous suppressants: Brimonidine or apraclonidine
3. Topical corticosteroids: Prednisolone acetate, dexamethasone phosphate, and fluorometholone
4. Osmotic agents: Glycerin (Osmoglyn-Alcon Laboratories) 2–3 mL/kg of body weight
5. Mannitol 25% solution (Alcon Laboratories) or isosorbide (Ismotic-Alcon Laboratories) 45% solution (220 mL bottle) 1.5 mL/lb of body weight

TABLE 13.4 Cycloplegic Agents

Ocular effect: Relaxes pupillary sphincter and ciliary muscle
Usage: For ocular inflammation from uveitis, trauma, postoperative period of filtering surgery, malignant glaucoma, and neovascular glaucoma
Atropine
Homatropine
Scopolamine
Cyclopentolate
Tropicamide

TABLE 13.5 Carbonic Anhydrase Inhibitors

Ocular effect: Decreases aqueous production
Usage: Effective in most glaucomas but causes systemic side effects, needs potassium replacement, side effects include tingling of hands and feet and lethargy
Acetazolamide
Methazolamide
Dichlorpheniramine

oriented and lie within the iris stroma. Prominent iris vessels can be seen after intraocular surgery, uveitis, iris tumors, trauma, postoperative inflammation from eye surgery. With time, inflammatory iris vessels will disappear with steroids, whereas iris neovascularization will continue if left untreated.

If neovascular glaucoma reaches the late stage, an elevated IOP and a cloudy cornea may be seen at presentation. The differential diagnosis is angle-closure glaucoma. The other entities to be considered are intraocular tumors, chronic retinal detachment, intraocular bleeding, and ghost cell glaucoma. Despite a cloudy cornea, one can visualize ectropion uveae and severe, prominent, iris neovascularization.

Medical Treatment

Prior to total angle closure with extensive PAS formation, aqueous suppressants such as brimonidine or apraclonidine can be used for medical treatment of neovascular glaucoma. These agents cause a decrease in aqueous production due to the open-angle glaucoma from the fibrovascular membrane formation. A cycloplegic agent like atropine sulfate and topical steroids will decrease inflammation. Strong cycloplegics will also increase the uveal scleral outflow.

If total synechial angle closure occurs, beta-blockers such as timolol maleate and carbonic anhydrase inhibitors are useful. Osmotic agents may also be needed to treat the elevated IOP in closed-angle neovascular glaucoma (Tables 13-3–13-6). Atropine and topical steroids will decrease inflammation and decrease the discomfort for the patient. Osmotic agents will clear the corneal edema. In severe neovascular glaucoma with vision, surgical management may be needed (see below). In end-stage neovascular glaucoma, with a blind, painful eye, patients will find relief with cycloplegics and topical steroids. A small minority may need retrobulbar alcohol injection (Tables 13-7–13-9).

Surgical Treatment

Rubeosis iridis is divided into three treatment categories: (i) Preglaucoma stage, (ii) open-angle glaucoma stage, and (iii) closed-angle glaucoma stage. The preglaucoma stage is rubeosis iridis at the pupillary margin, open angle, and no increase in IOP. PRP is the

TABLE 13.6 Osmotic Agents

Ocular effect: Osmotic ocular dehydration
Usage: Effectively lowers IOP, to break angle-closure attack, to clear up cloudy cornea in neovascular glaucoma or angle-closure glaucoma, potential serious side effects such as severe dehydration, anuria, acute pulmonary edema, cardiac decompensation, cannot be used chronically.
Mannitol
Glycerin
Isosorbide

TABLE 13.7 Treatment of Rubeosis Iridis

1. Elevated IOP → Yes → Aqueous suppressants, CAI, atropine, topical steroids → Clear media → PRP → **If IOP normal → Observe**
2. Normal IOP → Clear media → PRP → Regression of iris neo → **If IOP normal → Observe**
3. Elevated IOP → Unclear media → Panretinal cryopexy → Regression of iris neo → **Elevated IOP →** Anterior segment inflammation → Cycloablation with laser or cryotherapy → Filtration surgery (with or without Seton valve) → May need **vitrectomy + endolaser** in future
4. Elevated IOP → Clear media → PRP → **No regression of iris neo → Elevated IOP →** No anterior segment inflammation → Filtration surgery

TABLE 13.8 Treatment Goals

Lower IOP
Regression of rubeosis iridis
Treat glaucoma if any
Treat retinal ischemia with PRP or ablative procedure
Future role of bevacizumab in intractable neovascular glaucoma
Restoration of vision if possible

main treatment of choice for this group of eyes, if no view is available of the fundus. Possible risk factors for this stage are poorly controlled diabetes, inadequately controlled hypertension, and primary open-angle glaucoma as a baseline. While PRP may be effective in causing regression of the iris neovascularization, PRP does not reverse the PAS that have already formed in the angle.

In eyes with opaque media, where PRP is not possible, panretinal cryotherapy can be performed. This is done to the superior or inferior 180 degrees or opposite quadrants, such as superior temporal and inferonasal or superonasal and inferotemporal quadrants. Treat the areas between ora serrata and equator. Also, at this time, treat the ciliary body with five to eight spots (Fig. 13-3).

The open-angle glaucoma stage with rubeosis iridis has a more complicated course. At this stage, the IOP is elevated, and flare is seen in the anterior chamber. The treatment of this group involves surgical management. PRP is the first step, but if the ameliorative effects of PRP are not seen in a timely manner, goniophotocoagulation may be tried. Vessels are first treated in the angle, followed by the peripheral iris, and finally, the total iris may be treated. The laser parameters are 200-μm spot size, 0.2 second, and 200 MW of power, using argon green laser.

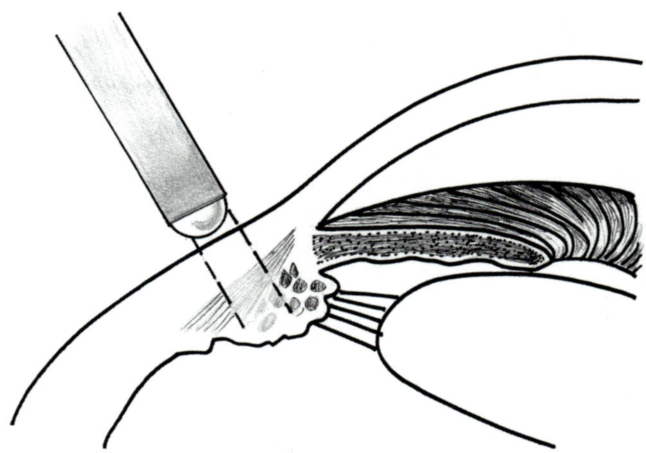

FIGURE 13-3. Cyclocryopexy.

TABLE 13.9 Other Considerations in Neovascular Glaucoma

1. Consider other forms of glaucoma
2. Optic nerve asymmetry or optic nerve damage, optic disc anomaly, optic nerve pit
3. Visual field defect
4. Monitor progress of retinal ischemia with fluorescein angiography
5. Vitrectomy may be necessary for visualization of the posterior pole.

Filtration Surgery

In patients who present with angle-closure glaucoma and rubeosis iridis, PRP and goniophotocoagulation have been tried, and the next step is filtration surgery. This stage is associated with anterior segment inflammation, PAS, ectropion uveae, and elevated IOP. Some glaucoma surgeons do not perform goniophotocoagulation prior to filtration surgery because goniophotocoagulation can create more inflammation in the preoperative period.

Filtration surgery for neovascular glaucoma has a low success rate of 11% to 33%.[16]

However, if PRP is added to the eye prior to filtration surgery, the success rate increases to 67%.[17,18]

Setons

As an alternative to filtration surgery with antimetabolites, Seton valves may be used. Molteno valves, Baerveldt and Krupin valves, and other shunts can be used. The most commonly used valve is the Molteno valve which is a silicone tube attached to a plate. The Molteno valve is sutured to the episclera. A cadaver scleral graft is used to cover the silicon tube and plate. Postoperative hypotony is a frequent complication, flat anterior chamber. Some surgeons tie the silicon tube with a suture which can be released later if additional IOP lowering is needed. Success rates of these Seton valves in controlling IOP are in the range of 75% according to Brown et al.[19] Molteno[20] has reported 87% success rate.

Cycloablation

Endolaser cyclophotocoagulation of the ciliary body and cyclocryotherapy can be used. According to Zarbin et al.,[21] endolaser cyclophotocoagulation has a 76% success rate. The technique is limited to the accessibility of the ciliary body and the ciliary processes. The eye should be aphakic or pseudophakic, and the pupil dilation must be large enough to permit the visualization of the ciliary processes.

Cyclocryotherapy is used as a last resort. The medical literature has reported high complication rate with 360-degree cyclocryotherapy. Krupin et al.[22] have reported postoperative incidence of phthisis bulbi to be 34% in neovascular glaucoma patients.

However, in our hands, we perform cyclocryotherapy only on 4 o' clock hours, and we have good IOP control without severe inflammation and phthisis bulbi. Caprioli et al.[23] have found that 360-degree cyclocryotherapy led to 55% of the patients with effective lowering of the IOP to <21 mm Hg, 29% had a cessation of glaucomatous visual field loss, and 70% experienced worse vision. Despite the side effects, cyclocryotherapy relieves pain in the neovascular glaucomatous patients. Thus, there is still a role of cyclocryotherapy in the management of severe pain in neovascular glaucoma.

REFERENCES

1. Higginbotham EJ, Yang CB. An approach to the management of neovascular glaucoma. In: Higginbotham EJ, Lee DA, eds. *Management of Difficult Glaucoma*. Cambridge, MA: Blackwell Scientific Publications; 1994:116.
2. Brown G, Margargal L, Schachat A, et al. Noevascular Glaucom: Etiologic considerations. *Ophthalmology*. 1984;91: 315–320.

3. Gartner S, Henkind P. Neovascularization of the iris (rubeosis iridis). *Surv Ophthalmol.* 1978;22:291–312.
4. Klein BEK, Klein R, Moss SE. Incidence of self reported glaucoma in people with diabetes mellitus. *BMJ.* 1997;81: 743–747.
5. Aiello LM, Wand M, Liang G. Neovascular Glaucoma and vitreous hemorrhage following cataract surgery in patients with diabetes mellitus. *Ophthalmology.* 1983;90:814–820.
6. Sivak-Callcott JA, O'Day DM, Gass JDM, et al. Evidence based recommendations for the diagnosis and treatment of neovascular glaucoma. *Ophthalmology.* 2001;108:1767–1776.
7. Hayreh SS. The role of panretinal photocoagulation in neovascular glaucoma associated with central retinal vein occlusion. In: Krieglstein GK, ed. *Glaucoma Update IV.* Berlin: Springer-Verlag; 1991:80–85.
8. Brown GC, Magargal LE, Simeone FA, et al. Arterial obstruction and ocular neovascularization. *Ophthalmology.* 1982;89:139–146.
9. Mills RP. Anterior segment ischemia secondary to carotid occlusive disease. *J Clin Neuro Ophthalmol.* 1989;9:200–204.
10. Iliev M, Domig D, Wolf-Schnurrbursch U, et al. Intravitreal Bevacizumab (Avastin) in the treatment of neovascular glaucoma. *Am J Ophthalmol.* 2006;142:1054–1056.
11. Al-Aswad L. Another role for Avastin? Neovascular glaucoma. http://www.revophthl.com/index.asp?page=1_959.htm. Accessed 24 April 2009.
12. Tamura T. Electron microscopic study on the small vessels in rubeosis iridis diabetica. *Jpn J Ophthalmol.* 1989;13:65.
13. John T, Sassani JW, Eagle RC. The myofibroblasts component of rubeosis iridis. *Ophthalmology.* 1983;90:721–728.
14. Wand M. Neovascular glaucoma. In: Ritch R, Shields MB, Krupin T, eds. *The Glaucomas,* vol 2. St Louis, MO: CV Mosby; 1989:1063–1110.
15. Mitsui Y, Matsuhara M, Kanagawa M. Fluorescence iridocorneal photography. *Br J Ophthalmol.* 1969;47:449–460.
16. Heuer DK, Parrish RK II, Gressel MG, et al. 5- Fluorouracil and glaucoma filtering surgery. *Ophthalmology.* 1989;93:1537–1546.
17. Herschler J, Agness D. A modified filtering operation for neovascular glaucoma. *Arch Ophthalmol.* 1979;97: 2339–2341.
18. Parrish R, Herschler J. Eyes with end-stage neovascular glaucoma: Natural history following successful modified filtering operation. *Arch Ophthalmol.* 1983;101:745–746.
19. Brown RD, Carins JE. Experience with the Molteno long tube implant. *Trans Ophthalmol Soc UK.* 1983;103: 297–312.
20. Molteno ACB. The dual chamber single plant implant-its use in neovascular glaucoma. *Asut NZ J Ophthalmol.* 1990;18:431–436.
21. Zarbin MA, Michels RG, de Bustros S, et al. Endolaser treatment of the ciliary body for severe glaucoma. *Ophthalmology.* 1988;95:1639–1648.
22. Krupin T, Mitchell KB, Becker B. Cyclocryotherapy in neovascular glaucoma. *Am J Ophthalmol.* 1978;86:24–26.
23. Caprioli J, Strang SL, Spaeth GL, et al. Cyclocryotherapy in the treatment of advanced glaucoma. *Ophthalmology.* 1985;92:947–954.

SUGGESTED READINGS

1. Allen RC, Bellows AB, Hutchinson BT, Murphy SD. Filtration surgery in the treatment of neovascular glaucoma. *Ophthalmology.* 1982;89:1181–1187.
2. Bagessen LH. Fluorescein angiography of the iris in diabetics and nondiabetics. *Acta Ophthalmol.* 1969;47:449–460.
3. Benson WE, Brown GC, Tasman W, et al. Complications of vitrectomy for nonclearing vitreous hemorrhage in diabetic patients. *Ophthalmol Surg.* 1988;19:862–864.
4. Brodell L, Olk RJ, Arribas NP, et al. Neovascular glaucoma: A retrospective analysis of treatment with peripheral panretinal cryotherapy. *Ophthalmology Surg.* 1987;18:200–206.
5. Carter JE. Chronic ocular ischemia and carotid vascular disease. *Stroke.* 1985;16:721–728.
6. Coppeto JR, Wand M, Bear L, et al. Neovascular glaucoma and carotid artery obstructive disease. *Am J Ophthalmol.* 1985;99:567–570.
7. Flanagan DW, Blach RK. Place of panretinal photocoagulation and trabeculectomy in the management of neovascular glaucoma. *Br J Ophthalmol.* 1983;67:526–528.
8. Gimbrone MA, Cotran RS, Leapman SB, et al. Tumor growth and neovascularization: An experimental model using rabbit cornea. *J Natl Cancer Inst.* 1974;52:413–427.
9. Gu XQ, Fry G, Lata GF, et al. Ocular neovascularization: Tissue culture studies. *Arch Ophthalmol.* 1985;103:111–117.
10. Hercules B. Gayed II, Lucas SB, et al. Peripheral retinal ablation in the treatment of proliferative diabetic retinopathy: A three-year interim report of a randomized, controlled study using the argon laser. *Br J Ophthalmol.* 1977;61: 555–563.
11. Jacoma EH, Conway BP, Campochiaro PA. Cryotherapy causes extensive breakdown of the blood-retinal barrier. *Arch Ophthalmol.* 1985;103:1728–1730.
12. Jocson VL. Microvascular injection studies in rubeosis iridis and neovascular glaucoma. *Am J Ophthalmol.* 1977;83: 508–516.
13. Michaels RG, Maumenee AE. Retrobulbar alcohol injection in seeing eyes. *Trans Am Acad Ophthalmol Otolaryngol.* 1973;77:164–167.
14. Ohrt V. Rubeosis iridis diabetica. *Acta Ophthalmol.* 1958;36:556–558.
15. Poliner LS, Christianson DJ, Escoffery RF, et al. Neovascular glaucoma after intracapsular and extracapsular cataract extraction in diabetic patients. *Am J Ophthalmol.* 1985;100:637–643.
16. Rice TA, Michels RG, Maguire MG, et al. The effect of lensectomy on the incidence f iris neovascularization and neovascular glaucoma after vitrectomy for diabetic retinopathy. *Am J Ophthalmol.* 1983;95:1–11.

CHAPTER 14

Informed Consent

WHAT CAN PATIENTS READ AND UNDERSTAND?

Informed consent forms assume that the patients can read and understand at levels of literacy that will allow them to make sense of the words describing the risks and benefits of the procedure.[1] Data from the National Assessment of Adult Literacy in 2003 show that prose literacy skills vary considerably based on ethnicity and age.[2] Over 19,000 adults participated in the tests. The average prose literacy scores are not different from 1992 and 2003. There are an estimated 11 million adults who are nonliterate in English. Of these, they belong to two groups: seven million who could not answer simple test questions and four million who could not take the test because of language barriers. Literacy skills are defined as[2]

1. below basic-simple/concrete literacy skills
2. basic-simple and everyday literacy skills
3. intermediate moderately challenging literacy activities
4. proficient-complex and challenging literacy activities.

Below basic or basic prose literacy skills
43% of all adults
32% whites
67% blacks
74% Hispanics
46% Asian/pacific islanders
61% adults aged 65 or older

Because consent forms are usually long, complicated, and hard to understand, the forms require "proficient" prose literacy skills—which most US adults do not possess.[1,2]

A health literacy study has enrolled 3,260 new Medicare enrollees in Cleveland, Houston, and Tampa.[3] Inadequate health literacy can be found in Medicare enrollees, aged 85 years or older compared with individuals aged 65 to 69 years. Overall, 33.9% of English-speaking and 53.9% of Spanish-speaking participants had marginal health literacy. Reading ability declined with age despite adjustment for years of school completed and cognitive impairment.[3]

Almost half of American adults read at or below the eighth grade level.[4] Illiteracy in the United States is the result of insufficient education.[4] A New England Journal of Medicine study in 2003 found that 54% of the Institutional Review Board (IRB) Web sites of 114 American medical schools had grade level readability standards.[5] The standards ranged from 5th grade to 10th grade reading levels. The mean grade level for the Web sites was 10.6 grade. The study authors concluded that the text of informed consent should be directed at the fourth grade level.[5] While most consent forms are not used in isolation, the fourth grade reading level text would lead to more effective understanding of the text.

Another study originating in Canada cites two cases where the absence of "plain language" in the informed consent led to lawsuits.[6] In one case, the physician did not tell the patient clearly about the risks and benefits of sterilization. The other was about oral surgery for a wisdom tooth extraction. In the latter case, the patient felt that the printed information in technical language fell short of meeting the requirements of informed consent. Canada, like the United States, has many patients with poor reading skills. In 1995, the International Adult Literacy Survey showed that 42% of the Canadians have inadequate reading skills and cannot read job applications and tables.[6] Thus, there is a critical relationship among the use of simple, layman's language, informed consent, and professional liability.

The need to communicate at the level of the patient is important. Once the need for surgery arises, how does one communicate this to the patient? In this conversation, the patient and the physician are in the room; sometimes there are family members present. The primary goal of the conversation is to establish the patient's understanding of the need for the procedure to regain sight, to speed recovery of vision, and to prevent adverse consequences. The benefits are usually discussed first and then the adverse outcome risks are discussed.

The next part of the conversation hinges on the relationship that the patient has with the physician: is it a long-standing relationship or a new interaction because the physician is a specialist, consultant retina-vitreous surgeon? No matter what, the physician and the patient need to feel comfortable with this relationship. Certain warning signs are not heeded: (i) the patient is very anxious and overanalytical and wants another opinion, (ii) denial or disbelief at the diagnosis or lack of trust in the treatment plan (see "Cross-cultural Considerations About Informed Consent" section in this chapter), and (iii) the need for more time to think about this diagnosis despite the severity and emergent nature of the disease such as a rhegmatogenous retinal detachment in a diabetic patient.

Once the clinician senses any lack of trust, in the diagnosis or the treatment plan, send the patient for another opinion. The patient will thank you for this action, in the end. Even if the treatment plan is simple or straightforward, do not perform the surgery if there is lack of trust. As we know, nothing is perfect, and there are no 100% guarantees.

In different cultures, the patient may have extreme fear and anxiety, but his entire family may believe in the diagnosis and treatment plan. Then, the surgeon can proceed in this situation knowing that the patient's immediate family and "community" are in support of the treatment plan.

MEDICAL-LEGAL BACKGROUND

Medical-legal issues are becoming more important as medical litigation is increasing.[7] In ophthalmology, cataract surgery is the most frequently performed surgery, and it has become the most common cause of ophthalmologic malpractice litigation. Cataract malpractice cases total one third of all cases against eye surgeons.[7–9]

In a 2004 study, a questionnaire was given to cataract patients about to undergo cataract surgery to determine the level of informed consent.[8] The questionnaires were given to the patients 24 hours in advance of the surgery.[8] Seventy patients in a hospital in Austria were the participants. Of this group, 40% felt that they had had no information about the surgery. Twenty-three percent believed that there were surgical procedures without risks. Seventy-six percent felt that there were no risks for their cataract surgery. Forty-four percent of the patients wanted the physician to make the decision about the surgery. Twenty-six percent wanted to make the decision of their surgery with their ophthalmologist. Thus, there is an overwhelming majority of these European patients who do not understand that there are risks to their surgery. While this was a study originated in Europe, there are lessons to be learned: provide informed consent so that the patient understands the risks of surgery.

In a 2003 study about vitreoretinal surgery, Kraushar[10,11] used a questionnaire to query the medical malpractice experiences of vitreoretinal specialists. The results showed that rhegmatogenous retinal detachment is the most common presenting diagnosis in these lawsuits. The most common type of surgical management for the rhegmatogenous retinal detachment was pars plana vitrectomy (40%). Negligent treatment (surgical or medical) (63%) was more common than negligent diagnosis (10%). Decreased vision after treatment (40%), failed surgery (13%), and no improvement in vision (10%) were the most frequently cited reasons for the malpractice litigation. Kraushar's conclusion was that vitreoretinal specialists are at risk for malpractice litigation because many of their patients have a poor prognosis of visual recovery and because most vitreoretinal surgery is more complex in nature than cataract surgery.

Rhegmatogenous retinal detachment has been the most common presenting diagnosis in most studies on ophthalmic malpractice litigation, and most of the patients with this diagnosis are treated by vitreoretinal specialists.[11] Many vitreoretinal patients present to the retinologist after penetrating eye trauma or failed treatment by another ophthalmologist. Thus, the patients who have had a poor outcome may be more prone to litigation. As emergency consultants, vitreoretinal specialists may not have enough time to create rapport, central to a good patient-physician relationship. In addition, as consultants, retinal surgeons are at risk for being included in lawsuits directed toward other physicians. These risks suggest the necessity of a thorough discussion of informed consent and the development of a good physician-patient relationship.[12]

The number of malpractice claims in ophthalmology is still constantly increasing.[7,9] Malpractice claims are initiated if there is evidence of negligence, injury, and proximate cause.[12] However, malpractice in this sense is often hard to prove, and therefore, inadequate or lack of informed consent is used as a secondary cause in more than 90% of all ophthalmologic malpractice cases.[11,12]

In the million-dollar verdict category, jury trials are 3% of malpractice payments. In Florida, the payments involving one million dollars or more, 7.5% followed a jury trial.[13]

INFORMED CONSENT

Informed consent is an important part of every surgeon's practice. Office procedures and outpatient surgical procedures necessitate that there is communication of the factual details of the procedure, the risks and benefits of surgery. The printed materials are proof and documentation that the ophthalmologist has provided the appropriate information to the patient. The patient, in signing the consent, is agreeing to the procedure. While the patient can still say that he is too confused, anxious, or unable to comprehend English, the signed informed consent with a witness is a useful document in the practice setting.

There are attorneys who advertise on the Internet for eye surgery complications. One example is Hill and Associates in Philadelphia, Pennsylvania, whose web site is www.eyesurgeryinjury.com.[14] This web site is the first of Google search engines because of paid advertising or software coding for the Google search engine. Hill and Associates state on the opening page

"If you have already had eye surgery and developed any of the following complications, you may or may not have grounds for a lawsuit for damages: (A) Did you fully understand the risks? (B) Were you misled about the outcome? (C) Was your injury or side effect the result of normal risk or medical negligence? Contact Hill & Associates, P.C. to determine if you have grounds for a medical malpractice lawsuit"[14] (Table 14-1).

TABLE 14.1 Medical-Legal Considerations of Informed Consent

1. Did the patient fully understand the risks?
2. Could the patient be misled about the outcome?
3. Could the patient ever say to the doctor that the side effect of the surgery is due to normal risk or medical negligence?
4. Could there ever be a discussion of wrongful death? Be careful of patients with multiple system disease or cardiovascular disease and/or diabetes.

"Did You Fully Understand the Risks?"

The attorneys will focus on the patient's understanding of all of the risks of the procedure. As a clinician and surgeon, it is important to discuss death as a side effect of anesthesia, especially in Type 1 diabetic patients. Type 2 diabetic patients with a history of hypertension and cardiovascular disease are at risk for ischemic heart disease complications and death perioperatively.[15] Tell the patient the risks, all of them. Do not skip the risk of death.[7]

"Were You Misled About the Outcome?"

Many surgeons have the nursing staff go over the informed consent and then the surgeon goes over the important caveats. Or, the risks of endophthalmitis are not explained in more than one sentence. This has to be told to the patient in terms of risk and benefit analysis: Is the benefit of improving vision worth the risk of the procedure?

Intravitreal injection of bevacizumab has a low risk of endophthalmitis, approximately 0.066% or 6/10,000 according to one 2009 study.[16] The risk of endophthalmitis with 0.87% of intravitreal triamcinolone injections is approximately 1 person in a 100 people or 8 people in a 1,000 people.[11] The incidence of endophthalmitis in pars plana vitrectomy is 0.046% or 5 people in 10,000.[12]

"Was Your Injury or Side Effect the Result of Normal Risk or Medical Negligence?"

The question asks if the physician exposed the patient to normal risk or was there medical negligence. Medical negligence can include errors of omission, that is, lack of informed consent. This question also considers the ultimate side effect, death. Wrongful death is in this category. In the category of "normal risk" and how to define risk, the clinician can provide articles or Internet links which state the statistics of the side effects. Always emphasize that while statistics only tell one side of the story, if the side effect happens to the patient, for that patient, the side effect will become 100%. Thus, some clinicians never reveal the numbers of 1 person in 10,000 but rather emphasize that "while the side effects are rare, but if it happens to you, the side effect is 100%."

Wrongful Death[19]

The Internet provides a trove of data for the patients and their families. It is useful to understand the patient's point of view. What does he think of the surgery and risks and benefits? Is the patient's expectation unrealistic, and can we as surgeons manage their unrealistic expectations?

The definition of wrongful death is a lawsuit which alleges that the victim dies as a result of the negligent conduct or misdeeds of another.[19] A wrongful death lawsuit would be brought against a person who negligently, recklessly, or purposefully caused, in whole or in part, the death of another person. A defendant can be held liable by evidence for the wrongful death of another even if there was no direct intention to kill the victim. Usually, to be successful in such an action, the plaintiff must prove the defendant was negligent or strictly liable for the victim's death. Common wrongful death cases arise as a result of auto accidents, industrial accidents, personal injury, and medical malpractice.[14]

While there is no protection against medical malpractice claims, the key to the physician's legal well-being lies in the informed consent and the ability to establish rapport with the family and patient. If the patient is satisfied with the care and understands why there is a need for surgery, usually, there is no lawsuit, even in adverse medical outcomes. Thus, inform the patient of the risks and possible problems after surgery.

ANESTHESIA RISKS

The surgeon is responsible for the well-being of the patient during the course of surgery. The eye surgery may be successful, but if the patient suffers severe life-threatening complications, the surgeon may be held liable for wrongful death. Diabetic patients are at increased risk for death in undergoing vitrectomy surgery. With general anesthesia, the risk for death is greater than with local, monitored intravenous anesthesia. The basis for the increased risk is the autonomic dysfunction that affects the hemodynamics of the diabetic patient about to have surgery[7,20] (Table 14-2).

Diabetic patients needing vitrectomy surgery are at the advanced stages of eye disease with increased ischemia affecting its microvasculature in the retina and other organs. Presumably, by the time the proliferative diabetic patient needs vitrectomy, he has abnormalities of the cardiovascular system and renal system.

These proliferative diabetic retinopathy patients manifest diabetic automatic neuropathy and autonomic dysfunction. Thus, these patients when anesthetized can experience hypotensive reactions where the systolic blood pressure can be below 90 mm Hg. Marked variability in heart rate and cardiac rhythm disorders during anesthesia are seen in patients with diabetes without known autonomic neuropathy.[20]

The ophthalmologist and the retina surgeon are concerned with patient survival during the surgery and the perioperative period. It is important that the diabetic patient has preoperative clearance with his internal medicine physician and anesthesiologist.

Even with local anesthesia, the draping of the mildly sedated patient can lead to fright, confusion, and obtunded behavior. Consequently, the partially sedated patient may thrash or flail his arms while the surgeon is operating with microsurgical instruments inside the globe. In these cases, mild confusion may mean hypoxia and eventual cardiovascular compromise leading to the worst possible side effect—death in the operating room.

Thus, for the informed consent, it is important to stress all the complications equally without minimizing any of the complications. To prevent any of the complications to the best of your ability, as the operating eye surgeon, obtain preoperative clearance and have some understanding of how much time the patient will be covered under the drapes, if local anesthesia is to be used. Perform the surgery as quickly and efficiently as possible. In these cases, the use of preoperative bevacizumab reduces inflammation and the severity of neovascularization, which may in turn lead to a quicker vitrectomy in the operating room.[16–18]

While the risks are more pronounced in patients with longer duration of diabetes and insulin-dependent diabetes, similar high risks for cardiovascular compromise occur in the advanced elderly patients who have Type 2 diabetes and concomitant heart disease and/or hypertension. Thus, it is important to be vigilant in the surgery of these patients.

In summary, diabetics who are about to undergo surgery, experience considerable risks: preoperative fasting, stress, and inadequate application of insulin. All the preoperative fasting can lead to metabolic derangement.[20]

One study examined 332 consecutive patients who had had a vitrectomy for diabetic retinopathy. It was thought that the 5-year survival rate was 68%. Fifty percent of patients

TABLE 14.2 Anesthesia Risks

1. Diabetes
2. Pregnancy
3. Heart disease
4. Amputation
5. Known autonomic dysfunction such as orthostatic hypotension
6. Peripheral neuropathy
7. Cancer
8. AIDS
9. Pediatric cases

with heart disease died within 3.5 years of the surgery. Patients without heart disease had a 5-year survival rate of 90%.[21]

Hypertensive and diabetic patients were evaluated as they underwent elective noncardiac surgery. Their preoperative status and intraoperative changes in mean arterial pressure (MAP) were recorded as predictors of postoperative ischemic complications. Of the 254 patients studied, before surgery and monitored during surgery, 30 (12%) had postoperative cardiac death, ischemia, or infarction. Twenty-four percent of the patients with a previous myocardial infarction or cardiomegaly had an ischemic postoperative cardiac complication. Even if the patient had no previous myocardial infarction or cardiomegaly, 7% still had an ischemic complication.[21]

This study concluded that patients with a previous infarction or radiographic cardiomegaly are at high risk for postoperative ischemic complications. Prolonged intraoperative increases or decreases of 20 mm or more in MAP also results in a significant increase in life-threatening surgical complications.[15,19–21]

Diabetic patients who have other associated diseases such as pancreatic transplant that requires long-term prednisone dosages are at higher anesthesia risks than their normal counterparts. Diabetic patients who have chronic drug addiction to illegal drugs require higher dosages of the anesthesia premedications. They may also need more intravenous anesthetic agents to create a pain-free state during local anesthesia. Some of these patients are elderly but have been taking sleeping medications or antianxiety drugs for many years. These patients will require large doses of anesthetic agents.

Cancer patients with diabetes about to have retinal surgery are at higher anesthesia risk than similar aged counterparts without cancer or diabetes. These patients may have had extensive radiation to the head and neck region and thus normal vascularization of the postoperative wound may not occur.[22–28] There may be problems with sclerotomy closure after vitrectomy.

Of equal concern is the cancer patient's complete blood count, which may show anemia of chronic disease. The cancer patient may be hypotensive and pose a cardiac risk.[23] These patients may need a visit to the anesthesiologist 1 week prior to surgery. They also need a visit to their internist to ensure a proper history and physical examination prior to anesthesia.[23]

AIDS patients with diabetes requiring vitreoretinal surgery, need preoperative clearance with their Infectious Disease consultants and hematologists.[23,24] They need to have the infectious disease precautions while at the hospital and in the operating room. Diabetic patients also do not have the same wound-healing qualities as their same-aged counterparts without diabetes.[19–21] Thus, informed consent is essential. The patients and their families must understand the risks and benefits of the surgery versus no surgery. The postoperative recovery may take longer than other vitreoretinal surgical patients without diabetes, cancer, or AIDS.[23–26]

An elderly diabetic patient with Alzheimer's Disease has to be treated with special care. If this person needs surgery for proliferative diabetic retinopathy, informed consent should be obtained with his family members in the room. If there is one person in the family with the power of attorney, he needs to be present for the informed consent.

In patients with mental illness, controlled by antidepressants or antischizophrenic medications, the clinician must be careful with the informed consent. Identify the family member with the power of attorney. Or, is there a social worker who can vouch for the informed consent? A witness has to be present in these cases. The surgeon should try to contact the family, establish rapport with them, and ascertain that the family also consents to the surgery. The family must agree on the surgery since the patient may not be able to verbalize his consent.

MONETARY AWARDS

Plaintiffs win less than half the medical malpractice lawsuits that go to trial. There are a low percentage of jury trials, but the million-dollar verdicts can occur with or without a jury trial.[27,28]

The median verdict for ophthalmology lawsuits in 1999 is $500,000 compared to the median jury award of $800,000 in the same year.[27] Whereas, the median jury award in 1993, 6 years earlier, was only $500,000. Nationally, there are 54 jury awards of at least $1 million in 2000, compared with 27 awards of at least $1 million in 1999. Thus, the number of claims is increasing and so is the dollar amount.[10,27,28]

CROSS-CULTURAL CONSIDERATIONS ABOUT INFORMED CONSENT

Informed Consent and Cultural Competence

Cultural competence in the context of medicine is the sensitivity to the cultural background and language of the patient. Understanding the need for a variety of communication skills is important in the process of informed consent. For example, verbal and nonverbal communication and written communication all play a role in the process of informed consent. Some cultures want a verbal description of the surgery about to be performed. The consent must be communicated to the patient's extended family since there might be a need to address the group of concerned family members to arrive at a consensus for surgery.

Whereas Western societies may favor verbal openness or directness about the type of surgery for the patient, other societies may prefer silence as a form of respect. Consequently, the patient and family, in being silent, may be showing signs of respect in their own cultural setting, but for the Western-trained physician, the silence may be confusing. As another by-product of the silence, the patient may never ask the questions that he may want to ask. If the surgery does not meet the expectations of the patient in the cross-cultural context, the patient may feel very confused and disappointed. For the Western-trained physician, confusion reigns as well: the patient never asks questions so how could the physician anticipate any concerns?

For the patient from another culture, he may feel that there are spiritual alternatives to health care. While this might not be true for patients ingrained with the practice patterns of Western medicine, spiritual healing is common in Native American, Asian, and South Asian cultures (Tables 14-3 and 14-4).

Native American Issues and Informed Consent

The Indian Health Service (IHS) has sterilized between 25% and 50% of Native American Women aged 15 to 44 years, between 1970 and 1976.[29,30] It is unclear how many of the Native American women had been sterilized in the 1960s. Forced sterilization occurred because there is a lack of informed consent or the consent is obtained while the patient is sedated during the preoperative setting for caesarean section or in severe pain during labor. In 1974, Dr Connie Pinkerton-Uri, a member of the Choctaw-Cherokee tribe, stated that there were only 100,000 total Native American women of child-bearing age and that the Native American population in the United States was dwindling.[30] She found that the women are unable to understand the consent forms which are written in 12th grade English. The women sign the consent forms because they are threatened with the loss of their children and/or welfare benefits. Cheyenne tribal judge, Marie Sanchez, questioned

TABLE 14.3 High Risk for Inadequate Informed Consent

1. Poor health literacy
2. Cultural barrier
3. Language barrier
4. Inability to understand the necessity of surgery

TABLE 14.4 Cultural Competency

Traditional vs. multicultural approaches to informed consent
1. Verbal and written communication vs. nonverbal communication
2. Individual patient vs. group identity
3. Nuclear family vs. extended family relying on the father
4. Verbal openness vs. silence as respect
5. Task oriented vs. trust oriented
6. Physical factors in illness vs. spiritual factors in illness
7. Reliance on data vs. reliance on relationships

50 random Cheyenne women and found that IHS doctors had sterilized 26 of them. Mary Ann Bear Comes Out, a member of the Northern Cheyenne tribe, wrote that the "data indicated the same rate of sterilization would reduce births from this group by more than half over a 5-year period."[30] The forced sterilization has affected the patients' families and friends. Many marriages have ended in divorce. Those affected female patients have long-standing psychological issues with shame, guilt, and drug abuse as a result of the inability to conceive children.[30]

In 1976, Congress passed the Indian Health Care Improvement Act that gave tribes the right to manage IHS programs. The Native American tribes have taken over many of the IHS facilities and have started their own health services.

Informed consent for Native Americans should address the fear of improper care. The possible risks and benefits to the patient should be explained as well as the possible alternatives to the proposed surgery.

African American Issues and Informed Consent

In different cultures, "medicine and informed consent" is a charged topic. The Tuskegee Syphilis Study (1932–1972) is a 40-year study that recruited 399 poor, mostly illiterate African American sharecroppers with syphilis to study for research related to the natural progression of the untreated disease. After 1947, penicillin became the standard of care for the treatment of syphilis. The researchers at the time continued to withhold penicillin from the study patients. Instead of treating all of the syphilitic patients or creating a control group of treated and untreated patients, all of the participants were prevented from attending syphilis treatment clinics available to other people in the area. In the period after World War II, when the revelations of Nazi human experimentation were known, the Tuskegee Study personnel continued their research without the study protocols according to the Nuremberg Code of Human Rights. The study continued until 1972 when a leak to the press results in its termination.[31]

The Tuskegee study began in 1932, since the standard medical treatments for syphilis were toxic and had questionable effectiveness. At the time, the remedies were mercurial ointments and bismuth. Part of the original goal of the study was to determine if patients are better off not being treated with such toxic remedies. The researchers wanted to understand each stage of the disease in hopes of developing treatments for each stage.

Ethical considerations were limited from the onset of the study. To ensure that the men would show up for the possible dangerous, painful, diagnostic and nontherapeutic spinal tap, the physicians would send the 300 patients a misleading letter entitled, "Last Chance for Special Free Treatment." The study required all participants to undergo an autopsy after death in order to receive funeral benefits. After penicillin had been discovered, researchers continued to deny such treatment to many study participants. Many patients were given placebo treatments so that researchers could observe the progression of the fatal disease.[31]

In 1947, penicillin was the standard therapy for syphilis. Several US government sponsored public health programs called "rapid treatment centers," whose purpose was to eradicate the disease. However, the study coordinators prevented their patients from participating.[32] When 250 of the subject men during World War II registered for the draft and were consequently diagnosed and ordered to obtain treatment for syphilis before they could serve in the armed forces, the Public Health Services (PHS) prevented them from getting treatment and thus serving the country.[32]

In 1966, Peter Buxtun, a PHS venereal disease investigator in San Francisco, sent a letter to the national director of the Division of Venereal Diseases to express his concerns about the ethics of the extended Tuskegee Study. The Center for Disease Control (CDC) which was in charge of the Tuskegee Study reaffirmed the need for the continuation of the study until completion as defined when all subjects had died and subjected to autopsy. The CDC sought and gained support for the continuation of the study from local chapters of the National Medical Association which represented African American physicians and the American Medical Association. By 1972, Buxtun finally went to the press, with the story appearing in the Washington Star on July 25, 1972 and front page headlines in the New York Times on July 26, 1972. As a result of public outrage, the CDC and PHS appointed an ad hoc committee to review the Tuskegee Study. The Committee found that the study was medically unjustified and ordered its termination. In 1974, Congress passed the National Research Act and created a commission to study the regulations governing studies involving human participants. On May 16, 1997, President Bill Clinton formally apologized and held a ceremony for the Tuskegee participants.

The Tuskegee Syphilis Study has damaged the trust of the black community toward public health efforts in the United States.[33] The historical distrust of government plays a role in the dissemination of rumors in the black community. For example, one such rumor was that the government is responsible for the HIV/AIDs crisis by introducing the virus into the black community.[33] Similarly, the Tuskegee Study has led blacks to distrust the concept of organ donation and the concept of preventive care. The cessation of the Tuskegee Study has led to the creation of the National Human Investigation Board, federal regulation requiring IRBs for the protection of human subjects in medical studies.[32,33]

Hispanic Issues and Informed Consent

The Hispanic American community includes people who have origins from Cuba, Central and South America, Mexico, Puerto Rico, and other Spanish-speaking countries. The majority of Hispanics are Catholic and believe that health is a gift from God. Prevention of illness is believed to be accomplished with prayer, the wearing of religious medals, amulets, or keeping relics or religious statues at home. Visiting shrines and offering medals and candles are commonplace in certain Hispanic communities.

Elders have an important status in society. An individual who is sick will turn first to family members for support. They may recommend simple, safe home remedies. In the traditional household, the head of the family is a male and makes all the major decisions. The mother is a revered position in the family; she is beloved and protected. Thus, in some Hispanic families, the daughter may be the one who helps the elderly patient and plays a pivotal role in the informed consent process. At times, if the mother is about to have surgery, the entire family may show up for the informed consent explanations because she is vital to the family unit. Hispanics are accustomed to the family as a support system postoperatively. This may be helpful in the postoperative care of diabetic traction retinal detachments where the recovery process may involve head positioning with gas bubble tamponades. In addition, the Hispanic patient who is ill is emotionally expressive. The patient will expect to be pampered when ill and the family is expressing their love for the patient by showing up in large numbers at the doctor's office.

In the management of diabetic retinopathy, most Hispanics see thinness as a problem and plumpness as an ideal state. Lifestyle management with diet and exercise in the Hispanic patient may not resonate well, and compliance may be an issue.

The curandero is a holistic healer who uses Aztec, Spanish, spiritualistic and homeopathic rituals. The curandero operates in a religious context as well, suing elements of Catholic and pentocostal rituals, penance, confessionals, artifacts, offerings of money, metal objects, wooden objects in the shape of the patient or in the shape of the involved body organ, and the laying of hands.

For translation purposes, ask a family member to translate or intervene as there are many cultural cues which are understood only in the context of patients' family. If no family member is available, use an interpreter to explain the medical terms and the purpose of the surgery, "restore vision so that you can see the new grandchild," "improve the vision so that you can return to being the homemaker and thus return to your central role as a mother." For pregnant diabetics with severe proliferative diabetic retinopathy, the explanation of her need for laser surgery would include "restore her vision so that she can see her new unborn child or take care of her other children while she is pregnant."

East Asian Culture and Informed Consent

For East Asian cultures, there is an emphasis on the extended family, respect for elders, and the patrilineal focus of respect. In cases of diabetes and diabetic retinopathy, where the focus of disease is not only ophthalmological but systemic, it is important to have the family understand the nature of the disease and how the diet may have impinged on the progression of the disease now needing surgery. There is a need for the family to understand the background explanation of the disease and how their family member arrived at this time and place, needing surgery.

In many elderly Asian patients, surgery is a last resort and they are accepting of consequences beyond their control. The grandmother or grandfather figure in the patient chair is a revered figure in the family and the decision may be made by the family council headed by the first-born son. Thus, informed consent is needed by the first-born son.

In some instances, the son, who is in charge, may want the more detailed explanation and may request that a shorter, "sugarcoated" version be given to the elderly relative, the patient. In Japan today, cancer diagnoses are still withheld from the female patients but only the husbands or sons know the details of the diagnosis.

For the East Asian community where English serves as a language barrier, it is best to have an interpreter, a family member, or a translator in the clinician's office. The translator serves to bridge the cultural gap. In some Buddhist cultures, corneal transplants are considered taboo since it is the placement of another person's soul into the patient.

The two main Chinese dialects are Mandarin and Cantonese. Mandarin is the official language of China. The written language is the same. Thus, the written literature about the surgery and informed consent can be useful for the explanation. The English version of the consent should be signed since this is the one that is uniform in your practice.

South Asian Issues and Informed Consent

In South Asian Indian culture, the older family members are often financially dependent on their children. They face a culturally different society, such as language barrier, culture mismatch, new lifestyle factors, and role reversal. Often, the husband's parents will join the family after they have retired or when help is needed. The grandparents' role in raising the children is highly respected. The son must be involved in the informed consent. If the son is unavailable, the next eldest, a daughter or another son, will be in charge.

The elderly parents or grandparents may not understand English. The main Indian language is Hindi, but there are other Indian languages: Telugu, Gujarati, Urdu, Kannada, Punjabi, Tamil, Bengali, Assamese Konkani, Marathi, Malayalam, Meitei, Mizo, Khasi, Garo, Oriya, and Kokborok. Usually, the family will come and serve as the translator. In a hospital setting, interpreters may be needed if the patient does not speak English and there are no family members available.

In the South Asian cultures, where religion is important, the physician can ask the patient and family about the surgery in that context. Many elders believe in Ayurvedic medicine, originating in India thousands of years ago. Ayurveda is derived from two Sanskrit works: ayu which means life and veda which means knowledge. Ayurvedic medicine explains how balance can be attained physically, mentally, and spiritually. Each individual is made up of three Doshas: Vata, Pitta, or Kapha. Each Dosha represents certain bodily

TABLE 14.5 Summary Informed Consent

1. Cross-cultural issues
2. Communicate with the patient at his literacy level
3. Talk about risks, such as death
4. Talk about blindness as a risk
5. If in doubt about informed consent, do it over, in front of family members and witnesses

activity, and the ratio of Doshas varies in each person. If there is an imbalance of one Dosha over the other, the Ayurveda will suggest lifestyle and nutritional guidelines, herbal supplements to rebalance the Doshas.

Hindu religion can affect certain health care decisions. "Karma" is a law of behavior and consequences in which actions of past life affects the circumstances in which one is born and lives in this life. The patient may believe that illness is caused by "Karma," despite complete understanding of the pathophysiologic causes of the illness. Thus, health is related to the connectedness of the body, mind, and spirit. The most elderly focus in preparing the soul for life after death.

The cultural and religious background of the Asian Indian elders lead to family centered decisions rather than individual based decision making in the informed consent process. Some families may ask that the patient be kept uninformed about the diagnosis and the details of the surgery. This is culturally acceptable.

Because family is important, it is expected for several members of the family to show up with the patient for the doctor's visit. On the day of informed consent, there will be several family members who will be there to show respect for the patient. However, the first-born son or his wife will be the one who will need to understand the informed consent. That person is the one who will finally convince the father or mother to sign the consent in the native language.

Take-Home Message

The take-home message of this chapter is that the clinician must inform the patient of the risks and benefits. Be thorough and be honest with the patient. Establish rapport with the patient and family prior to surgery. Other modes of communication such as nonverbal cues or verbal communication in addition to the printed text of the informed consent may make the process more congruent to the cultural construct of the patient and his family. In our practice, if there are a lot of questions on the part of the patient and family, despite our lengthy discussion of risks and benefits, we send them for a second opinion at the university eye clinic or to another retinal specialist. Involve as many second and third opinions to be placed in the chart. Each of the second-opinion consultations serve as additional patient education opportunities for the patient. The patient may need more time to accept his surgical diagnosis and prognosis. Let the patient ultimately make the decision about the surgery (Table 14-5).

REFERENCES

1. http://www.forensic-psych.com/articles/artCulturallyCompetentConsent.php. Accessed 23 February 2009.
2. http://nces.ed.gov/naal. Accessed 23 February 2009.
3. Gazmararian JA, Baker DW, Williams MV, et al. Health illiteracy among medicare enrollees in a managed care organization. *JAMA*. 1999;282:545–551.
4. National Work Group on Literacy and Health. Communicating with patients who have limited literacy skills. *J Fam Pract*. 1998;46:168–176.
5. Paasche-Orlow MK, Taylor HA, Brancati FL. Readability standards for informed-consent forms as compared with actual readability. *N Engl J Med*. 2003;348:721–726.
6. Gordon D. MDs failure to use plain language can lead to the courtroom. *CMAJ*. 1996;155:1152–1154.
7. Blackston JW, Bouldin MJ, Brown CA, et al. Malpractice risk prevention for primary care physicians. *Am J Med Sci*. 2002;324:212–219.

8. Kiss CG, Richter-Mueksch S, Stifter E, et al. Informed consent and decision making by cataract patients. *Arch Ophthalmol.* 2004;122:94–98.
9. Kraushar MF, Turner MF. Medical malpractice litigation in cataract surgery. *Arch Ophthalmol.* 1987;105:1339–1343.
10. Kraushar MF. Medical malpractice experiences of vitreoretinal specialists: Risk prevention strategies. *Retina.* 2003;23: 523–529.
11. Kraushar MF. Medical malpractice litigation in the management of vitreoretinal diseases. *Arch Ophthalmol.* 1987;105:187–190.
12. Kraushar MF, Turner MF. Medical malpractice litigation in ophthalmology: The New Jersey experience. *Ophthalmic Surg.* 1986;17:671–674.
13. Vidmar N, Mackillop K, Lee P. Million dollar medical malpractice cases in Florida: Post-verdicts and pre-suit settlements. http://papers.ssrn.com/sol3/papers.cfm?abstract_id=880736. Accessed 1 March 2009.
14. www.eyesurgeryinjury.com. Accessed 1 March 2009.
15. Charlson ME, MacKenzie CR, Gold JP, et al. The preoperative and intraoperative hemodynamic predictors of postoperative myocardial infarction or ischemia in patients undergoing noncardiac surgery. *Ann Surg.* 1989;210:637–648.
16. Artunay O, Yuzbasioglu E, Rasier R, et al. Incidence and management of acute endophthalmitis after intravitreal bevacizumab (Avastin) injection. *Eye.* 2009; February epublished: http://www.ncbi.nlm.nih.gov/pubmed/19218994?dopt=Abstract. Accessed 1 March 2009.
17. Moshfeghi DM, Kaiser PK, Scott IU, et al. Acute endophthalmitis following intravitreal triamcinolone acetonide injections. *Am J Ophthalmol.* 2003;136:791–796.
18. Aaberg TM Jr, Flynn HW Jr, Schiffman J, Newton J. Nosocomial acute-onset postoperative endophthalmitis survey. A 10-year review of incidence and outcomes. *Ophthalmology.* 1998;105:1004–1014.
19. www.wrongful-death.com. Accessed 1 March 2009.
20. Knuttgen D, Weidemann D, Doehn M. Diabetic autonomic neuropathy: Abnormal cardiovascular reactions under general anesthesia. *J Mol Med.* 1990;68:1168–1172.
21. Helbig H, Kellner U, Bornfeld N, Foerster MH. Life expectancy of diabetic patients undergoing vitreous surgery. *Br J Ophthalmol.* 1996;80:640–643.
22. Payne WG, Naidu DK, Wheeler CK, et al. Wound healing in patients with cancer. http://www.pubmedcentral.nih.gov/articlerender.fcgi?artid=2206003. Accessed 1 March 2009.
23. Cornell K, Waters DJ. Impaired wound healing in the cancer patient: Effects of cytotoxic therapy and pharmacologic modulation by growth factors. *Vet Clin North Am Small Anim Pract.* 1995;25:111–131.
24. Lord RV. Anorectal surgery in patients infected with human immunodeficiency virus: Factors associated with delayed wound healing. *Ann Surg.* 1997;226:92–99.
25. Irvine AR, Lonn L, Schwartz D, et al, Retinal detachment in AIDS. *Br J Ophthalmol.* 1997;81:180–183.
26. Brem H, Tomic-Canic M. Cellular and molecular basis of wound healing in diabetes. *J Clin Invest.* 2007;117: 1219–1222.
27. Kraushar MF, Robb JH. Ophthalmic malpractice lawsuits with large monetary awards. *Arch Ophthalmol.* 1996;114: 333–337.
28. Linebarger EJ, Hardten DR, Shah GK, Lindstrom RL. Phacoemulsification and modern cataract surgery. *Surv Ophthalmol.* 1999;44:123–147.
29. Dillingham B. Sterilization of native Americans. *Am Indian J.* 1977;16.
30. Lawrence J. The Indian Health Service and the sterilization of native American Women. *Am Indian Q.* 2000;24: 400–419.
31. Parker L. Bad blood still flows in Tuskegee Study. *USA Today.* Retrieved 12–4–2008.
32. Heller J. Syphilis victims in US study went untreated fro 40 years. Syphilis victims got no therapy. *New York Times.* 26 July 1972:1, 8.
33. Thomas SB, Quinn SC. The Tuskegee Syphilis Study, 1932 to 1972: Implications for HIV education and AIDS risk education programs in the Black community. *Am J Pub Health.* 1991;81:1498–1505.

SUGGESTED READINGS

1. Festinger L. *Conflict, Decision and Dissonance.* Stanford, CA: Stanford University Press; 1964.
2. Festinger LA *Theory of Cognitive Dissonance.* Stanford, CA: Stanford University Press; 1957.
3. Fortney JA. Assessing recall and understanding of informed consent in a contraceptive clinical trial. *Stud Fam Plann.* 1999;30:339–346.
4. Heckhausen H, Gollwitzer P. Thought contents and cognitive functioning in motivational vs volitional states of mind. *Motiv Emotion.* 1987;11:101–120.
5. Jonas E, Schulz Hardt S, Frey D, Thelen N. Confirmation bias in sequential information search after preliminary decisions: An expansion of dissonance theoretical research on selective exposure to information. *J Pers Soc Psychol.* 2001;80:557–571.
6. Kraushar MF. Malpractice and the physician patient relationship. *Compr Ther.* 1987;13:3–4.
7. Kraushar MF. Recognizing and managing the litigious patient. *Surv Ophthalmol.* 1992;37:54–56.
8. Kraushar MF, Steinberg JA. Informed consent: Surrender or salvation? *Arch Ophthalmol.* 1986;104:352–355.
9. Lanckton AV. The contours of informed consent. *Surv Ophthalmol.* 1996;40:391–394.
10. Leydhecker W, Gramer E, Krieglstein GK. Patient information before cataract surgery. *Ophthalmologica.* 1980;180: 241–246.
11. Morgan LW, Schwab IR. Informed consent in senile cataract extraction. *Arch Ophthalmol.* 1986;104:42–45.
12. Priluck IA, Robertson DM, Buettner H. What patients recall of the preoperative discussion after retinal detachment surgery. *Am J Ophthalmol.* 1979;87:620–623.
13. Robinson G, Merav A. Informed consent: Recall by patients tested postoperatively. *Ann Thorac Surg.* 1976;22: 209–212.
14. Rosenberg M, Abelson R. *An Analysis of Cognitive Balancing.* New Haven, CT: Yale University Press; 1960.

CHAPTER 15

Guidelines for Nursing Staff and Medical Assistants

The physician's staff is crucial to the successful delivery of care in diabetic retinopathy. The staff member is the first person meeting the new diabetic patient on the telephone or in the office. The receptionist, with her sunny telephone voice, is the "voice" of the practice. Thus, the entire staff should be educated about the needs of the diabetic patient with vision loss (Tables 15-1 and 15-2).

WHAT IS THE MISSION STATEMENT?

What do we as physicians stand for? Ask each of your new hires to articulate what should be the mission of the office in serving diabetic patients. What do patients want? "They want to get better" is the single most common answer. How do we convey this message as physicians and as staff members? To "get better" means that the vision will improve. Obviously, the improvement of vision may take weeks or months depending on the status of the patient's diabetic retinopathy. What can the staff do to facilitate the patient's sense of well-being despite his fears and anxiety about vision loss? To translate this into concrete terms: How can the staff make the patient feel that today's visit to the retinal specialist is a "step in the right direction" in his search for quality health care in recovering eyesight? (Tables 15-3 to 15-14).

Suggestions for the staff include diabetic education materials in the waiting room, a videotape monitor with helpful diabetic videos, and a corner bookcase of diabetic cookbooks, all to allay the anxieties while the patient is in the waiting room. At the exit interview, there should be a written handout tailored to the patient and his diagnosis. Helpful Web sites and local addresses of diabetic organizations and the American Diabetes Association can be distributed at the exit interview, prior to making the patient's return appointment (see Appendix B). The patient has to feel that his questions are answered and that the office will be receptive to his future telephone calls and questions.

The Mission[1]

Service is the mission. We, as physicians, serve by making the diagnosis and providing treatment. We do this with integrity, commitment, and compassion. The staff reflects our values by supporting the patient's treatment plan, by educating the patient, and by acting as "care coordinators" of the patient and his needs. For example, the nurse or medical assistant is the person who gathers all of the patient's lab tests and collates the nephrologist's report, cardiologist's report, and podiatrist's report prior to the scheduled surgery.

As a physician and leader in the office, you want your mission to become the mission of all of the staff members. Everyone in the office, from the bookkeeper/biller to the receptionist, understands that the most important goal is improving vision for the diabetic patient. Everyone plays a role in that mission. The nurse takes the phone calls about

TABLE 15.1 Concepts for Staff Education

Background diabetic retinopathy
Nonproliferative diabetic retinopathy
Proliferative diabetic retinopathy
Diabetic macular edema

TABLE 15.2 Goal of the Office

1. Education of the Staff
2. Health Literacy of the Staff
3. Compassionate Service: Art and Science of Medicine
4. Teamwork: The physician and staff are part of a team.

diabetic complications. Or, the medical assistant gives appropriate reading materials for the patient and family members. The biller can help with questions about insurances or home health care services for the patient, so that the patient can continue his path toward vision rehabilitation. The entire office is there to serve the patient during his journey toward recovery of vision.

COMPASSION AND EMPATHY

For all new hires, we have them experience the sensation of "loss of vision," by letting them walk blindfolded in a dark hallway or a dark room. This exercise usually reminds the young staff members what our diabetic patients may be experiencing when they come to a vitreoretinal specialist's office for the first time. The need for compassion and empathy is important for everyone who works in health care.

Providing the best service is an important goal for the office staff. The diabetic patient has special needs in that he or she may need water, a cup of orange juice, or peanut butter crackers in the instances of hypoglycemia. The elderly patients may need a wheelchair or cane. An extra staff member may be needed to help them ambulate to the bathroom or to the examination room.

CROSS-CULTURAL CONSIDERATIONS

As the United States' population becomes more diverse, the physician's office must respond to the changing needs of the patient population.[2] With non–English speaking patients, where there is no translator, the challenge of providing service is enormous.

TABLE 15.3 Mission Statement

1. Integrity, Commitment, and Compassion
   a. Delivery of health care
   b. Committed to excellence of diagnosis, treatment, and service
   c. Compassionate care
2. Educate the patient
3. Teamwork approach to diabetic retinopathy
   a. The patient must want to do his part of compliance with treatment plans.
   b. The physician and his office must educate the patient to increase his motivation for compliance.

TABLE 15.4 Telephone Triage: A Script

Your receptionist: Hello. This is Dr John Doe's office. How can we help you today? (Say this with a smile.)
Patient: I would like to make an appointment. My doctor, Dr Joe Smith, says that I have a vitreous hemorrhage or bleeding in the eye.
Your receptionist: Yes, we have a cancellation today. You can come at 2 PM today or if you would like, you can be squeezed in at 9 AM tomorrow. (Free up time for emergencies such as this patient with a diabetic vitreous hemorrhage.)
Patient: I am really nervous. Can you squeeze me in tomorrow?
Your receptionist: Yes I understand. Please give us your name and telephone number so we can input the information into the computer. We will see you 9 AM tomorrow. (Be reassuring, kind, calm.)
Please bring all your eyedrops and pills for hypertension or diabetes. Bring in all your medications or a list of medications. Bring any lab tests that you might have from your visits with Dr Smith. Bring sunglasses because your eyes will be dilated and you will want sunglasses afterwards. The sunglasses will help you drive home. Bring your medical insurance card, as well. You can come a few minutes early to fill out our forms. The entire examination may take 2 hours or more, since we are squeezing you in. There might be a delay.
Patient: I can wait. I am so nervous that I want to be squeezed in. By the way, will I need to bring someone to drive me home?
Your receptionist: If that makes you feel more comfortable, yes. But if you want to drive home, it will be okay. Usually, after 20 minutes, you can drive home with sunglasses.
Patient: Thank you.
Your receptionist: Thank you. See you tomorrow. (Say this with a smile.)

In these instances, the Google Web site will translate any word or phrase into the language of the patient. Type in "diabetes" in French and then the word is translated on the Google Web site. This is possible for the Arabic and Asian languages as well.

When there is an interpreter, the ease of communication is enhanced. Thus, it is important to provide bilingual handouts if possible. This can be done with the Google Web site. At least the translator will have access to your English language handouts.

In some cultures, the female patient will want a female attendant in the room. Be prepared to ask the family member if the patient would like a female assistant during the examination.

DEALING WITH DENIAL AND DIABETES

Some patients find that the diagnosis of diabetes is overwhelming and become difficult to treat. In some cases, these patients may be going through the grieving cycles described by Kubler-Ross in her 1969 seminal work, *On Death and Dying*.[3] She describes the five stages of grieving as a patient confronts death: denial, anger, bargaining, depression, and acceptance.[3] While diabetes is well treated in America, the patient may feel that the diagnosis implies a loss of control and thus triggering the feelings of denial and anger.

TABLE 15.5 First Telephone Encounter with a New Patient

1. Establish rapport with the patients with sunny, happy, welcoming telephone voice.
2. Ask about name, telephone number, or whatever demographics that you need in order to schedule patients
3. Tell them that the office visit may take 2 hours. Always underpromise and overdeliver. If you tell them 1 hour and the visit actually lasts 1½ hours, the patients will be angry. If you tell them that it will take 2 hours and they leave after 1½, the patients are ecstatic. It is all about expectations.
4. Ask about the medicines and a medicine list. Ask about lab tests. Ask about insurance last.
5. The encounter has to be soothing and calming.
6. Having a gruff pit bull as your receptionist is not useful. You want a kind nurse or nurse's aide to answer the phone asking about patients. A pit bull receptionist serves as a barrier to more patient appointments.

TABLE 15.6 Information for a New Diabetic Patient

1. Handouts about the definition of Type 1 and Type 2 diabetes mellitus
2. Diabetic recipes
3. Nutritionist information
4. Food pyramid
5. List of blood tests that are commonly needed by the ophthalmologist
   a. Cholesterol, triglycerides
   b. Fasting blood sugar
   c. Hemoglobin A1c
   d. Electrolytes, renal function
   e. Complete blood count
6. List of diabetes complications and the eye
   a. Diabetic retinopathy
   b. Glaucoma
   c. Cataract
   d. Corneal problems
7. Common symptoms of diabetic retinopathy
   a. Loss of vision
   b. Decreased vision at near or decreased vision when reading or using the computer
   c. Total loss of vision
   d. Waxing and waning of vision loss
   e. Central loss of vision when reading

It is important for the staff and the physician to be sensitive to these issues. For the staff, the patient may present with intense anger and refuse to keep appointments or refuse to cooperate. For the physician, the patient could also show anger or try to bargain with the doctor in terms of the treatment plan. For example, the patient may say, "I do not want laser under any circumstances because my cousin had laser and went blind." This patient is bargaining with the ophthalmologist. Thus, as part of the health care team, we should be cognizant of the patient's psychological issues.

STAFF EDUCATION

The essentials of diabetes education involve population demographics and the definition of the disease and its complications (see Chapter 1). There are approximately 23 million diabetics in the United States, of which 6 to 8 million are undiagnosed and 16 million are diagnosed. It is interesting to note that a third of the diabetic population is unaware that they have the disease and is therefore unaware of the need to see an ophthalmologist or optometrist. Thus, for ophthalmologists and vitreoretinal specialists involved in the clinical practice of diabetic retinopathy, the physician and staff could play a larger role in the education of the diabetic patient.

Diabetes is a metabolic disease involving (i) the inability to produce insulin, which is Type 1 diabetes or (ii) the inability to produce enough insulin, which is Type 2 diabetes. There is an epidemic of Type 2 diabetes because of the rise of obesity in teens. While the

TABLE 15.7 Patients Who Should Be Expedited

1. Abrupt loss of vision
2. Painful headache or eye ache with loss of vision with nausea and vomiting
3. Loss of vision lasting 10 minutes and then the vision returns
4. Partial loss of vision in one or both eyes
5. Sudden double vision

TABLE 15.8 Patients with Special Emotional Needs

1. Children and teenagers with new diagnosis of diabetes
   a. This group may be emotionally unprepared for the diagnosis because of their developmental age
2. Adults with new diagnosis of diabetes
   a. New diagnosis entails explanations and educational materials
3. Elderly patients who live alone with diabetes
   a. Patients who do not have a family support system may need more interaction by the social worker
   b. May need home health aids if they have vitrectomy surgery
4. Patients with sudden visual loss
   a. Anxiety with loss of vision in a sighted world
   b. Angle-closure glaucoma or neovascular glaucoma because of diabetic retinopathy

epidemiologic studies of the past 20 years have shown that after 15 years of diabetes, there is a significant incidence of diabetic retinopathy. However, as one third of the diabetic population is unaware that they have diabetes, their late diagnosis may mean that their true duration of diabetes is greater than that previously documented on a medical record. Thus, in clinical practice, it is common to see significant diabetic macular edema in a patient who is newly diagnosed with diabetes. Diabetes can occur in anyone with a family history, obesity, or hyperlipidemia. There are high-risk groups such as Native Americans, Hispanics, Asians, South Asians, and African Americans.

There are many complications of diabetes, but for the ophthalmologist, the most common complications fall into three categories: (i) background diabetic retinopathy or nonproliferative diabetic retinopathy, (ii) proliferative diabetic retinopathy, and (iii) diabetic macular edema. Diabetic macular edema can occur in any stage of diabetes. Nonproliferative diabetic retinopathy is the type that involves hard exudates, cotton-wool spots, hemorrhages, and microaneurysms, everything up until the occurrence of retinal neovascularization. Once neovascularization occurs anywhere in the retina, it is proliferative diabetic retinopathy. It is this proliferative diabetic retinopathy that requires laser and possible vitrectomy. These stages of diabetic retinopathy can accelerate with poor systemic control of diabetes.

Diabetic retinopathy and diabetic kidney disease (diabetic nephropathy) tend to be associated with one another. If the patient has eye disease, he will have kidney disease, since there are microscopic vessels in both of these organs, and as we know, diabetes affects the microvasculature. There is a link between diabetic retinopathy and heart disease as well. People with diabetic retinopathy are twice as likely to have a heart attack or stroke and three times as likely to die from it.

TABLE 15.9 Diabetic Retinopathy: Concepts and Definitions for Staff

1. Diabetic retinopathy affects the smallest vessels in the back of your eyes.
2. Diabetic retinopathy is a microvascular disease.
3. When blood sugar has been high for many years, the walls of the blood vessels fall apart and blood and fluid leaks out onto the retina, causing vision loss.
4. The retina is like the inside lining of the eye, the film inside a camera. This inside lining gets damaged with the leakage of blood and blood proteins.
5. Development of diabetic retinopathy is related to cholesterol levels and the overproduction of human growth hormone and the hormone leptin found in fat cells.
6. Eventually, the blood vessels become so abnormal, full of leaking holes, that new blood vessels form, "neovascularization of the retina." These new blood vessels are abnormal and cause more blood leakage and more vision loss occurs.
   a. Treatment is with laser or bevacizumab, an intravitreal injection of a monoclonal antibody. This is available at your retinal specialist's office.

TABLE 15.10 Prevention: Points for Patients

1. See an ophthalmologist (eye MD) or eye care practitioner (optometrist) who has a lot of experience at looking at retinas for regular checkups.
2. To get a good look at the retina, a dilated exam will be done (eyedrops will be used to "dilate" or "open up the pupil" so that the ophthalmologist or optometrist will look inside).
3. Yearly eye exams with early laser treatment will prevent blindness.
4. If you do have diabetic retinopathy, your ophthalmologist or retinal specialist will perform a fluorescein angiogram. This involves a special digital camera which takes photos of your eye and analyzes the blood circulation around the retina. After a few photos, the ophthalmologist or retinal specialist will inject a special dye (fluorescein) into your arm, where it will travel through your blood vessels to the blood vessels of your eye. While the dye is traveling into the retina, more photos will be taken to examine the retinal blood vessels and determine if any retinal damage has occurred.
5. Laser could be the next step if you have diabetic retinopathy.

The American Diabetes Association survey found that 68% of those with diabetes are not aware of their increased risk for heart disease and stroke. Sixty percent do not know that they are at high risk for high blood pressure and abnormal lipids in the blood, both of which increase the overall risk of heart disease and stroke.

There is a high rate of cardiovascular disease (CVD) in diabetic patients. The risk factors of CVD are obesity, lack of physical exercise, hypertension, high triglyceride levels, and low HDL cholesterol levels. These risk factors are present in people with Type 2 diabetes, as well.

One of the main reasons that diabetes damages the body is that diabetes affects the tiniest blood vessels. The resulting microvascular disease will adversely change the physiology of the eye, kidney and heart.

Researchers find that the risk in people with Type 2 diabetes is twice as high as that in people without diabetes. Thus, diabetic patients must monitor their blood sugars, their cholesterol, and triglyceride levels. In addition, the diabetic patients must actively pursue steps to reduce heart disease and stroke: lose weight, exercise a minimum of 150 minutes/week, and raise the good cholesterol levels by exercise.

It is important for the staff to understand that (i) diabetic patients have a higher risk of developing eye conditions that can lead to blindness, (ii) diabetic retinopathy is the most common cause of blindness in people between 21 and 64 years of age, (iii) regular eye exams and early diagnosis can prevent significant vision loss from diabetic retinopathy,

TABLE 15.11 Laser for Diabetic Retinopathy: Points for Patients

1. Diabetic Macular Edema
   a. The retinal specialist aims the laser, which is a high-energy beam of light, at the blood vessels leaking blood and sealing them so that they stop leaking.
   b. For some forms of macular edema, the vision might not improve, but the laser will stabilize the vision so it will not get worse.
   c. Yearly dilated examinations are important to pick up this condition before visual loss occurs.
2. Proliferative Diabetic Retinopathy
   a. If you have proliferative diabetic retinopathy, the type of eye finding where all the blood vessels leak and new abnormal ones are created which leak even more, the retinal specialist will use a "scatter laser treatment" also known as "panretinal photocoagulation" to stop the bleeding.
   b. The laser treatment uses a laser to destroy many different parts of the retina where the abnormal blood vessels are growing wildly. It is thought that the laser, which destroys some parts of the retina, prevents further signals that lead to new vessel growth. Researchers feel that the laser may thin the retina, thereby increasing the amount of oxygen that can get to the good retina, and may induce parts of the eye to produce certain chemicals that prevent the growth of new vessels.

TABLE 15.12 Vitrectomy Surgery for Serious Diabetic Retinopathy: Points for Patients

1. If you have a lot of bleeding inside your eye from proliferative diabetic retinopathy, then you may need a "vitrectomy" to improve your vision.
2. In this procedure, you will be given a local or general anesthetic. You may or may not stay overnight in the hospital, depending on your overall health and eye-surgery findings.
3. During the vitrectomy, the retinal surgeon will make a tiny incision in your eye and will remove the bloody vitreous gel, which is the gel inside your eye, next to your retina. The gel gets replaced with a saline solution. This is okay since most of the vitreous is mostly liquid anyway.
4. At the same time, the surgeon will repair your retina if it is damaged.
5. When you go home, your eyes may be red and sensitive for a few days. You will have to wear an eye patch and plastic or metal eye shield at bedtime to protect your eye for a few days or weeks depending on the severity of your surgery. You will be given antibiotic drops to use in the operated eye.
6. If you need the procedure done in both eyes, your doctor will schedule the second eye after the first one heals.

and (iv) patients with diabetes are more likely to have glaucoma and tend to develop cataracts earlier than those patients without the disease.

The staff should be trained in the vocabulary of diabetes and diabetic retinopathy. For example, terms such as fasting blood glucose, hemoglobin A1c, lipid profiles, total cholesterol, and triglycerides are needed to understand the systemic and ophthalmic condition of the diabetic patient. It is the staff who obtains these laboratory data from the family care practitioner or internal medicine physician.

Hemoglobin A1c or "glycated hemoglobin" is a blood test that provides a snapshot of your blood glucose levels for the past 3 or 4 months. High levels show that the patient has had difficulty controlling his blood sugar for a while, before this test. Normal levels are less than 6%. For every 1% decrease in hemoglobin A1c, the level of diabetic retinopathy improves 35%.

TABLE 15.13 Other Eye Conditions: Points for Patients

1. Patients with diabetes are likely to develop other eye conditions than other people without diabetes.
2. Glaucoma
   a. Fluid from inside the eye does not drain through normal channels. Instead, fluid builds up inside the eye, increasing the pressure inside the eye, eventually destroying the optic nerve.
   b. The diabetic patient is twice as likely to develop this common form of glaucoma, called "open-angle glaucoma."
3. Neovascular Glaucoma
   a. In diabetic patients with new vessel formation, the type of diabetic retinopathy called "proliferative diabetic retinopathy," neovascular glaucoma occurs because the abnormal blood vessels grow over the normal drainage system inside the eye. High-intraocular pressure can occur, and pain can occur in the late stages. In the early stages, the patient may not know that he has this type of glaucoma until he sees the ophthalmologist or retinal specialist. This needs medications, laser surgery, and other forms of surgery. This type of glaucoma may require the services of a glaucoma-trained ophthalmologist.
4. Cataracts
   a. Cataracts occur when the lens of the eye becomes cloudy or opaque. Then, there is mild to severe vision loss. Although cataracts occur in nondiabetic patients over the age of 65, they occur earlier in diabetic patients. They can occur in children with uncontrolled Type 1 diabetes. Cataracts can be easily treated with surgery. The cloudy lens becomes replaced with an "intraocular implant," a new, tiny plastic lens that fits inside the eye.

TABLE 15.14 Drugs That Are Contraindicated with Diabetes

1. Chromium
   a. The exact amount of chromium needed in your diet is 15 to 50 μg a day. If you take too much, chromium will be accumulated in your liver where it can be toxic. Some studies have shown excess chromium can cause cancer.
   b. On study in China showed that people with Type 2 diabetes, who were chromium deficient, are given large doses of chromium. They improved hemoglobin A1c, blood glucose, and cholesterol while reducing their insulin requirements. However, most patients in America do not have chromium deficiency.
2. Cinnamon: No evidence that this works.
3. Aspirin: No evidence that this works.
4. Pancreas formula: Mixture of herbs, vitamins, and minerals to help diabetes. No evidence this formula works.
5. Gymnema Sylvestre: Part of alternative medical treatment called Ayurvedic medicine. This has never been tested in a controlled study in humans. No evidence that this works.

HEALTH LITERACY

The staff member is the first to greet the patient. Thus, the staff must be able to communicate about diabetes in simple, everyday terms. Some patients are illiterate in English despite being born in America. Or, the level of education makes it hard for the patient to understand informed consent. In this instance, the staff must make the explanations aimed at a "third-grade" level of education. All this can be done smoothly with the medical assistant or nurse who understands that educating these patients is important for treatment compliance and a successful visual outcome.

CLINICAL CORRELATION

Telephone triage for a new patient with a complaint of sudden vision loss in one or both eyes.

Staff response: This patient has to be seen urgently. Squeeze the patient into today's schedule. Ask the physician when is the best time or bring the patient immediately to the office and tell him that there is going to be a wait since he is being "squeezed into the schedule." Warn him that he may be in the office for about 2 to 3 hours when you add in the waiting time and the possibility of laser.

CLINICAL CORRELATION

Telephone triage for an established patient who has had declining vision for 6 months (see Tables 15-4 to 15-7).

Staff response: This patient has had worsening vision over 6 months. Waiting a day or two longer will probably not hurt the patient adversely. He already has waited 6 months.

The appointment can be tomorrow or the next day.

CLINICAL CORRELATION

Telephone triage for an established patient who has pain, nausea, vomiting, the worse headache of his life, and loss of vision. His visual loss began as a halo around street lights.

Staff response: It could be angle-closure glaucoma in this patient. This is one of the few emergencies in ophthalmology, and the patient must be seen immediately. This has to be underscored for the patient. If he cannot come in to the doctor's office, instruct him to go to the nearest emergency room with ophthalmologists on call (see Table 15-8).

CLINICAL CORRELATION

Telephone triage for a post-op patient with a new painful red eye. Surgery was last week.

Staff response: This is another emergency because he has had surgery last week. A painful red eye after surgery makes all ophthalmologists suspect endophthalmitis. When the patient arrives at the office, he may have such severe pain that he does not want anyone to look at his eye unless he is the ophthalmologist. If the patient does show such pain, make sure that the physician sees him immediately.

CLINICAL CORRELATION

Telephone triage for a post-op laser patient with a new painful red eye, nausea, and vomiting. Laser was done yesterday.

Staff response: This is another emergency because he has had laser surgery yesterday. He may have angle-closure glaucoma by the complaint of pain, red eye, nausea, and vomiting. This is angle-closure glaucoma until proven otherwise.

After panretinal photocoagulation, there can be mild choroidal effusion or choroidal folds, enough to push the lens-iris diaphragm forward, causing an angle-closure glaucoma picture. This is rare but can happen in eyes which have a narrow angle at a baseline evaluation. Or, the patient could have had combined mechanism glaucoma and now the closed angle component is causing the pain, redness and nausea, and vomiting (see Table 15-11 to 15-13).

CLINICAL CORRELATION

New patient: 43-year-old female presents to office with a referral from a primary care physician. She is newly diagnosed with diabetes.

Staff response: General diabetes education handouts can be passed out to the patient. The handout lists the Web site of the American Diabetes Association, food groups, nutritional food pyramid, and definitions about diabetes. Cookbooks are shown to the patient.

Examination room: The patient can have a written summary written by the physician, or there can be a scribe who will hand the patient the summary of findings. The fundus photos serve as a visual prop for the patient, reminding him that he does have a complication of diabetes, that is, diabetic retinopathy.

Exit interview: The staff reiterates and summarizes the doctor's findings. A piece of paper summarizing all the diagnoses is handed out to the patient. A large manilla envelope can be given to the patient to hold all the patient materials. The envelope can have the next appointment written in large block letters if the patient has vision impairment.

CLINICAL CORRELATION

Candidate for employment. A candidate for employment is introduced to the staff. The young woman is 21 years old and has never had any experience with diabetes. She is the only child. Her parents are alive and well (see Table 15-6).

Caveats: A young person who never has any exposure to disease or sick people may not be the best person for the job. She is the only child so that her personal interactions may be more inwardly directed or introspective. Watch her interactions with the other staff members during the interview. Have her try the front desk for an hour and watch her reactions. Some candidates for employment are not able to exhibit compassion toward the elderly. A good question is Do you have a favorite relative? Did you have a good relationship with your grandfather or grandmother?

Ask her what the mission of a doctors' office should be. Listen carefully to the answers. Have various senior staff members ask her the same question.

CLINICAL CORRELATION

Lost to follow-up. A 60-year-old smoker, diabetic for 10 years and having missed 24 months of follow-up, presents with acute loss of vision. He comes without an appointment.

Chief complaint: "I can't see out of my left eye since a week ago." The staff pulls out the old chart, updates his demographics, his allergy and medication record, and his primary care practitioner's name, address, telephone number, and fax. The staff tries to obtain last lab tests which show fasting blood glucose, hemoglobin A1c, and lipid profiles. A medical record release is signed by the patient for the release of last lab results only.

Vision testing: The technician will do a careful pinhole examination of vision. If the patient is 20/200 or worse, the physician is alerted, so that appropriate testing can be ordered during his visit. Perhaps, the ophthalmologist will want to order a visual field prior to dilation drops.

Examination room: The staff writes notes for the patients and writes down the patient's questions so that the physician indeed answers all of them prior to the patient's leaving the office. Fundus photographs usually help with the explanation for this long-lost patient. Vitreous hemorrhage is present. Laser is necessary to treat high-risk characteristics of proliferative diabetic retinopathy. The staff asks about his need for water before getting settled in the laser room. The consent is read to him by a staff member, and the physician goes over the consent once more prior to signing.

Exit interview: The patient needs to have a letter typed to the referral physician upon discharge since he has a serious condition requiring laser. The patient receives a packet of papers to take to his internist and a packet of instructional handouts for himself. They are appropriately labeled in large print.

CLINICAL CORRELATION

Aphasic, elderly, nursing home patient with diabetes. Eighty-year-old diabetic female from a local nursing home comes, with an attendant, with loss of vision in one eye. She has had a stroke and is somewhat aphasic.

Staff interactions: Paperwork to be handled for the nursing home has to be done by the staff, alleviating delays when the patient is exiting the office. Vision and dilation may have to be done in an area where there is wheelchair access to the slit lamp. Attend to the patient's immediate needs, such as going to the bathroom, need for orange juice, or water. Because this patient is elderly, in a wheelchair, the staff should be thinking of ways to make her more comfortable since she may not be able to articulate all of her thoughts because of her expressive aphasia (see Tables 15-9 and 15-10).

Exit interview: The staff must interact with the attendant. The papers have to be signed. A typed summary can be generated for the nursing home. The return appointment must be clearly stated in the nursing home orders. Staple the doctor's business card to the sheets of paper destined for the nursing home to facilitate communication between the nursing home and office.

CLINICAL CORRELATION

Non–English speaking patient. A non–English speaker comes with a written sheet of paper stating, "diabetic retinopathy." There is no physician's address. The patient and husband only speak Arabic.

Staff response: Our staff is not fluent in Arabic. We log onto the computer, www.Google.com, type in "diabetes translate to Arabic." Immediately, google, cut and paste any sentence, and have it translated for free.

We write on a sheet of paper that we could not translate Arabic but gave them the address and telephone number of the local emergency room of a county hospital which had Arabic translators. We map directions on a printed sheet of paper and give it to them. We hand the telephone to them with an Arabic translator on the other end of the telephone line. The patient and husband smile and say thank you. They leave with gratitude because we show them compassionate care.

Follow-up The staff calls to make sure that they arrive at the hospital and are seen. If this is not possible because they are hard to reach en route to a busy, county hospital emergency room, the staff calls the patient's house and leaves a message.

Comment: While we are not able to provide all services, we make the effort to get the patients to a place where they could be served. We are proud of our staff's efforts to help people with multicultural needs.

CLINICAL CORRELATION

Cross-cultural issues in a new patient. A 45-year-old Asian female who speaks Chinese is a new patient with the diagnosis of diabetes and sudden loss of vision.

Cross-cultural considerations: Chinese is one of the languages that our office speaks. Our handouts are bilingual and are given to her. One of our medical assistants provides translation although the patient speaks enough English to understand the diagnosis.

Examination room: The patient likes seeing her fundus photographs and fluorescein angiogram. The images explain the need for laser for diabetic macular edema. The explanation is done through the photographs.

Laser room: The patient appreciates the medical assistant who is fluent in Chinese. Having an interpreter is helpful in anxious patients who need laser. The presence of an interpreter makes the situation go smoothly especially during the actual laser procedure.

Exit interview: The patient is satisfied with the care and the availability of patient materials in two languages. She tells us that she would send her aged mother to our office for an evaluation of unexplained vision loss.

CLINICAL CORRELATION

A 16-year-old female is newly diagnosed with insulin-dependent diabetes but has decreased vision. She is at the office with her mother.

Staff response: Recognize that this 16 year old is a teenager and carries a new diagnosis of diabetes. She must have fear and anxiety but being a teenager, she may be a difficult patient. Or, the patient, while a teenager, may act childlike because of the strangeness of the situation. She may act younger than her stated years because of her personal anxiety about her diagnosis of diabetes and fear of vision loss. The staff should be sensitive to the issues of teens and children. She should be treated with care and compassion since she is probably nervous about being in an ophthalmologist's office. She may sense her parent's anxiety as well. The staff should communicate to the teen and her parent about the diagnosis of diabetes, the possible side effects on insulin, complications of diabetes, compliance, and diabetic diets. Nutritionist referrals can be provided as well.

In addition, the 16 year old is a minor and the parent has to sign the forms permitting her to be seen. The mother can be included in all the discussions with the doctor and patient. Handouts are given to the patient. The patient, while a teenager, may act childlike because of the strangeness of the situation. She may act younger than her stated years because of her personal anxiety, newness of the diagnosis of diabetes, and fear of vision loss. The staff should be sensitive to the issues of teens and children.

Chief complaint: The chief complaint, in the words of the patient, describes why the patient is seeking medical attention. Her concerns inform the rest of the examination.

Vision testing: The vision part of the examination is very important because it sets the tone for the doctor's visit: Why doesn't the patient see 20/20? The answer to the question sets in motion the rest of the examination and the type of ancillary testing to be done at the office visit.

Examination room: A same sex assistant may be helpful to alleviate fears and anxiety. The patient has no diabetic macular edema or microaneurysms. Her refractive error shifts toward myopia during this early stage of insulin treatment. Reassurance is given.

During this time, the explanation of the diagnosis about her diabetic retinopathy can be reinforced by the staff nurse, technician, after the physician has seen the patient. The medical assistant can use the same words that the physician uses so the concepts are reinforced and repeated. This is the time for the staff member to write down the patient's comments and questions so that they can be answered at the close of the visit. Write down the diagnosis for the patient to take home. The piece of paper is a useful reminder of what has transpired during the office visit.

Exit interview: For the first visit, an exit interview with the physician and staff is useful. The patient has the opportunity to ask questions, and the medical assistant is ready to take notes. In addition, the medical assistant can reiterate the physician's statements and write down the diagnosis for the patient. The piece of paper serves as a reminder to the patient about medications or future appointments. An informational packet can be given. Make sure all questions are answered. The mother and daughter may have different issues.

For this case, have a separate exit interview with the mother since she may want to talk to the staff or health care team about her fears without her daughter hearing them.

A separate interview with the daughter in another room may be useful since the daughter may have questions that she does not want the mother to hear. The adolescent patient may appreciate the time to go over her personal issues with a medical assistant or nurse.

CLINICAL CORRELATIONS

Optometric referral of a patient with clinically significant macular edema. A 40-year-old male with decreased vision is referred by a physician. The patient has been noncompliant with medications, diet, or exercise.

Staff response: The patient is noncompliant and needs reinforcement about the complications of diabetes, such as diabetic retinopathy. Handouts can be prepared ahead of time for this category of patients. Be prepared for two types of patients: one who denies that anything is wrong and one who is grateful for information. For both, the staff needs to provide patient education and note on the medical record that explanations were given to the patient. For the patient who denies the serious nature of his disease and subsequent diabetic retinopathy, telephone reminders for office appointments may be necessary.

Chief complaint: The patient says that he cannot see. This is the time to ask what type of job the patient has. If he is a software engineer, vision is very important. If he works with his hands, he may not notice a change in vision until the loss of vision is severe in both eyes. Is the patient exhibiting other risk factors? The medical assistant can alert you to his history of smoking.

Vision: Is the vision good enough to pass the driver's license test? If not, the patient may be at the threshold of failing the visual requirements for the driver's test. The staff or medical assistant can inform the physician about the possible concerns of this patient.

Fundus photography: The presence of diabetic macular edema with hard exudates and hemorrhages can be demonstrated on photographs. The pictorial demonstration of diabetic retinopathy can underscore the importance of the office visit for the noncompliant patient. For the first time, the patient can see the correlation of poor blood sugar control and eye disease.

Exit interview: The photos will remind the patient to change his noncompliant habits. A written note about the diagnosis is given to the patient. The education materials and return appointment can be placed together with the photographs so that the patient can review the data at his leisure.

CLINICAL CORRELATION

A 50-year-old white female presents with adult onset diabetes and complains that she cannot see to read. The vision loss was sudden and abrupt.

Staff response: The abruptness of vision loss is disturbing. This patient needs to be seen immediately. Expedite her being seen quickly.

Diagnosis and management with staff interface: The patient has a vitreous hemorrhage and needs to have laser. Here the staff and medical assistants have to be careful to reiterate the retinal surgeon's diagnosis and his treatment plan. Photographs of the patient's retina with proliferative diabetic retinopathy can be shown to the accompanying family members. Informed consent is important. Having a witness to the informed consent may be useful.

Exit interview: Patient handouts are to be given. The diagnosis of proliferative diabetic retinopathy and its treatment options can be written down for the patient. The fundus photograph of the retinal neovascularization and vitreous hemorrhage can be included in the materials to be sent home with the patient.

Staff follow-up: After laser, the staff should call up in 24 hours to find out if the patient is comfortable and should answer additional questions, if any. The retinal specialist can also talk with the patient if there are more in-depth questions.

REFERENCES

1. Lencioni P. *The Five Dysfunctions of a Team: A Leadership Fable.* San Francisco, CA: Jossey-Bass; 2002.
2. Fadiman A. *The Spirit Catches You and You Fall Down.* New York: Farrar, Straus and Giroux; 1997.
3. Kubler-Ross, E. *On Death and Dying.* New York: Scribner & Sons; 1970.

APPENDIX A

Photo Atlas of OCT and Diabetic Retinopathy

Case 1. JJ is a 65-year-old female with new diagnosis of Type 2 diabetes, visual field normal OU, no family history of glaucoma. V 20/20 OD, 20/25 OS.

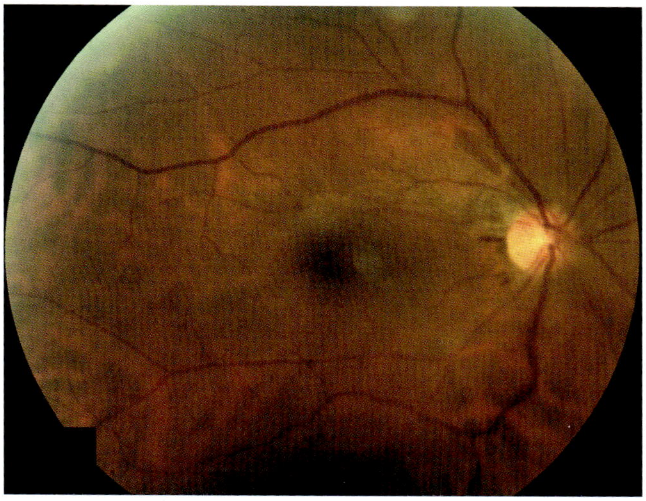

Case Figure 1-1 Color Photo OD: Venous engorgement, flame shaped hemorrhages at the optic disc.

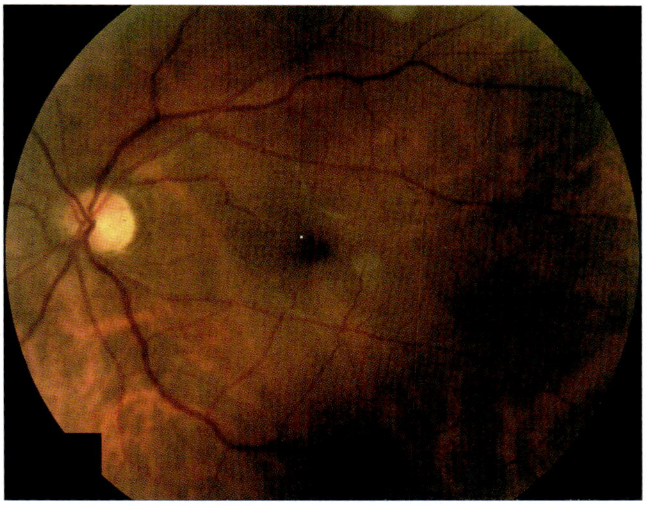

Case Figure 1-2 Color Photo OS: Arteriovenous nicking, gliosis seen superior to the macula, few microaneuryms.

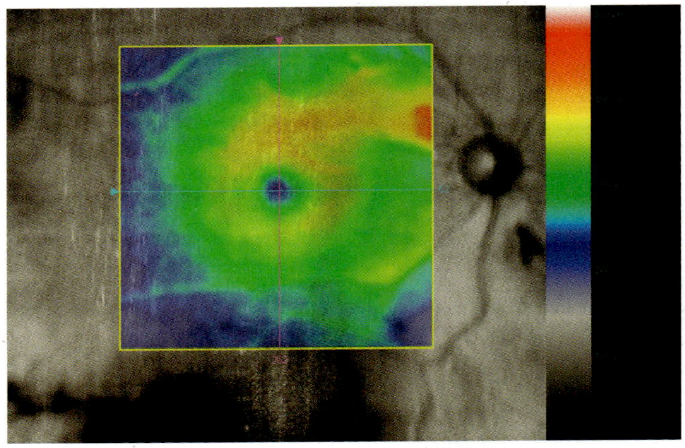

Case Figure 1-3 Macular Cube OD: The map shows that there is macular edema.

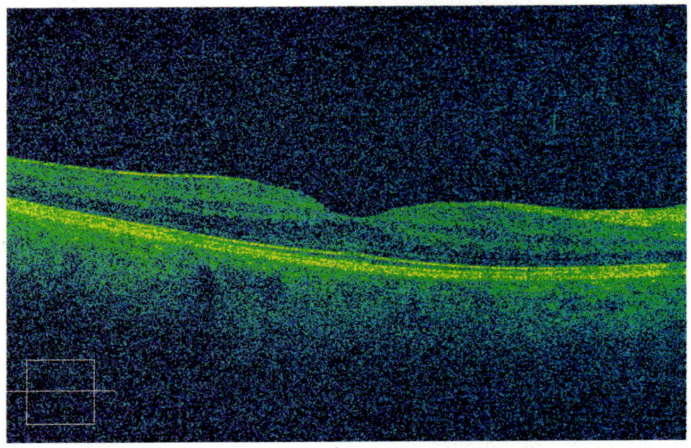

Case Figure 1-4 Horizontal Section OD: Note the elevation of the retinal pigment epithelium at the fovea and the overlying edema at Henle's layer at the fovea, and the thickening of the internal limiting membrane (ILM) at the right side of the scan.

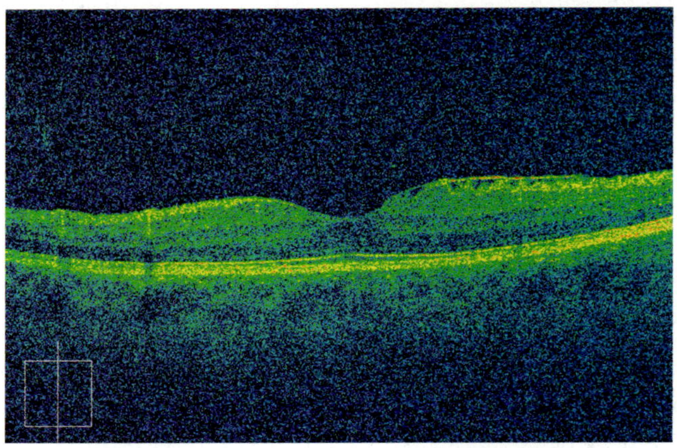

Case Figure 1-5 Vertical Section OD: There is ILM abnormality on the right hand side of the scan, causing gliosis, and irregularity of the nerve fiber layer and ganglion cell layer. On the left side of the scan, there is abnormality macula.

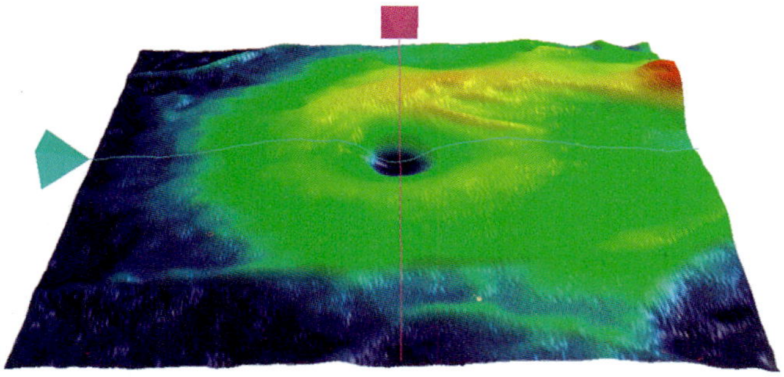

Case Figure 1-6 OD: Right side of the scan shows surface irregularity corresponding to the nasal macula.

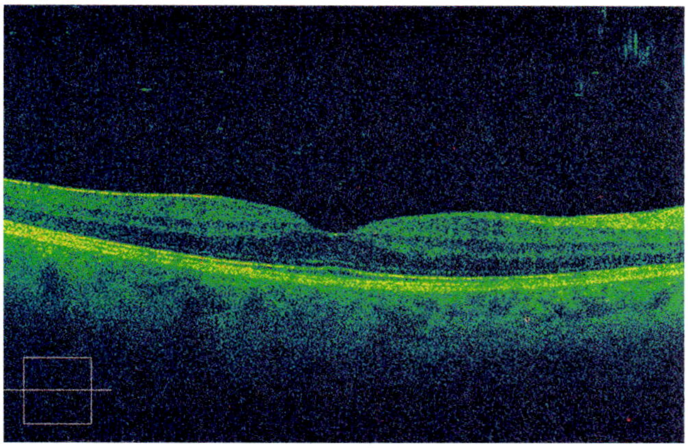

Case Figure 1-7 5-Line Raster OD: Macular edema is shown, magnified.

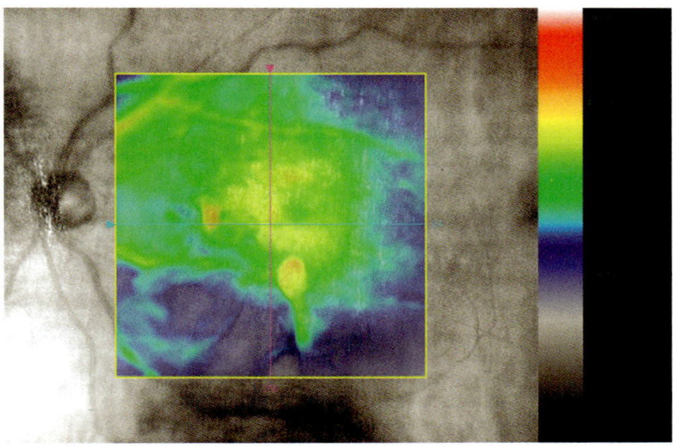

Case Figure 1-8 Macular Cube OS: Irregularity of the macula.

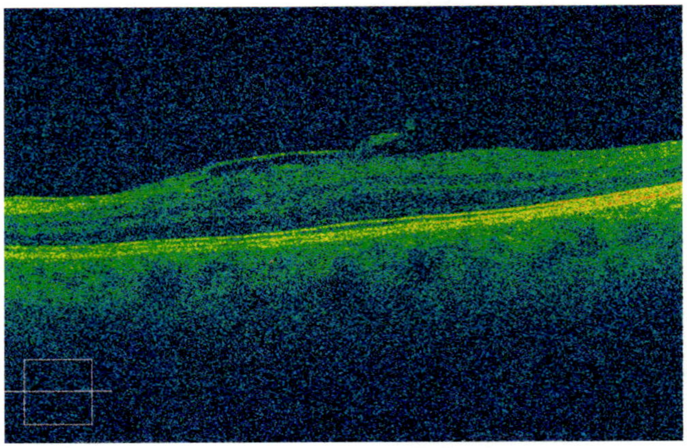

Case Figure 1-9 Horizontal Section OS: Macular edema with abnormal ILM interface with vitreous.

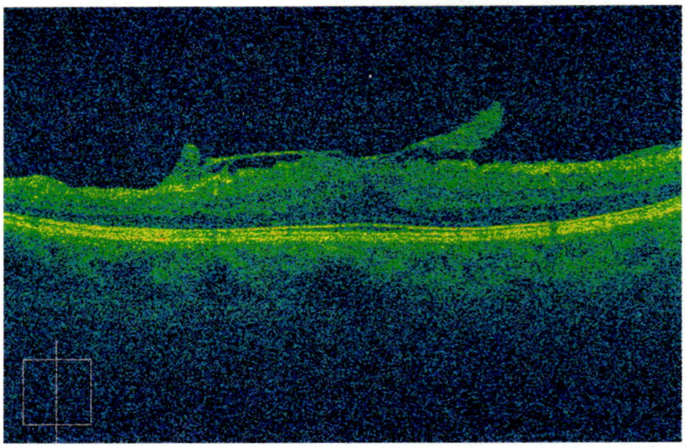

Case Figure 1-10 Vertical Section OS: Massive amount of macular edema with surface abnormalities.

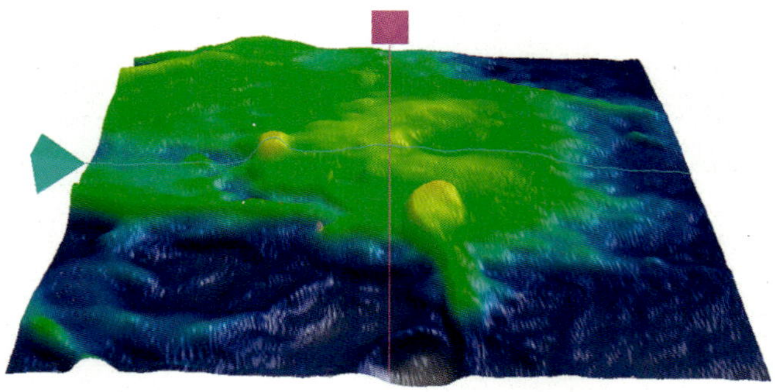

Case Figure 1-11 OS: 3D image shows irregularity of the macula.

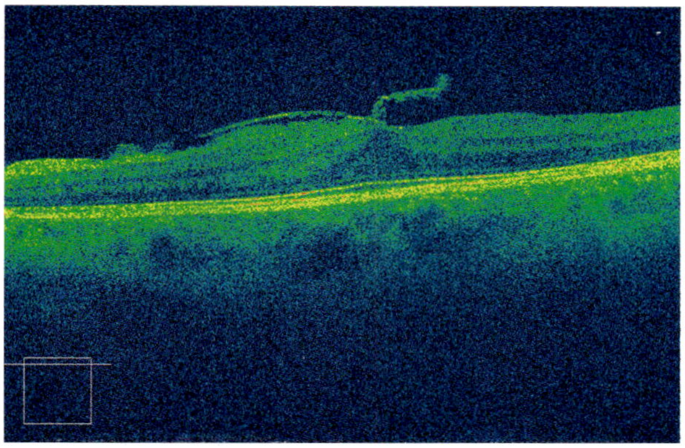

Case Figure 1-12 5-Line Raster OS: Massive focal macular edema with overlying surface changes at the ILM.

Case 2. EM is a 56-year-old Filipino female with newly diagnosed diabetes, HbA1c = 6.65, FBS = 150 mg/dL, newly diagnosed with toxoplasmosis IgG 1.72 (normal 1.10) with decreased vision OD, V 20/30 OD, 20/15 OS.

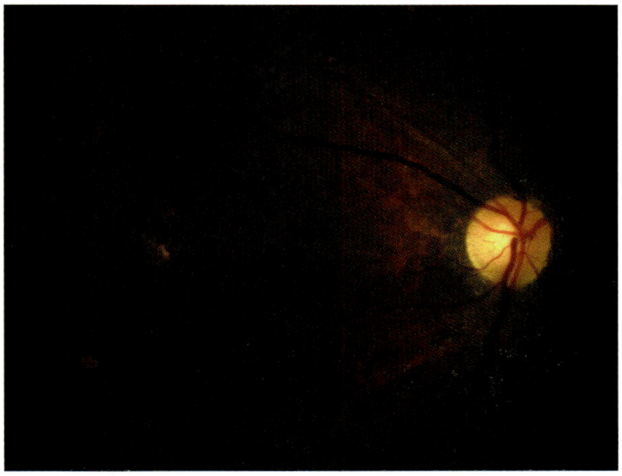

Case Figure 2-1 Color Photo OD: Arteriovenous nicking, arteriolar narrowing, dot hemorrhage at temporal macula.

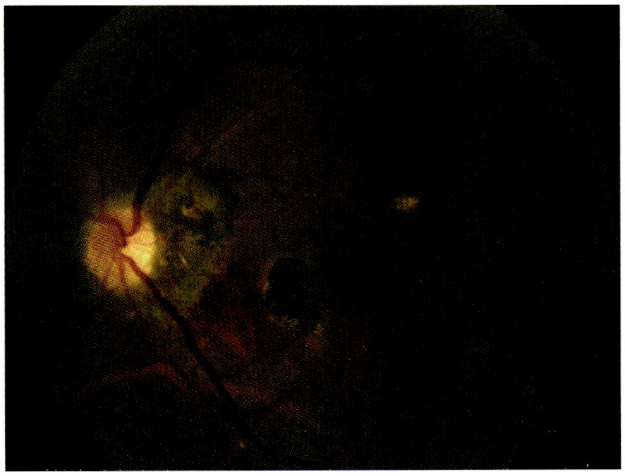

Case Figure 2-2 Color Photo OS: Toxoplasmosis scar of the optic nerve, and inferonasal to fovea. There is a yellow lesion superotemporal to the macular. Diabetic hard exudates are seen at the edge of the temporal macula.

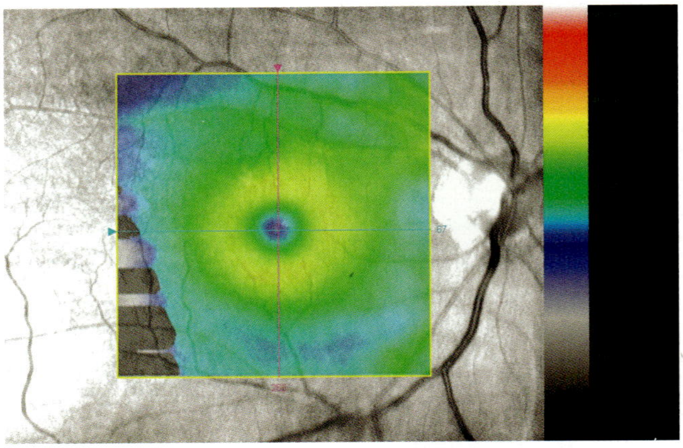

Case Figure 2-3 Macular Cube OD: Massive thickening.

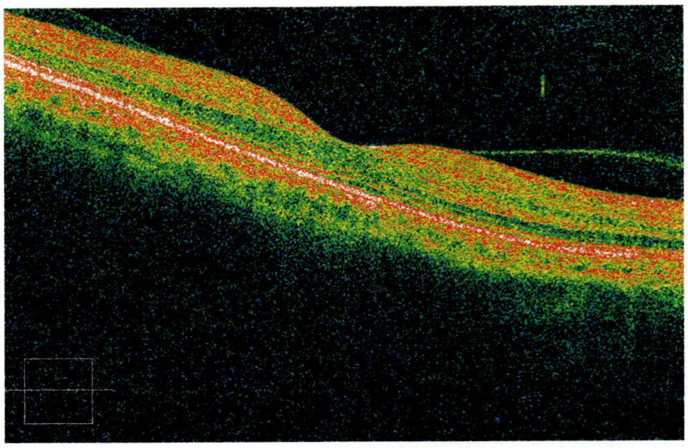

Case Figure 2-4 Horizontal Section OD: All layers of the macula are thickened.

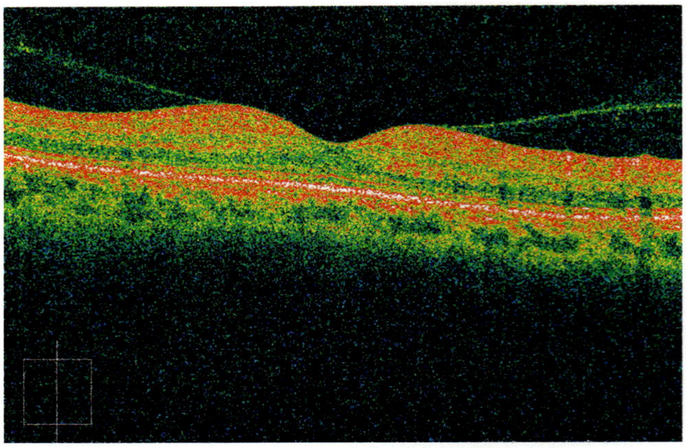

Case Figure 2-5 Vertical Section OD: The vitreous is tense over the thickened macula.

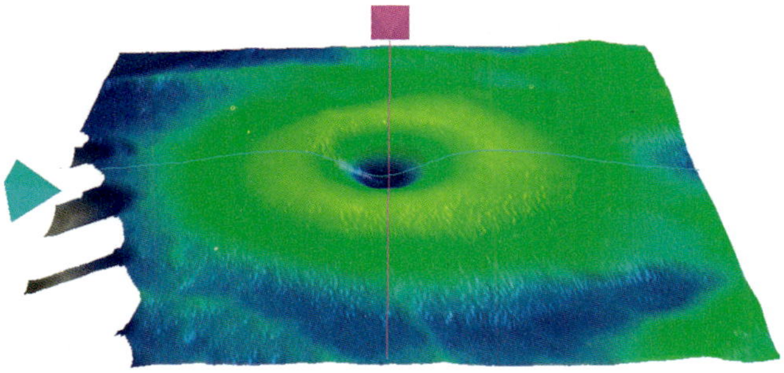

Case Figure 2-6 OD: 3D scan shows abnormal topography.

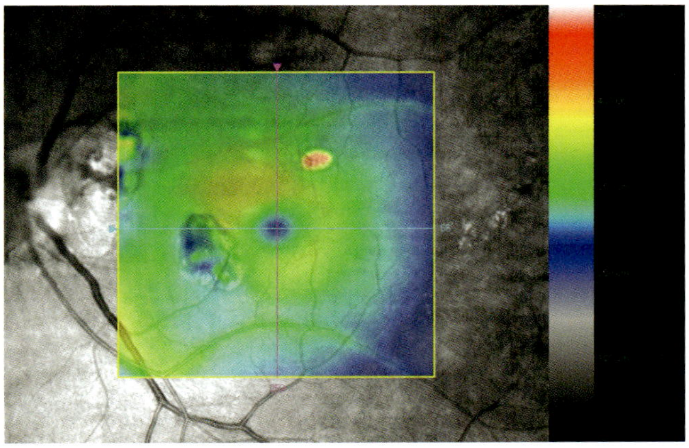

Case Figure 2-7 Macular Cube OS: Abnormal topography.

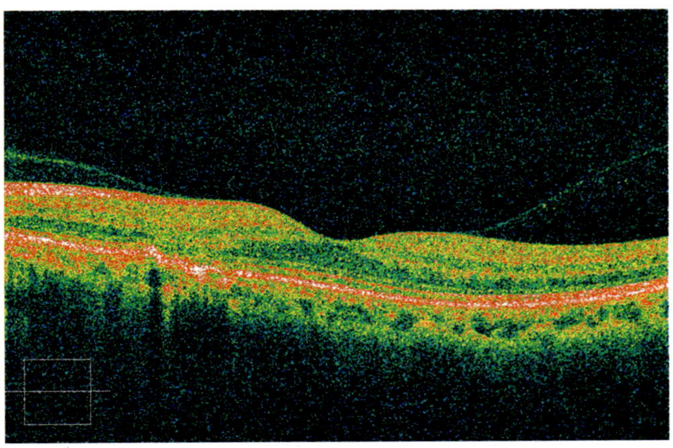

Case Figure 2-8 Horizontal Section OS: All layers of the macula are thickened, especially on the left side of the scan. Note asymmetry of the vitreous interface.

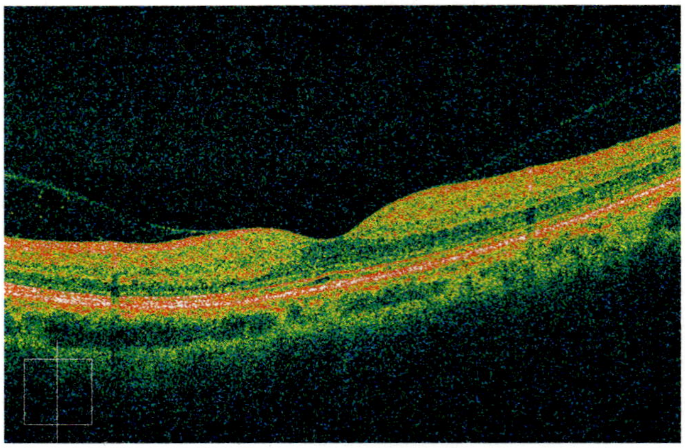

Case Figure 2-9 Vertical Section OS: The vitreous is distorted on the left side, macular edema.

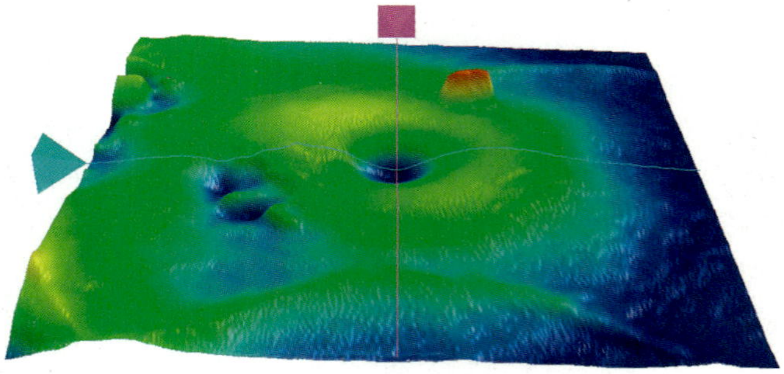

Case Figure 2-10 OS: 3D scan shows abnormal topography with a toxoplasmosis lesion playing a role in the diabetic macular edema.

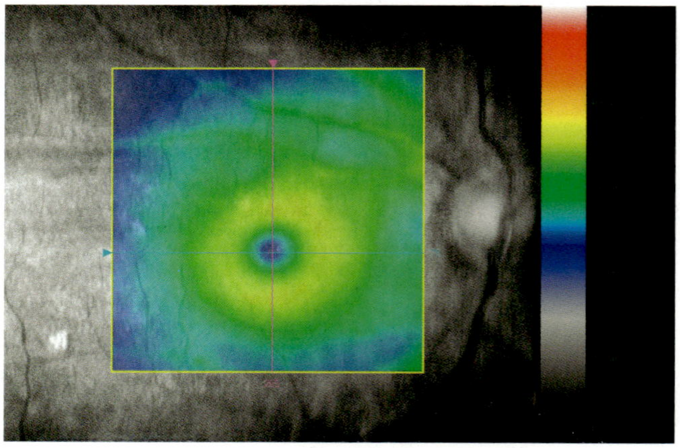

Case Figure 2-11 OD Macular Cube: Abnormal reflex with thickening at the nasal edge of the macula, right side of the scan.

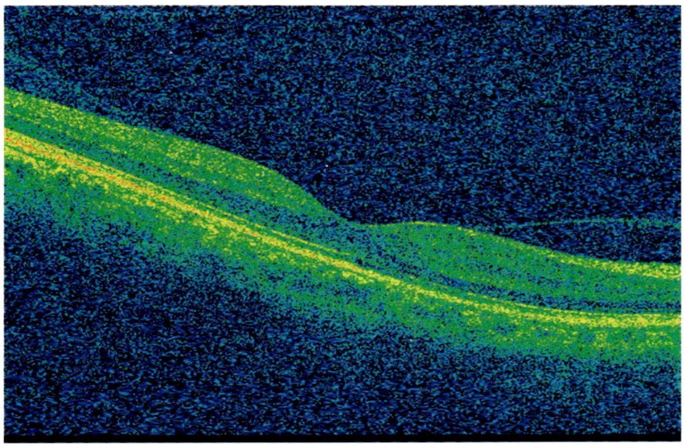

Case Figure 2-12 Horizontal Section OD: Macular edema with some changes at the retinal pigment epithelium in the fovea.

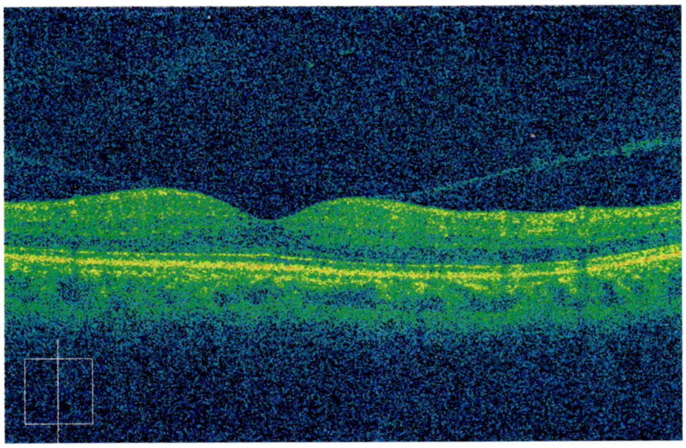

Case Figure 2-13 OD: 3D scan shows the height of the macular edema.

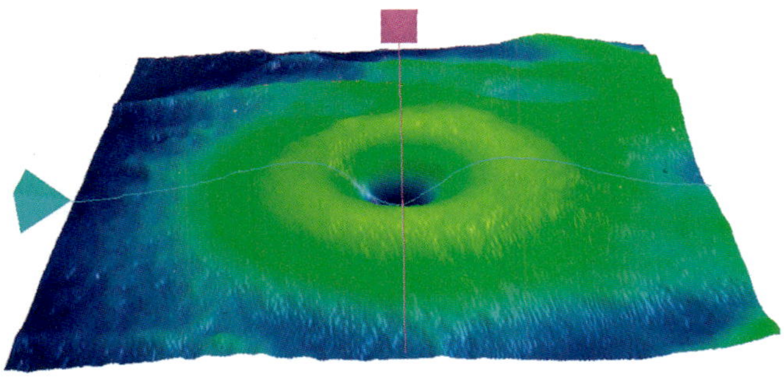

Case Figure 2-14 Vertical Section OD: Abnormal vitreous interface and macular edema are seen.

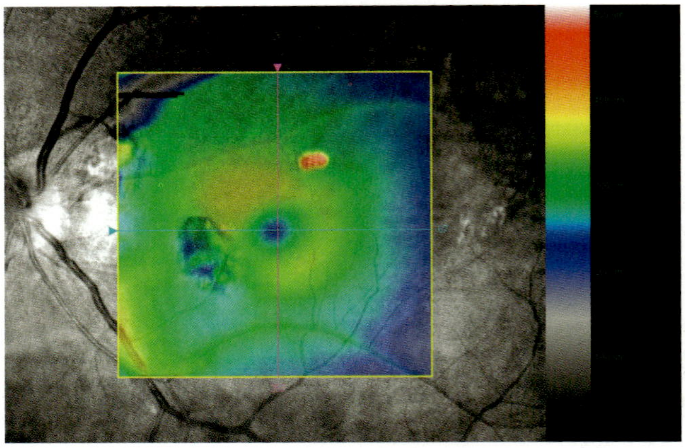

Case Figure 2-15 OS Macular Cube: Abnormality of the macula with toxoplasmosis lesion and diabetic macular edema.

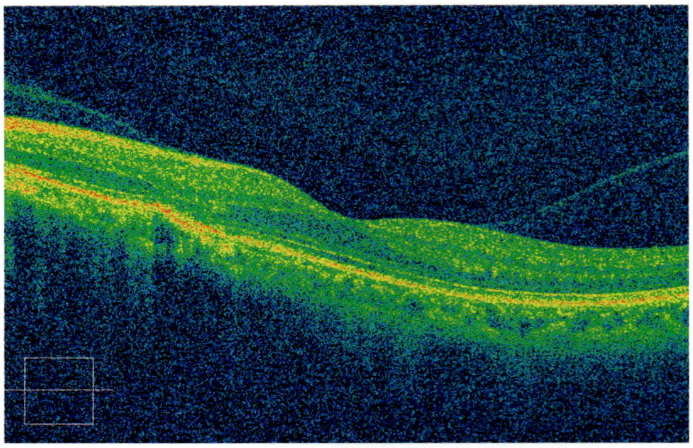

Case Figure 2-16 Horizontal Section OS: Nasal macula corresponds to the chorioretinal lesion from the toxoplasmosis, and the macular edema is centered over the fovea extending temporally. Retinal pigment epithelial (RPE) layer is swollen.

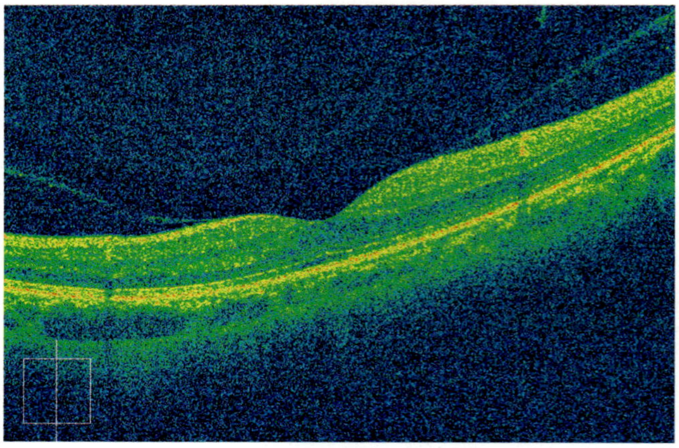

Case Figure 2-17 Vertical Section OS: Note the abnormality at the RPE layer subfoveally.

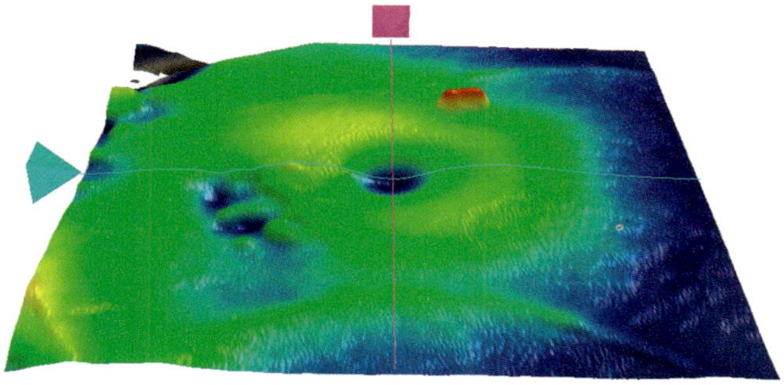

Case Figure 2-18 **OS:** 3D scan shows the extent of the edema in the four quadrants of the macula.

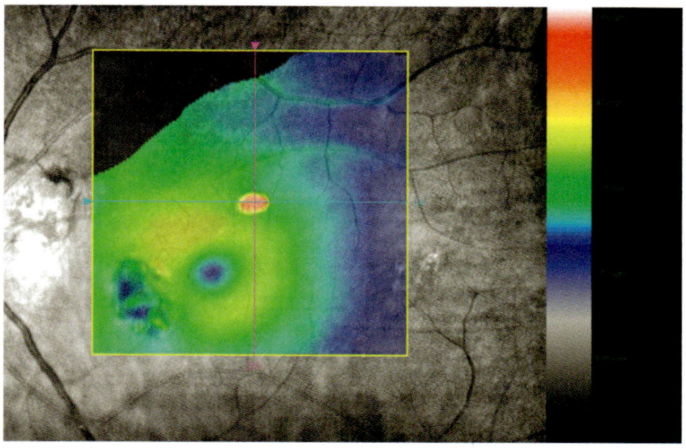

Case Figure 2-19 **OS:** Macular cube of presumed toxoplasmosis lesion superior to OS macula.

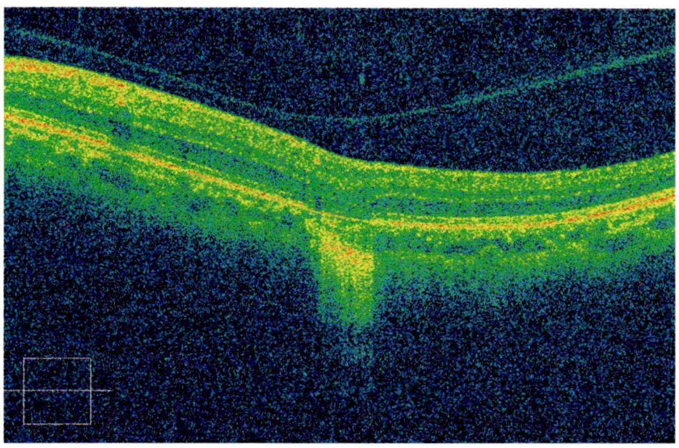

Case Figure 2-20 Non-macular OCT through the presumed toxoplasmosis lesion.
Horizontal Section OS: Macular Cube.

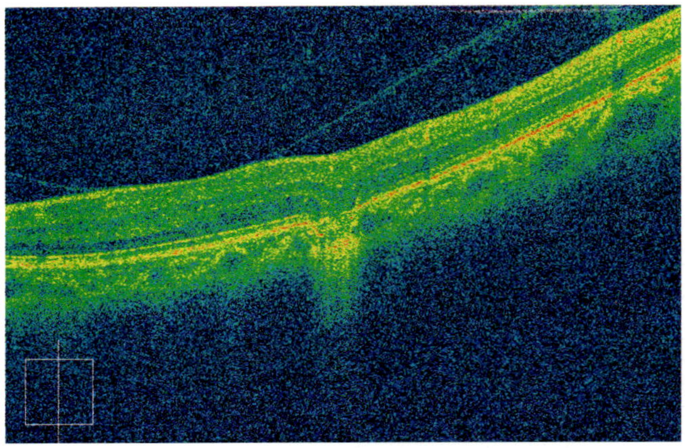

Case Figure 2-21 Vertical Section OS: Macular Cube.

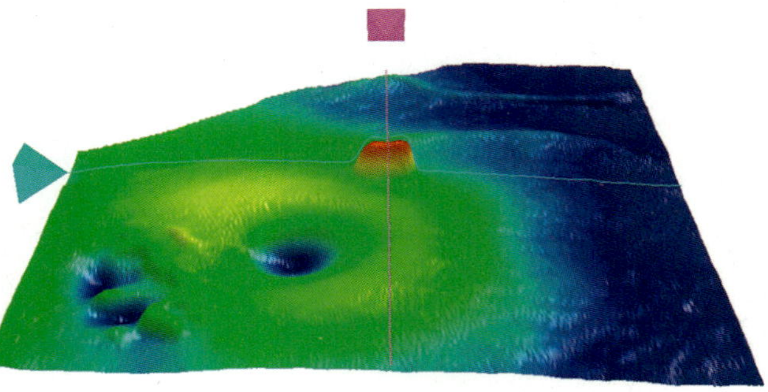

Case Figure 2-22 OS: 3D scan: Note the massive elevation of the presumed toxoplasmosis lesion, above that of the elevation of the macular edema OS, superotemporal to the macula. Note the pitting of the dark hyperpigmentated, old toxoplasmosis lesion inferonasal to the macula.

Case 3. RC is a 57-year-old African American male with a 20-year history of Type 2 diabetes with decreased vision OD >OS, V 20/25 OD, 20/20 OS, HbA1c = 8.4%, FBS = 177 mg/dL.

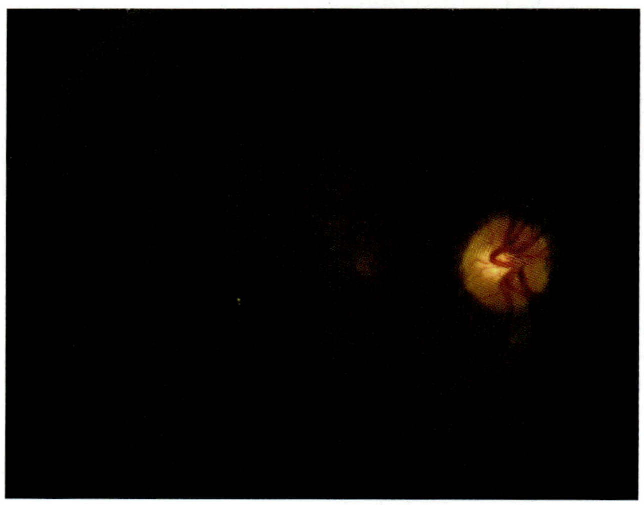

Case Figure 3-1 Color Photo OD: Arteriolar narrowing, venous engorgement, arteriovenous nicking, macular edema seen.

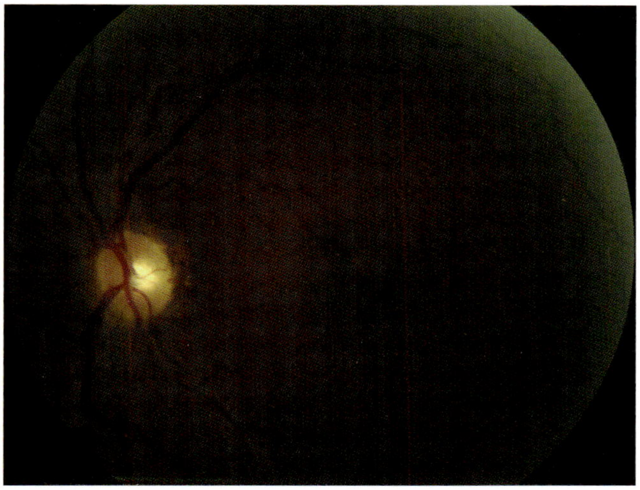

Case Figure 3-2 Color Photo OS: Arteriolar narrowing, marked venous engorgement OS >OD, arterio-venous nicking, nerve fiber layer defects seen along the superior and temporal arcades, macular edema seen.

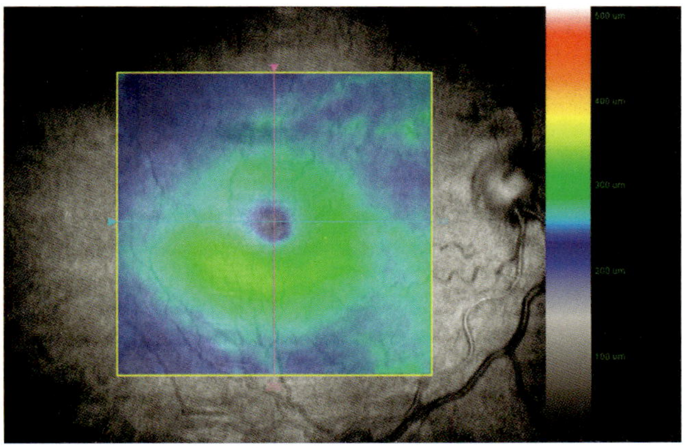

Case Figure 3-3 Macular Cube OD: Macular edema seen inferotemporally.

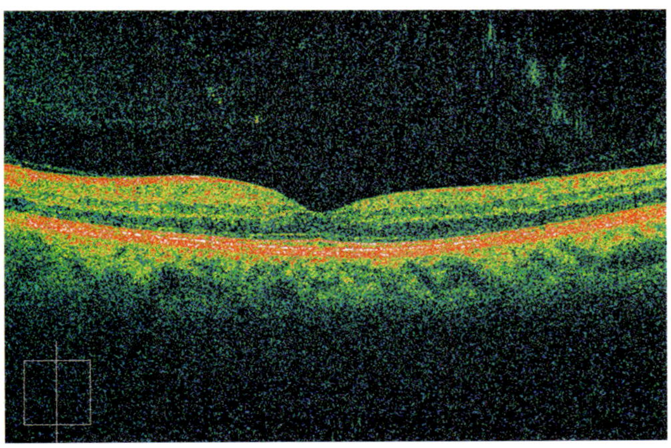

Case Figure 3-4 Vertical Section OD: Macular edema seen at the fovea, abnormal vitreous overlying the macula.

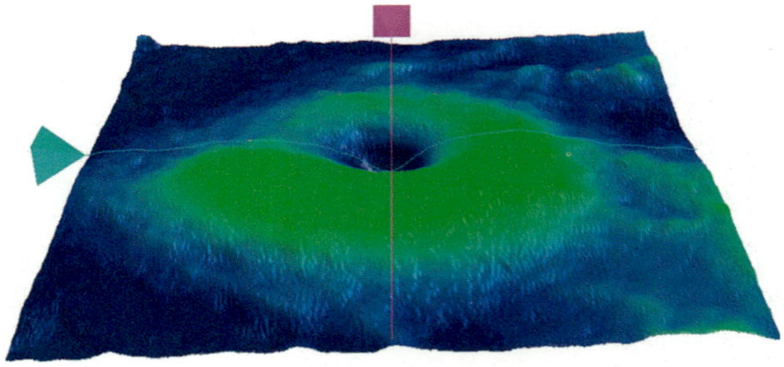

Case Figure 3-5 OD: 3D image shows topographical elevation denoting the macular edema.

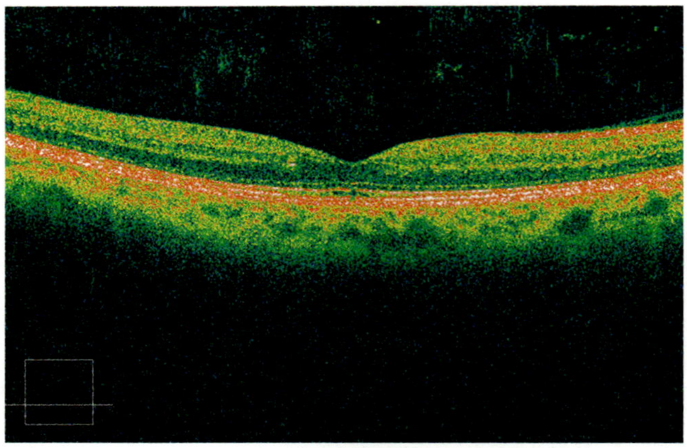

Case Figure 3-6 5-Line Raster OD: Irregular external plexiform layer at the fovea shows edema.

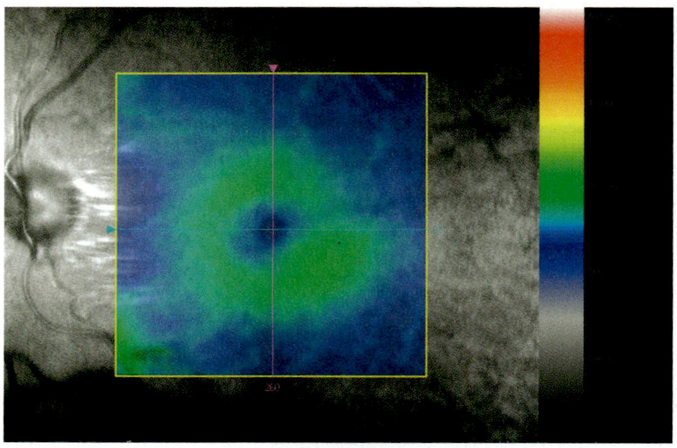

Case Figure 3-7 Macular Cube OS: Macular edema inferotemporally.

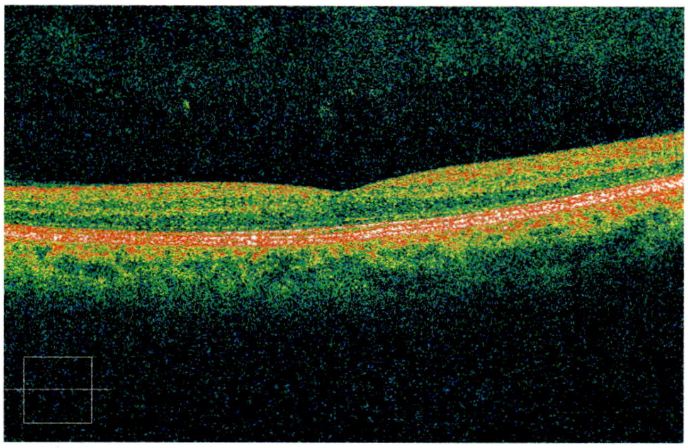

Case Figure 3-8 Horizontal Section OS: Abnormal external plexiform layer.

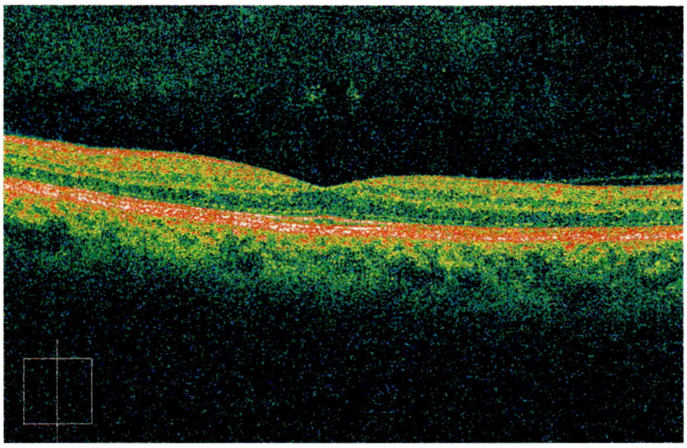

Case Figure 3-9 Vertical Section OS: Macular edema under the fovea, note the abnormal ILM to the right of the scan.

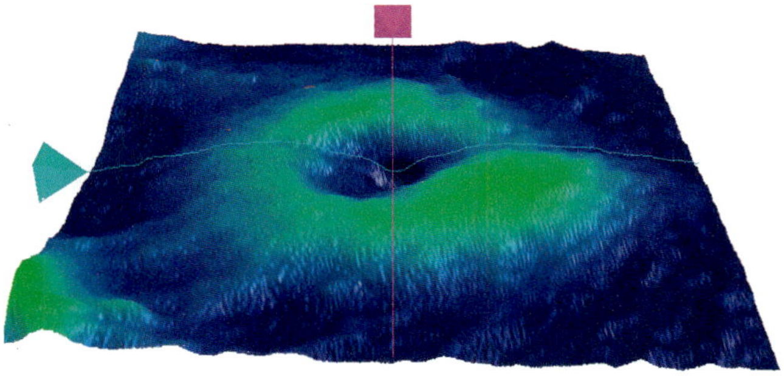

Case Figure 3-10 OS: 3D image shows irregular contour temporal to the macula.

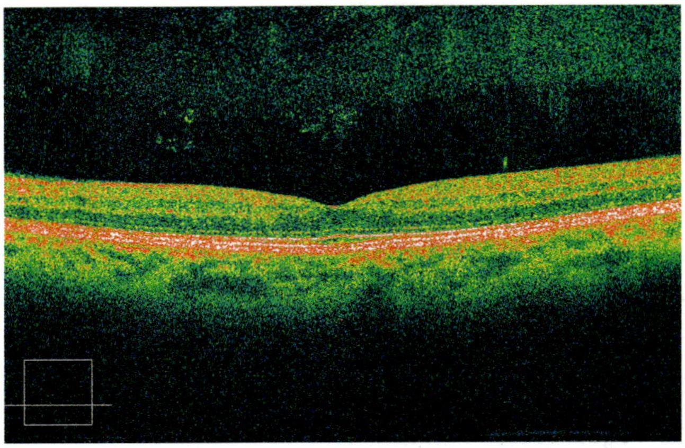

Case Figure 3-11 5-Line Raster OS: Abnormal external plexiform layer, abnormal retinal pigment epithelium, and abnormal vitreous with posterior vitreous detachment.

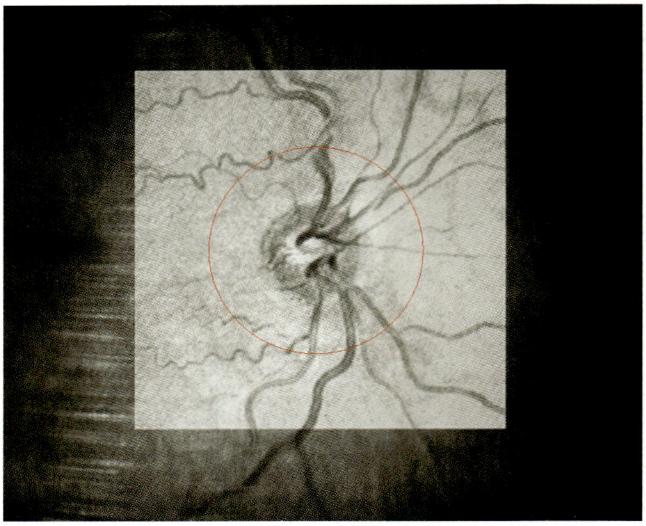

Case Figure 3-12 OD Optic Disc: Note tortuosity of the arterioles, venous engorgement.

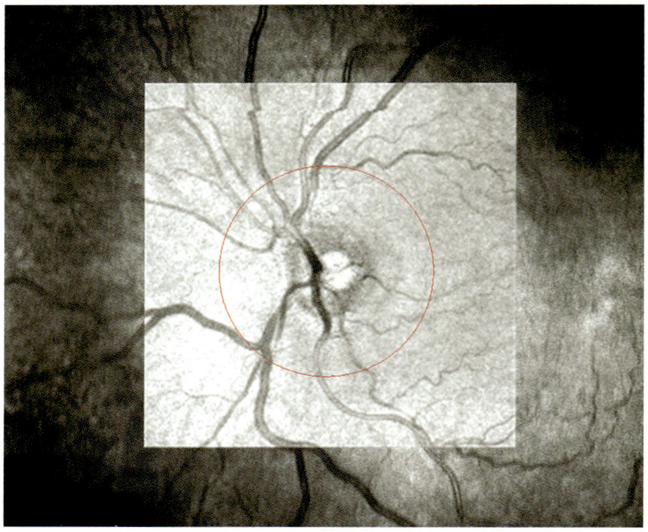

Case Figure 3-13 OS Optic Disc: Note the abnormality of the optic disc temporal rim, tortuosity of the arterioles and venules.

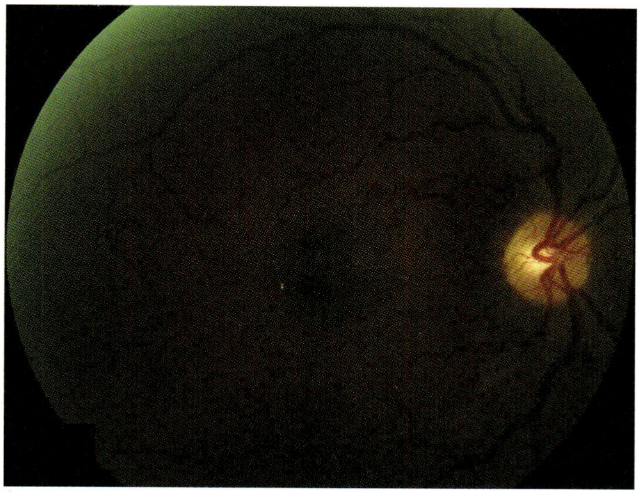

Case Figure 3-14 Color Photo OD: Arteriolar narrowing and tortuosity.

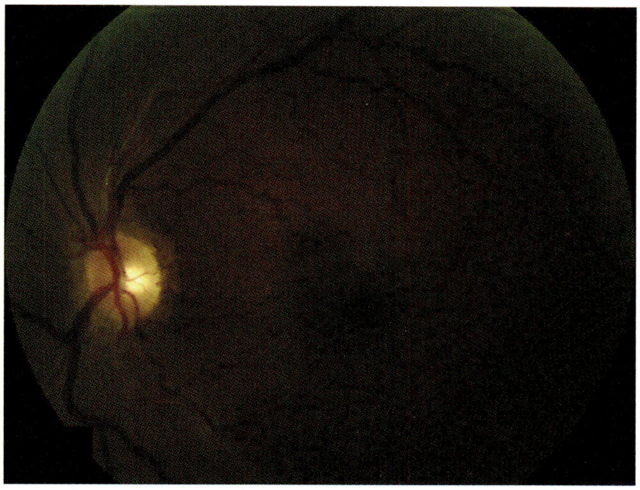

Case Figure 3-15 Color Photo OS: Venous tortuosity OS greater than OD, arteriolar narrowing, and tortuosity.

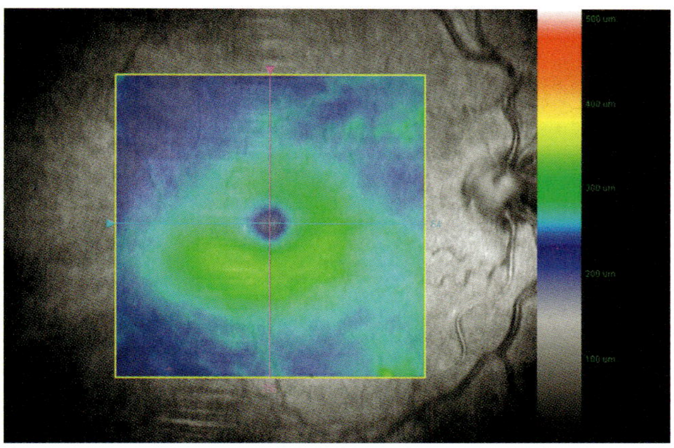

Case Figure 3-16 Macular Cube OD: Macular edema pronounced inferiorly.

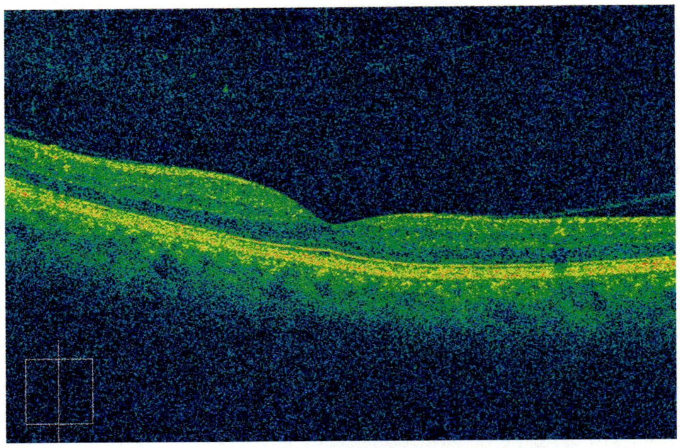

Case Figure 3-17 Vertical Section OD: RPE abnormality under the fovea and edema at the external plexiform layer.

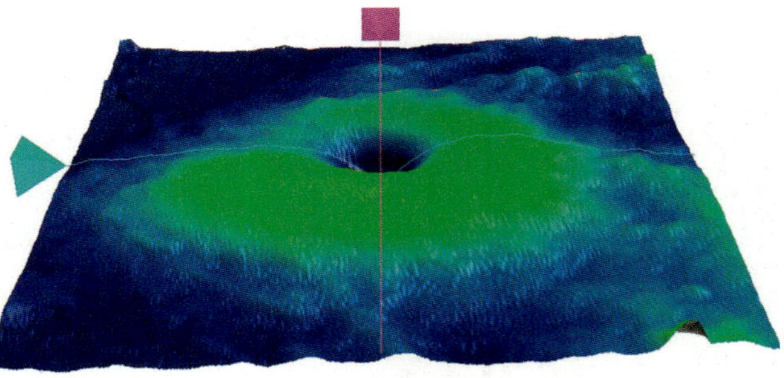

Case Figure 3-18 OD: 3D image with "grainy texture" to the topography of the macular edema.

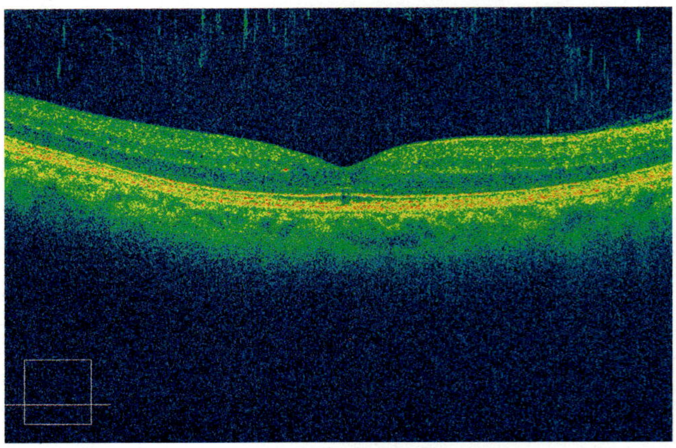

Case Figure 3-19 5-Line Raster OD: Abnormal vitreous and edema at the external plexiform layer with RPE changes, as well.

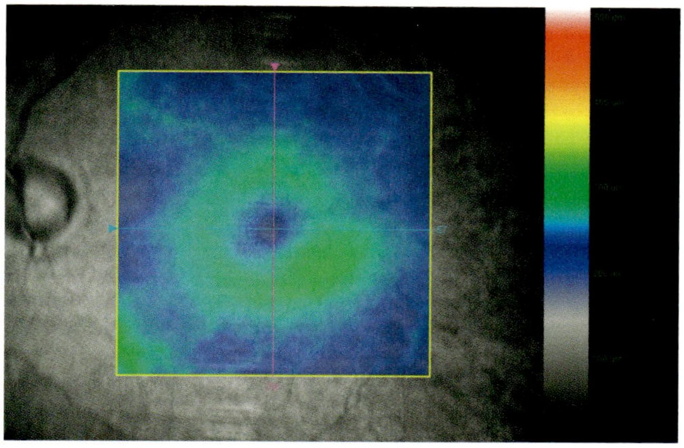

Case Figure 3-20 Macular Cube OS: Macular edema inferotemporal, ovoid foveal pit suggesting asymmetric macular edema.

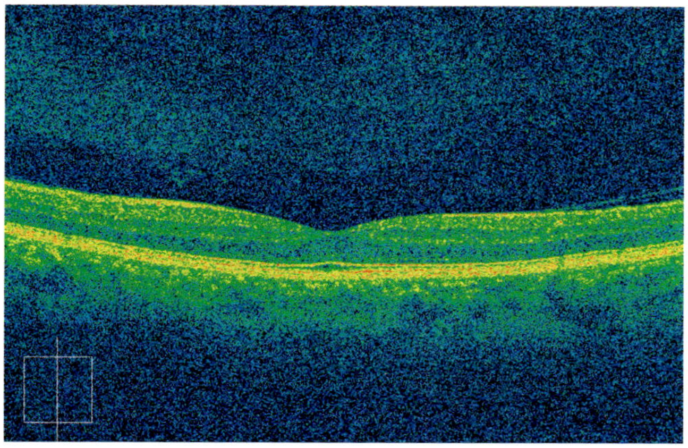

Case Figure 3-21 Vertical Section OS: Macular edema with RPE changes.

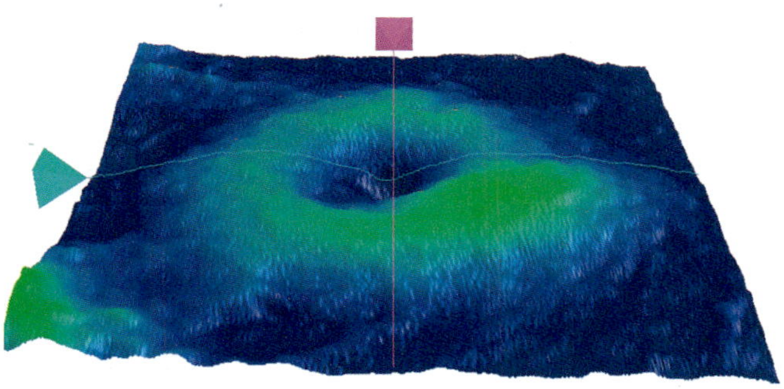

Case Figure 3-22 OS: 3D scan showing tilted oval foveal pit, showing the edema pushed temporally.

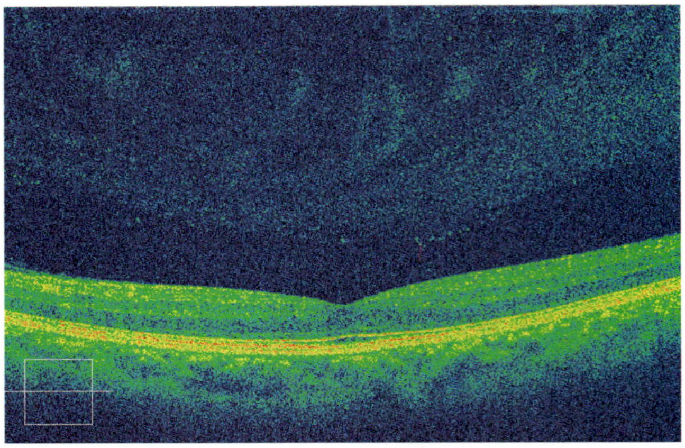

Case Figure 3-23 5-Line Raster OS: Focal RPE changes under the foveal macular edema with overlying posterior vitreous detachment.

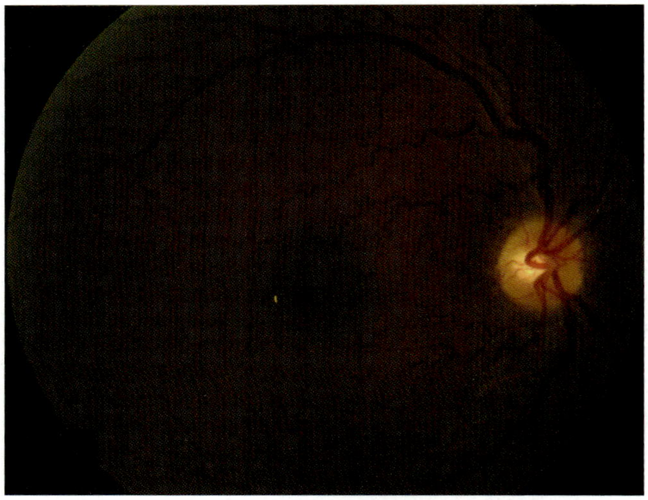

Case Figure 3-24 Color Photo OD: Arteriolar narrowing and worsening venous tortuosity one month later.

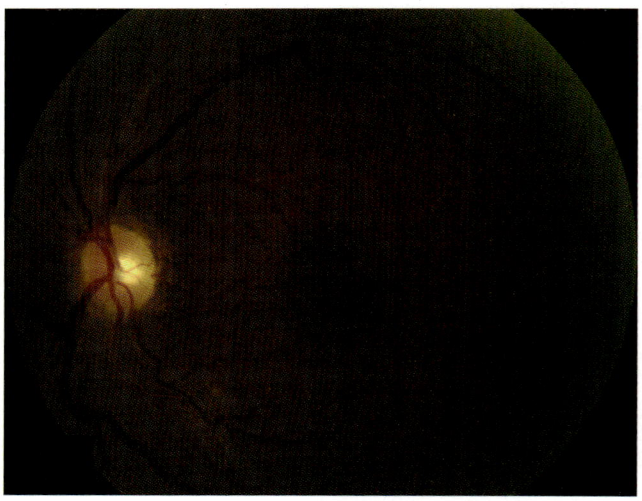

Case Figure 3-25 Color Photo OS: Arteriovenous nicking and arteriolar narrowing. Venous tortuosity is also worsening.

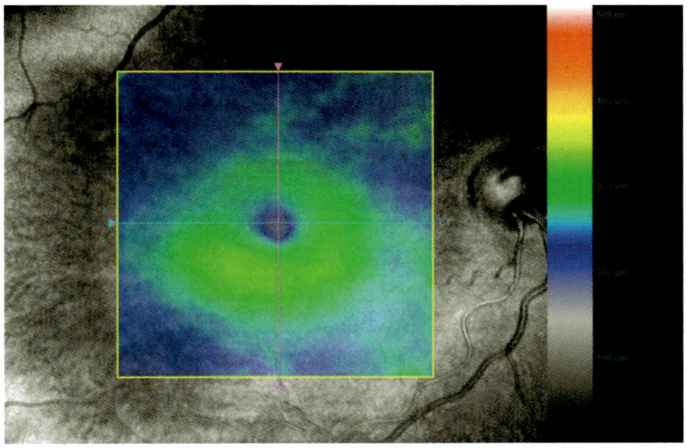

Case Figure 3-26 Macular Cube OD: Total asymmetry of edema, and the area of the edema is larger two months later than at presentation in Case Figure 3-1.

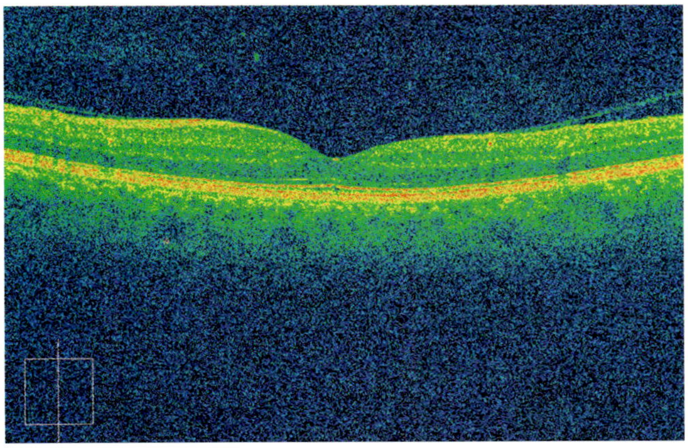

Case Figure 3-27 Vertical Section OD: Increased elevation of the external plexiform layer two months later. ILM attachment noted to be nasal to the macula.

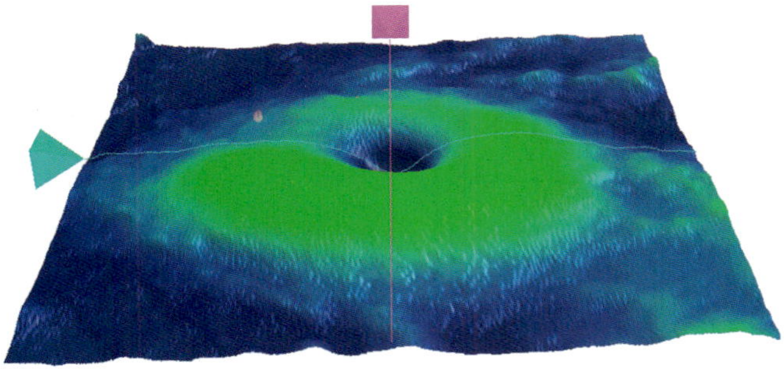

Case Figure 3-28 OD: 3D scan: Irregular surface and increased elevation of the macular edema noted today versus two months ago at presentation.

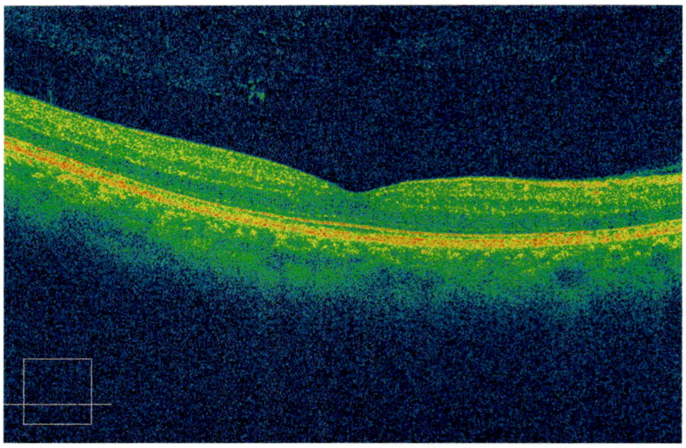

Case Figure 3-29 **5-Line Raster OD:** Edema noted today versus two months ago at presentation.

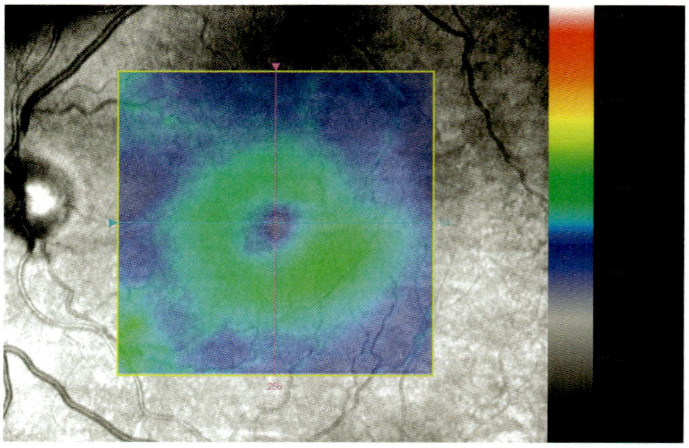

Case Figure 3-30 **Macular Cube OS:** Irregularly shaped area of the macular edema.

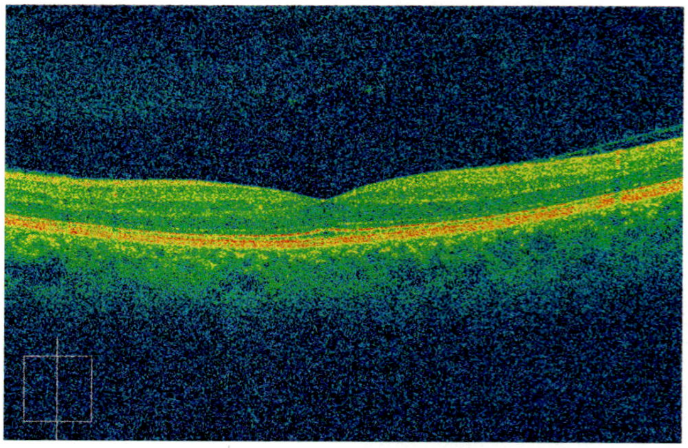

Case Figure 3-31 **Vertical Section OD:** Increased elevation of the external plexiform layer and RPE layer.

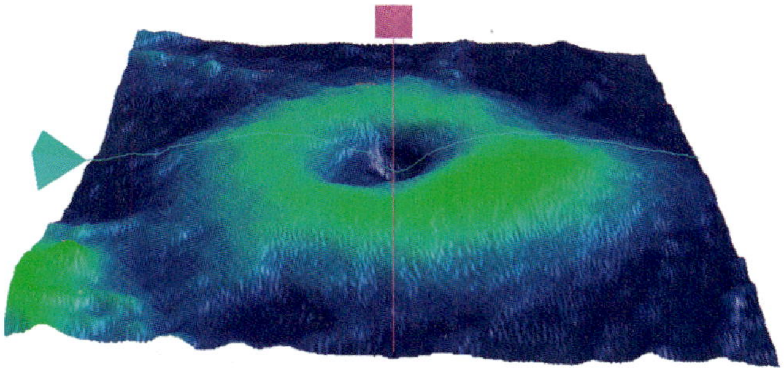

Case Figure 3-32 OS: 3D scan: There is abnormal foveal topography and tilting of the foveal pit.

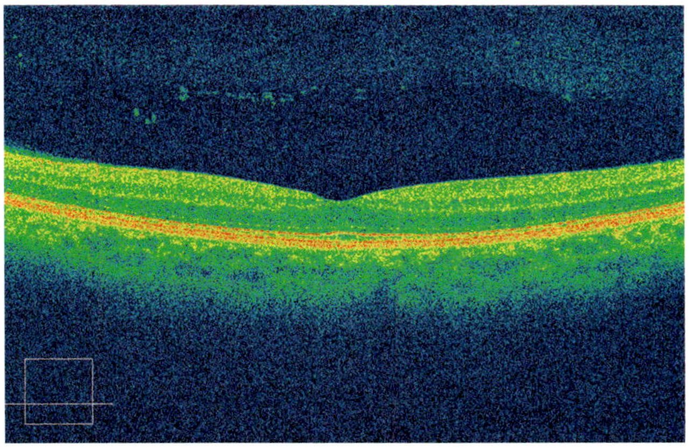

Case Figure 3-33 5-Line Raster OS: Note the irregularity of the surface of the ILM and macula interface. There is foveal edema as well.

Case 4. JB is a 53-year-old white male with hypertension and diabetes for one 1 year, V 20/25 OD, 20/20 OS.

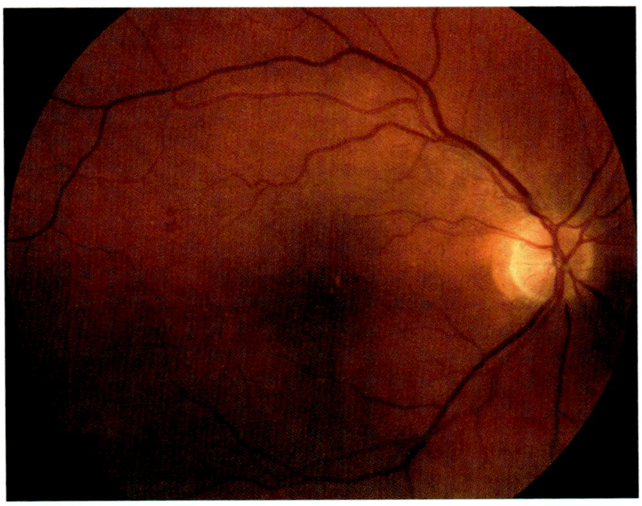

Case Figure 4-1 Color Photo OD: Small number of hard exudates in the macula and superotemporal to the macula. Few dot blot dot hemorrhages superotemporally to the macula.

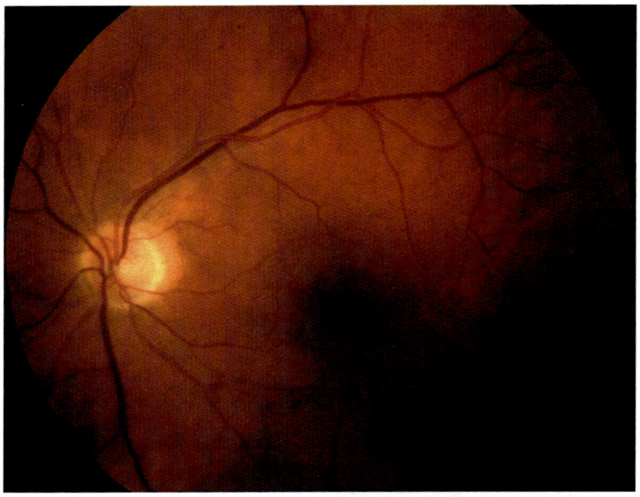

Case Figure 4-2 Color Photo OS: Arteriovenous nicking and venous tortuosity, inferior arcade versus superior arcade.

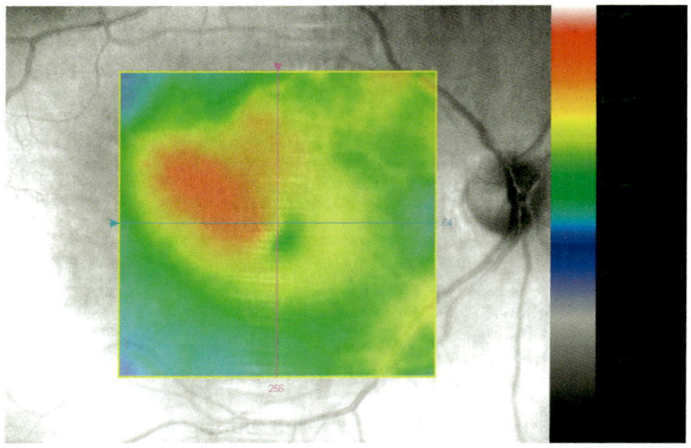

Case Figure 4-3 Macular Cube OD: Macular edema temporal to the fovea.

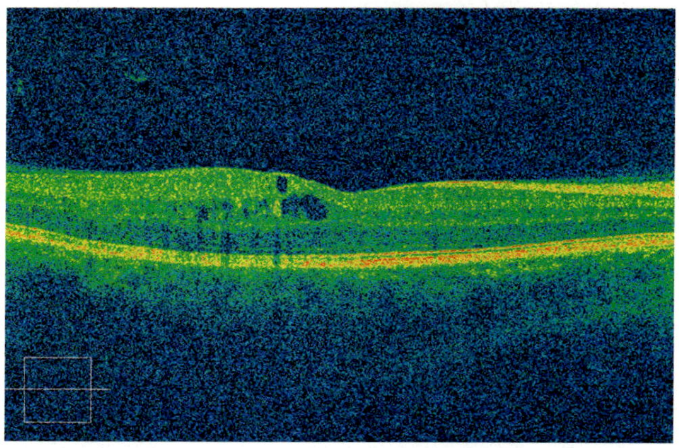

Case Figure 4-4 Horizontal Section OD: Note the cystic changes of the macula, located in the external plexiform layer.

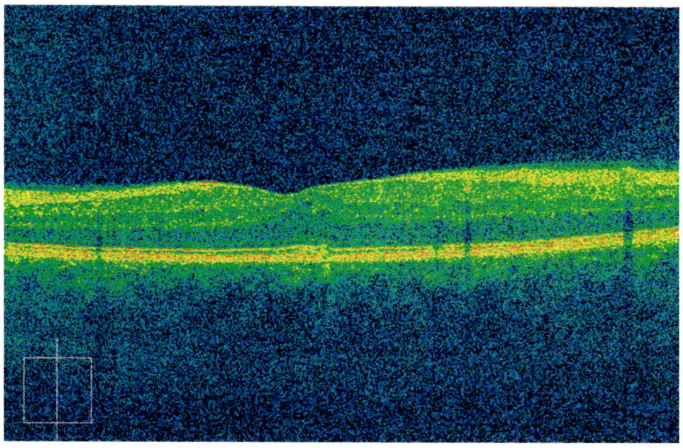

Case Figure 4-5 Vertical Section OD: Small cyst seen in the fovea.

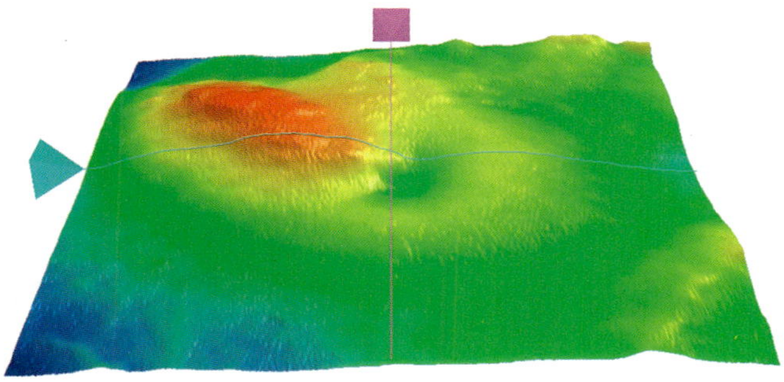

Case Figure 4-6 OD: 3D scan showing lopsided macular edema with foveal pit forming a shallow crater in an oval formation.

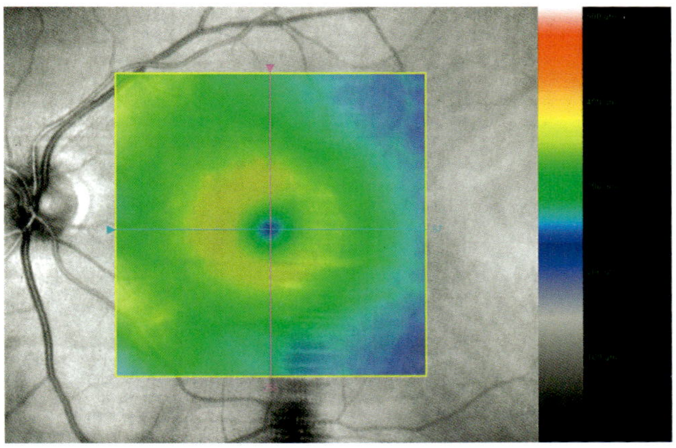

Case Figure 4-7 Macular Cube OS: Edema is now shifted towards the nasal macula.

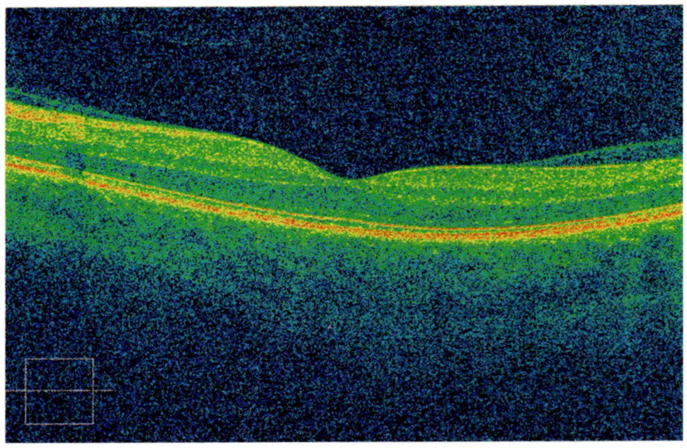

Case Figure 4-8 Horizontal Section OS: Note the cystic changes of the macula, located in the external plexiform layer, shifted to the nasal macula.

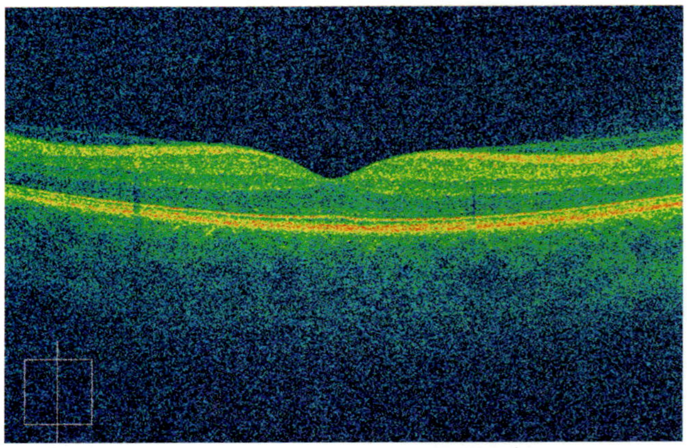

Case Figure 4-9 Vertical Section OS: Small abnormalities at the foveal pit and RPE in the fovea.

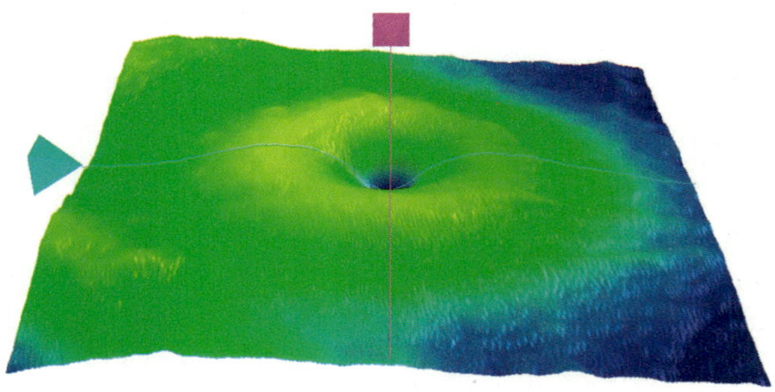

Case Figure 4-10 OS: 3D scan showing surface irregularity of the macula.

Case 5. HN is an 87-year-old Asian female with 9 years of Type 2 diabetes with decreased vision, V 20/30 OD, 20/30 OS. She had macular laser with another ophthalmologist and now refuses laser.

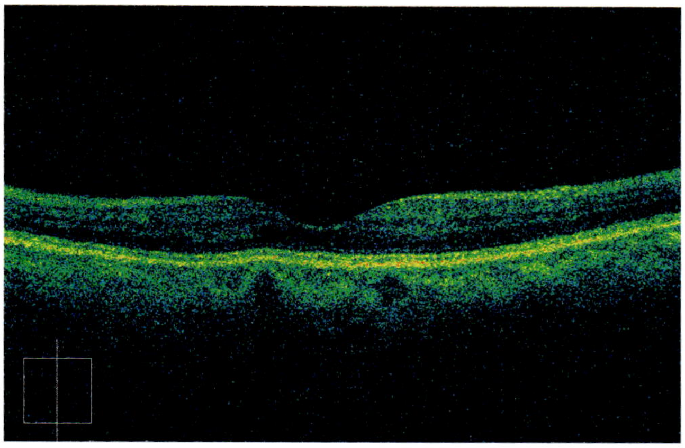

Case Figure 5-1 Macular Cube OD
Vertical Section OD: Macular edema noted temporally at the fovea.

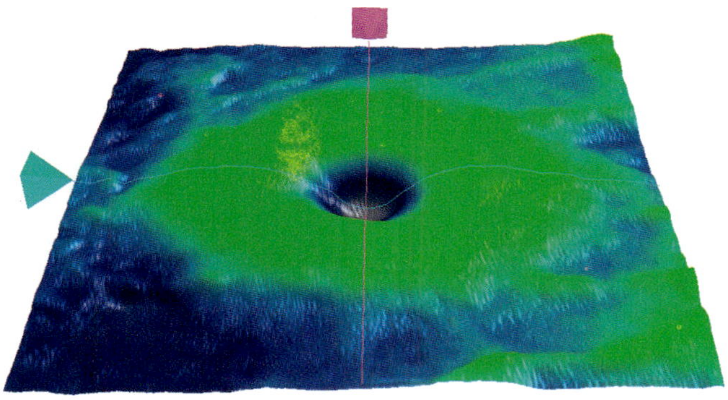

Case Figure 5-2 **OD:** 3D showing irregular contour of the macula reflecting macular edema,

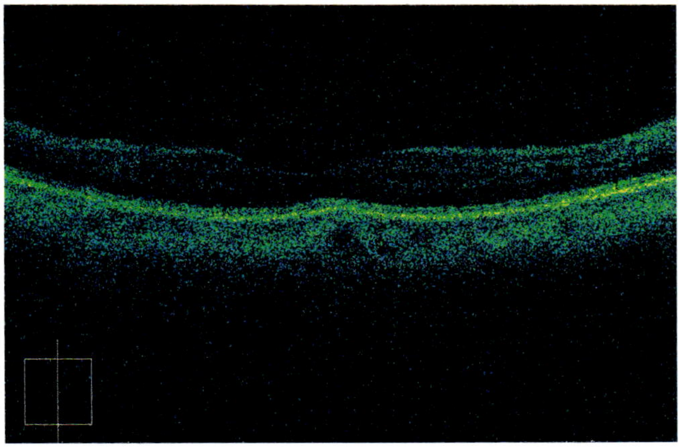

Case Figure 5-3 **Vertical Section OS:** Abnormal architecture of the macula with distortion of the ten retina layers due to the edema.

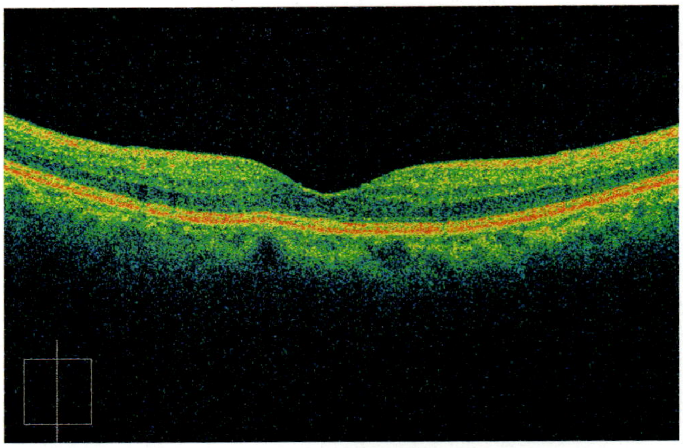

Case Figure 5-4 Vertical Section OD: 1 month later, worsening edema is noted. Note the beginning abnormality of the RPE under the fovea.

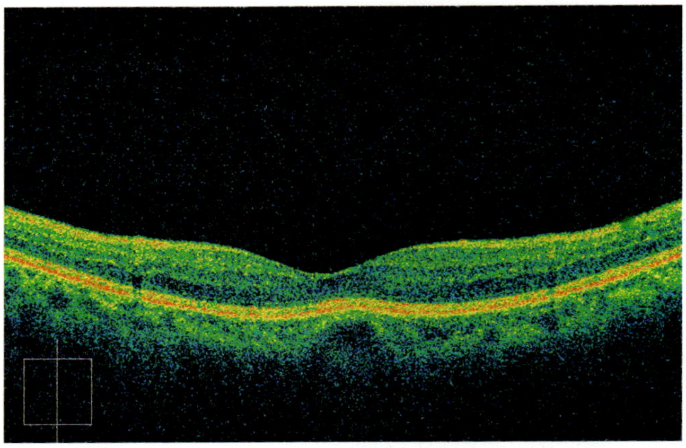

Case Figure 5-5 Vertical Section OS: 1 month later, 10–14–2008, worsening edema at the external plexiform layer is noted.

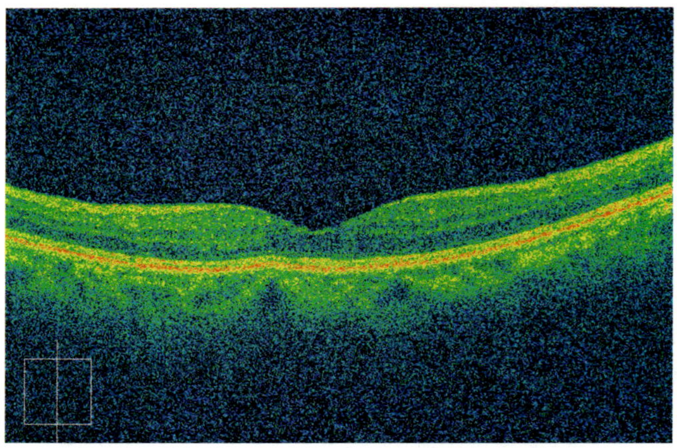

Case Figure 5-6 Vertical Section OD: 6 months later, the ILM is ragged. The macular edema is worse.

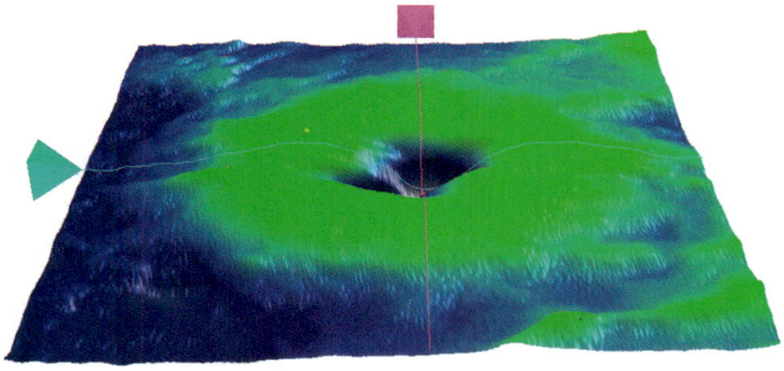

Case Figure 5-7 OD from 6 months later: 3D scan showing the loss of the smooth contour of the macula and some "folds" due to the macular edema.

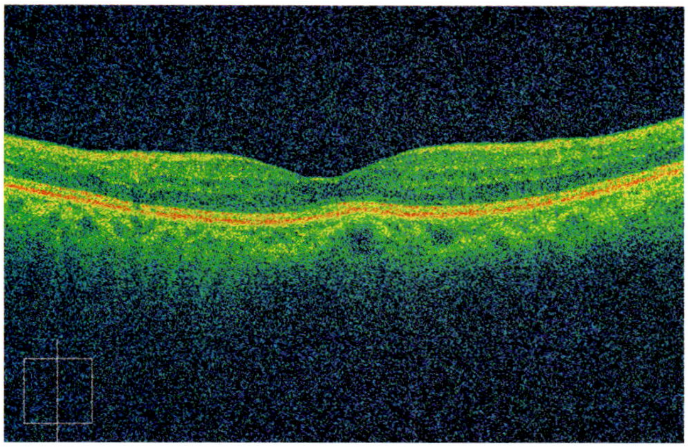

Case Figure 5-8 Vertical Section OS: 6 months later, temporal macula shows abnormal architecture of the ten layers of the retina.

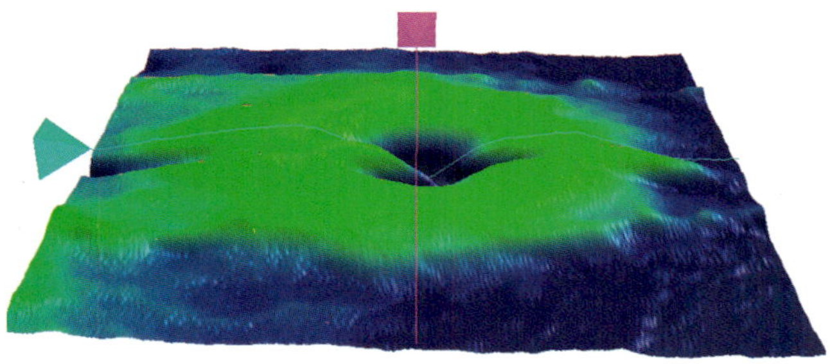

Case Figure 5-9 OS: 3D scan showing "folds" due to the macular edema, and the foveal pit is nc longer, rounded but misshapen.

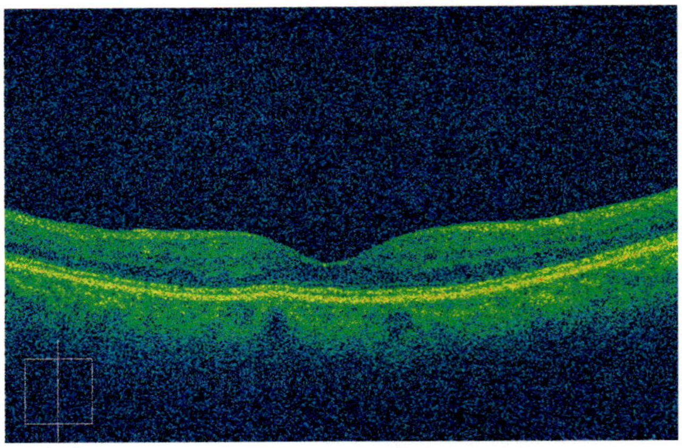

Case Figure 5-10 Vertical Section OD: 8 months after presentation, the ILM is thickened, and the separate layers of the retina are less clearly defined. The macular edema is worse.

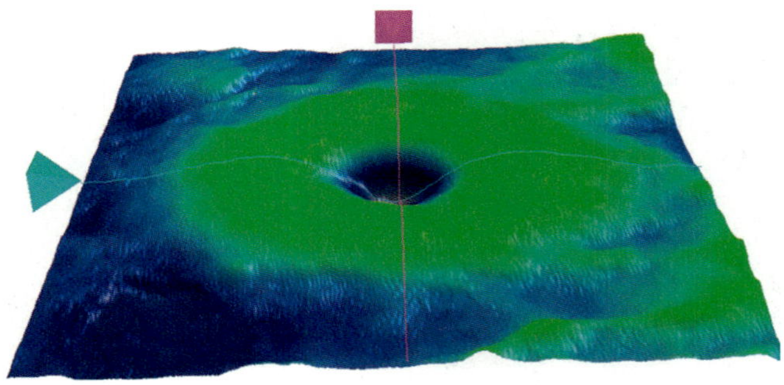

Case Figure 5-11 OD: 3D scan shows lumpy quality to the contour of the surface of the macula, 8 months after presentation.

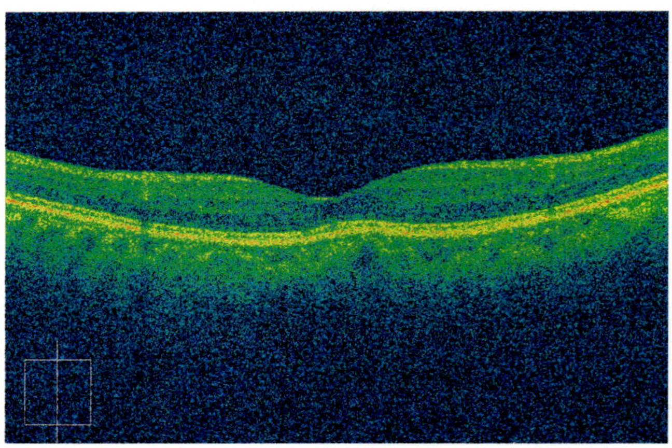

Case Figure 5-12 Vertical Section OS: 8 months after presentation, nasal and temporal macula show abnormal architecture of the ten layers of the retina and thickening of the nerve fiber layer. The RPE shows a lack of smoothness under the fovea.

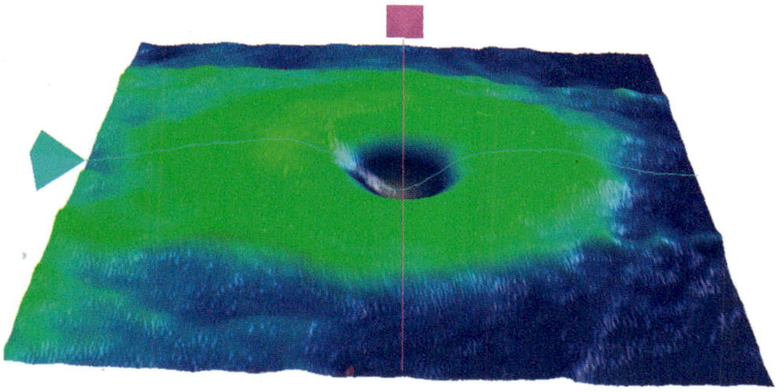

Case Figure 5-13 OS: 3D scan shows the elevation of the macular edema forming a superior and inferior "ridge-like boundary" to the macula. The scan allows the edema to be almost palpable to the viewer, 8 months after presentation.

Case 6. MT is 55-year-old African American female with 5 years of Type 2 diabetes, V 20/25 OD, 20/30 OS.

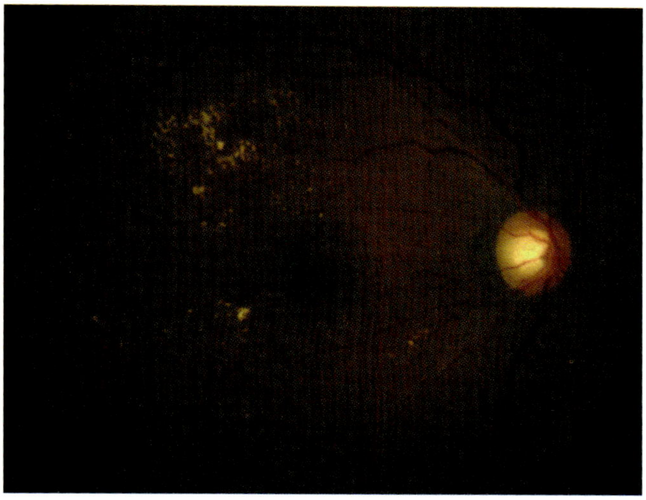

Case Figure 6-1 Color Photo OD: Hard exudates rings, dot blot hemorrhages, macular edema, mild venous engorgement, optic disc with some sloping of the cup.

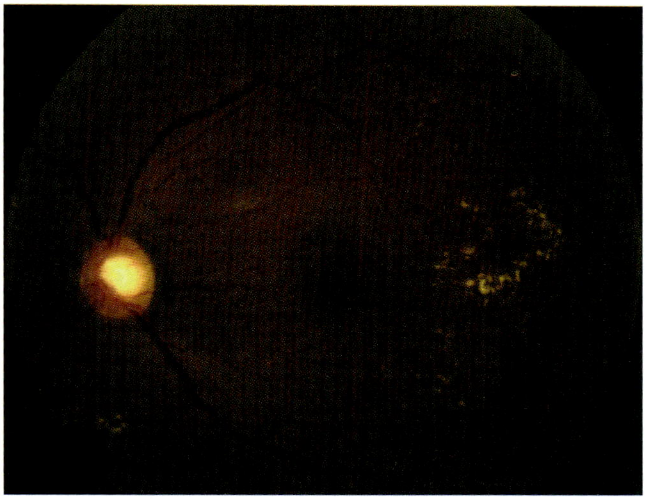

Case Figure 6-2 Color Photo OS: Hard exudates rings, dot blot hemorrhages, macular edema, optic disc cupping more pronounced, venous engorgement worse in the inferior arcade than in the superior arcade.

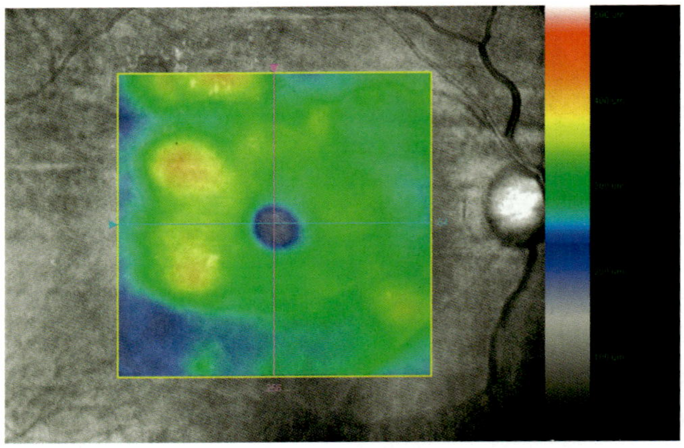

Case Figure 6-3 Macular Cube OD: Macular edema pronounced at the temporal macula. Note the optic nerve cupping at the far side of the scan on the right.

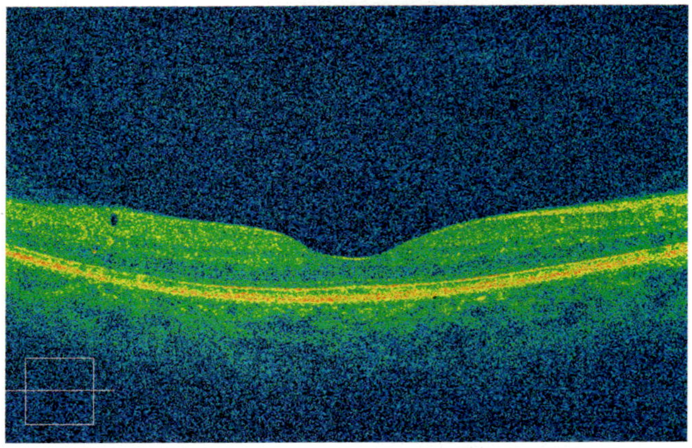

Case Figure 6-4 Horizontal Section OD: Abnormal architecture of the macula temporally with cystic edema seen as well.

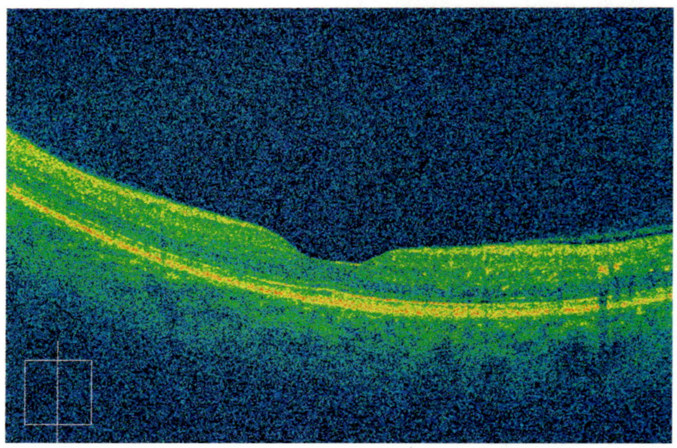

Case Figure 6-5 Vertical Section OD: Thickening of the nerve fiber layer with edema seen at the external plexiform layer.

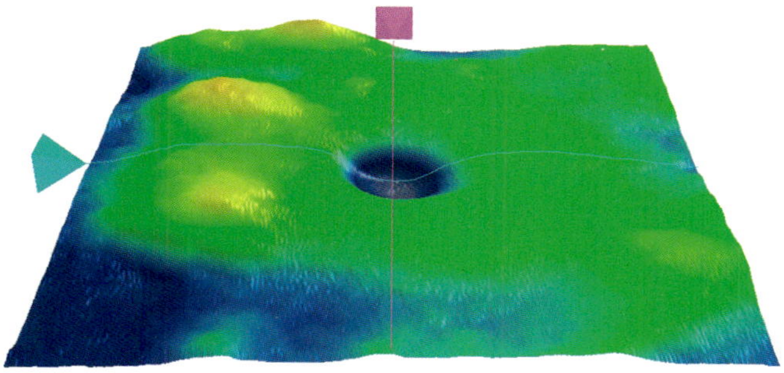

Case Figure 6-6 OD: 3D scan with gross contour abnormality temporal to the macula.

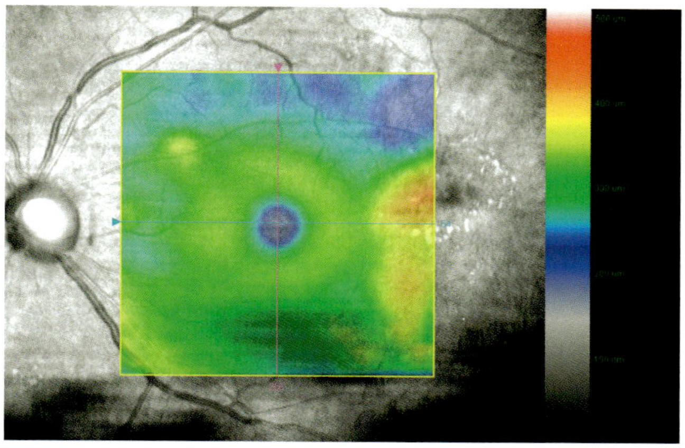

Case Figure 6-7 Macular Cube OS: Macular edema pronounced at the inferior macula and the hard exudate ring temporally.

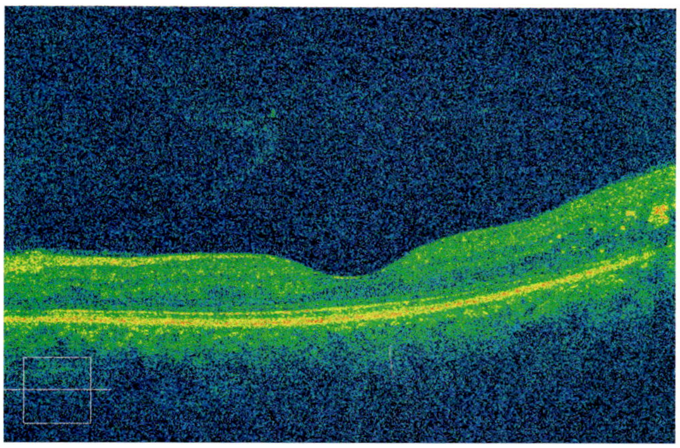

Case Figure 6-8 Horizontal Section OS: Abnormal architecture of the macula nasally and temporally with thickening of the ILM, nerve fiber layer. Note the cystic formation at the nasal and temporal macula.

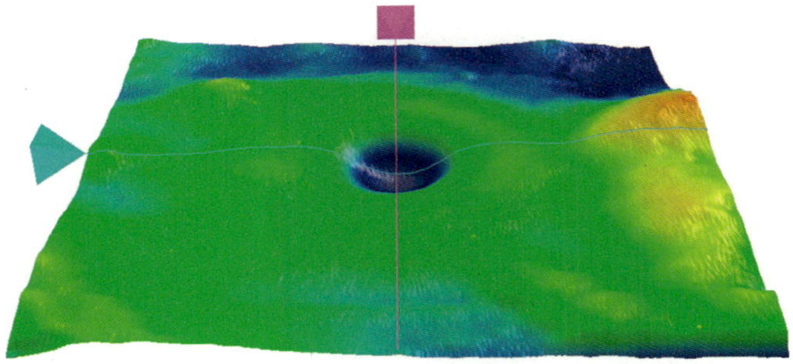

Case Figure 6-9 OS: 3D scan showing various hills and valleys corresponding to the edema instead of the normal, smooth contour of the macula.

Case 7. PS is a 53-year-old White male with HbA1c = 12%, FBS = 350 mg/dL, 18 years duration of diabetes, Type 1 diabetes for the past 15 years, with poor compliance. His vision is V 20/25 OD, 20/25 OS.

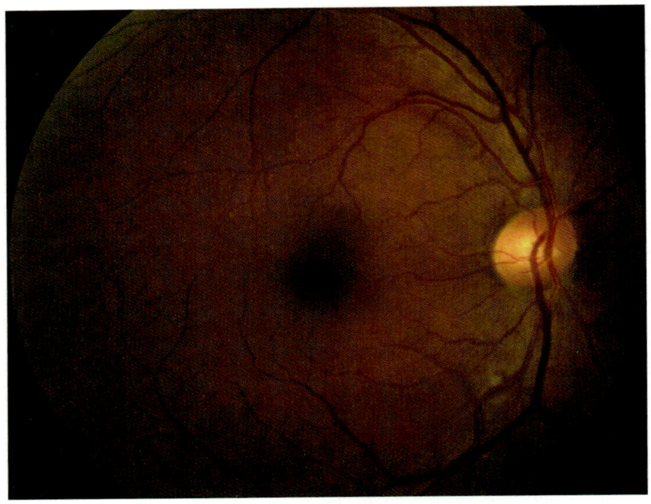

Case Figure 7-1 Color Photo OD: Cotton- wool spot along the inferior arcade, few dot hemorrhages.

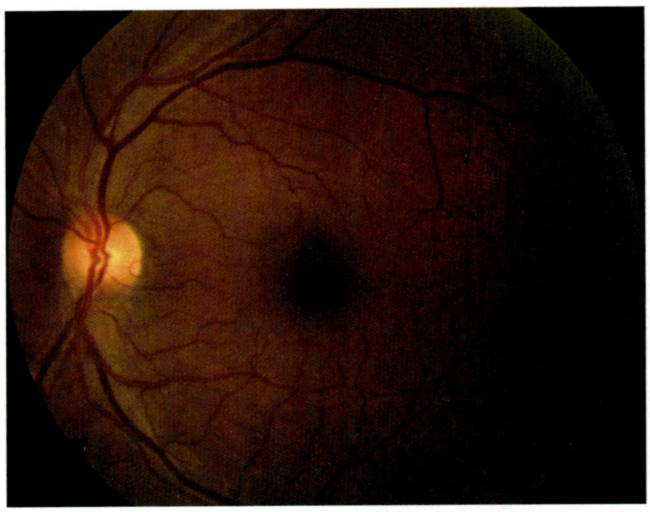

Case Figure 7-2 Color Photo OS: Cotton- wool spot is seen at the edge of the inferonasal arcade, few dot hemorrhages.

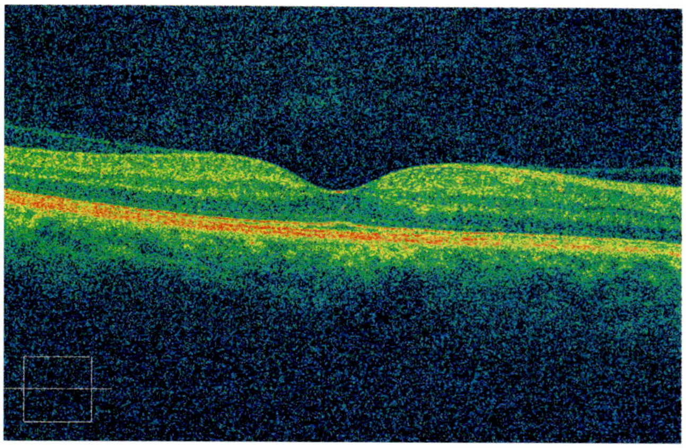

Case Figure 7-3 Horizontal Section OD: Shaggy or shadows at the posterior edge of the external plexiform layer nasally, consistent with macular edema.

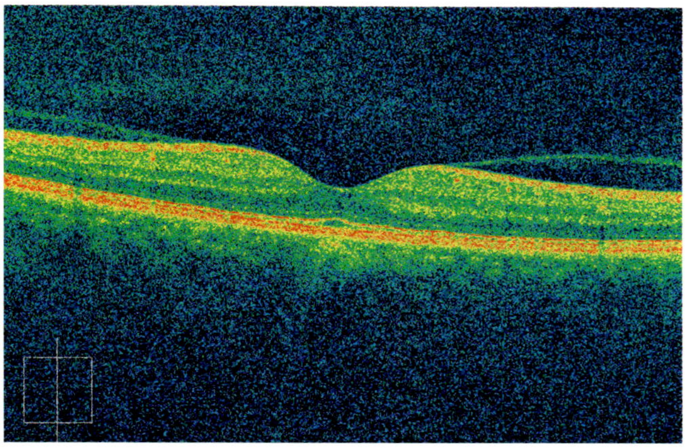

Case Figure 7-4 Vertical Section OD: Temporal macula is irregular wavy like pattern of the interface of the internal and external plexiform layers denoting macular edema. Also, the RPE is abnormal.

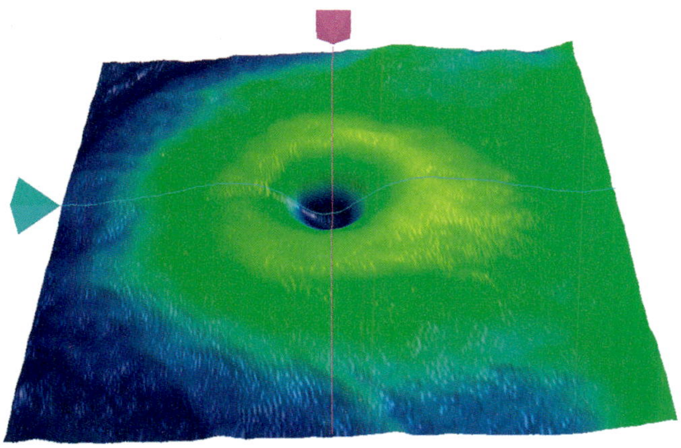

Case Figure 7-5 OD: 3D scan showing irregular surface of the macula.

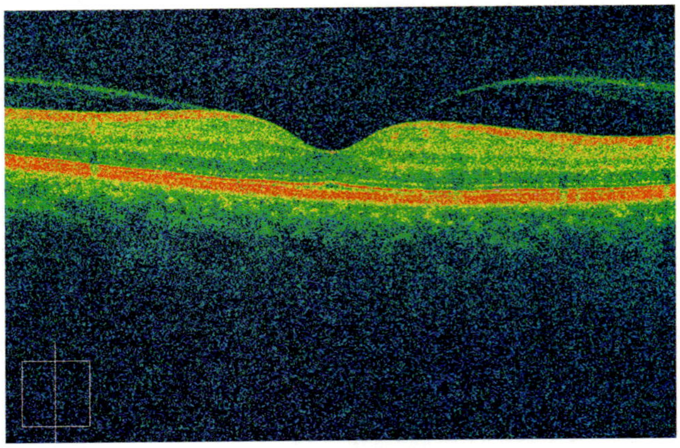

Case Figure 7-6 Vertical Section OS: Nasal and temporal macula with abnormal ILM and nerve fiber layers. Note the posterior vitreous is attached to the ILM.

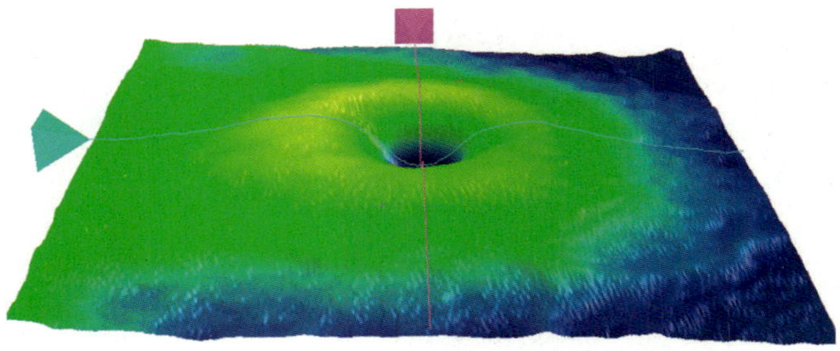

Case Figure 7-7 OS: 3D scan showing irregular surface of the macula with ovoid foveal pit.

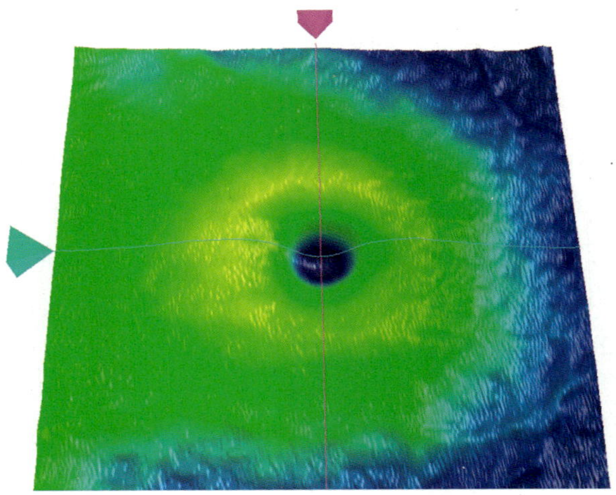

Case Figure 7-8 OS: 3D scan rotated upwards showing irregular surface of the macula nasally.

Case 8. EY is a 64-year-old female with one 1 year duration of Type 2 diabetes with V 20/40 OD, 20/40 OS.

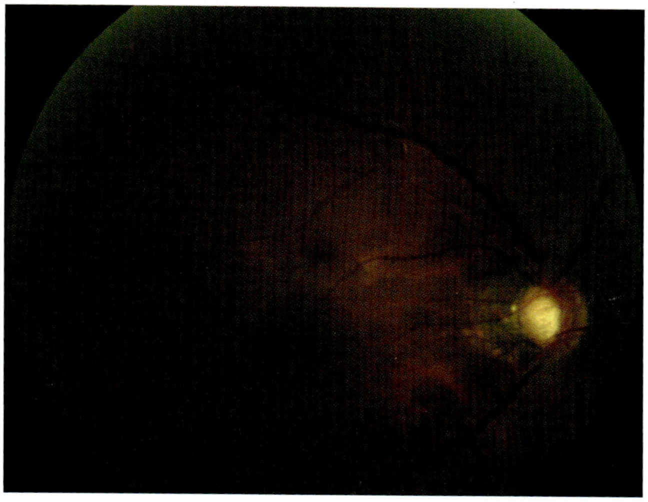

Case Figure 8-1 Color Photo OD: Macular edema with hemorrhage superior to the macula, glaucomatous cupping is noted.

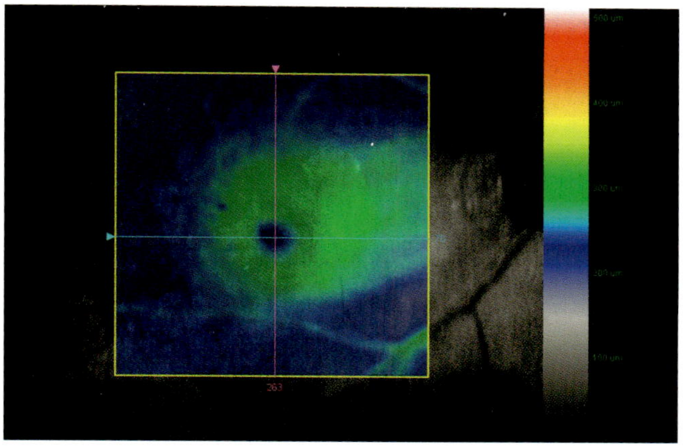

Case Figure 8-2 Macula Cube OD: Edema is noted around the fovea.

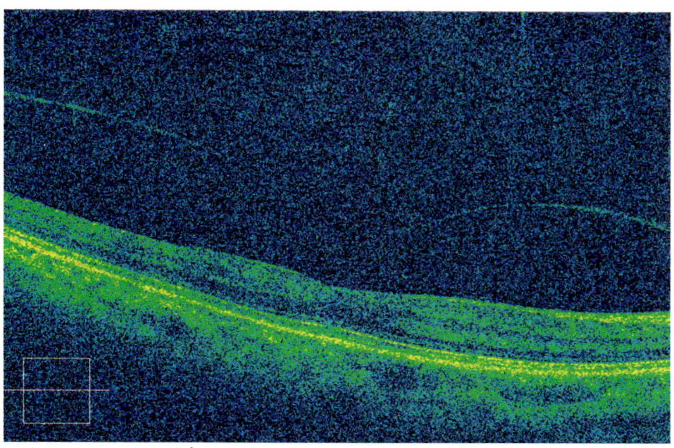

Case Figure 8-3 Horizontal Section OD: Edge of the vitreous body is seen in this scan. Macular edema is also seen.

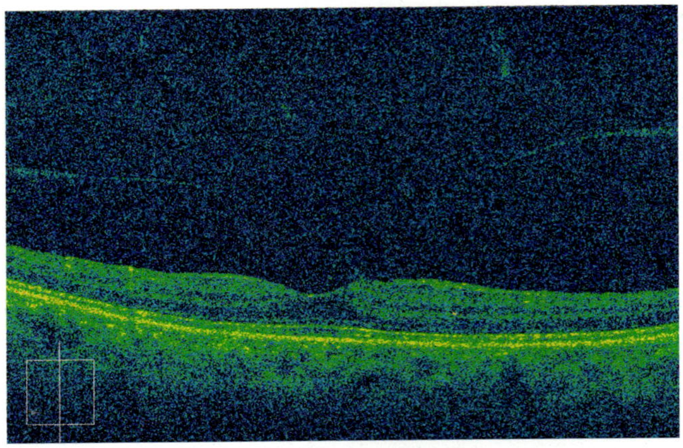

Case Figure 8-4 Vertical Section OD: Edge of the vitreous body is seen in this scan, which appears to be attached to part of ILM in the foveal region. Macular edema is seen at the fovea.

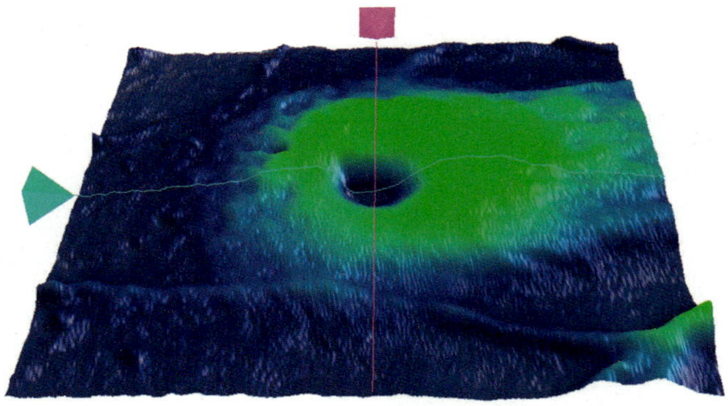

Case Figure 8-5 OD: 3D scan shows edema spreading from the disc towards the fovea and spilling over to the temporal area of the macula.

Medical Equipment, Supplies and Patient Education Materials

OPTICAL COHERENCE TOMOGRAPHY (OCT)

Heidelberg Engineering Spectralis OCT

U.S. Corporate Office
1499 Poinsettia Ave., Suite 160
Vista, CA 92081–8543
Tel: (800) 931–2230
Fax: (760) 598–3060
http://www.heidelbergengineering.com/products/spectralis-oct/

Zeiss Cirrus OCT

Carl Zeiss Meditec, Inc.
5160 Hacienda Drive
Dublin, CA 94568
Tel: (925) 557 4100
Fax: (925) 557 4298
info@meditec.zeiss.com
www.meditec.zeiss.com/us

Optovue OCT

Optovue, Inc.
45531 Northport Loop W.
Fremont, CA 94538
Tel: (510) 623–8868
Toll-Free: (866) 344–8948
www.optovue.com

FUNDUS CAMERA

Topcon Fundus Camera

Topcon Medical Systems, Inc.
37 West Century Road
Paramus, NJ 07652
Tel: (201) 599–5100, (800) 223–1130
Fax: (201) 599–5250
http://www.topconmedical.com/

OIS Digital Fundus and Fluorescein Camera

221 Lathrop Way, Suite I
Sacramento, CA 95815
Tel: (916) 646–2020, (800) 338–8436
Fax: (916) 646–0207
info@oisi.com
www.oisi.com

Zeiss Fundus Camera

Carl Zeiss Meditec, Inc.
5160 Hacienda Drive
Dublin, CA 94568
Tel: (925) 557–4100
Fax: (925) 557–4101
info@meditec.zeiss.com
www.meditec.zeiss.com

Kowa Fundus Camera

Kowa/Optimed, Inc.
20001 S. Vermont Avenue
Torrance, CA 90502
Tel: (310) 327–1913
Fax (310) 327–4177
http://medical.kowa.com/

Handheld Fundus Camera

Kowa
Kowa/Optimed, Inc.
20001 S. Vermont Avenue
Torrance, CA 90502
Tel: (310) 327–1913
Fax: (310) 327–4177
http://medical.kowa.com/

ELECTROPHYSIOLOGY EQUIPMENT

LKC Technologies, Inc.

2 Professional Drive, Suite 222
Gaithersburg, MD 20879
Tel: (301) 840.1992, (800) 638–7055
Fax: (301) 330.2237
sales@LKC.com

Diagnosys LLC

Suite 500, 175 Cabot Street
Lowell, MA 01854
Tel: (978) 458–1600
Fax: (978) 458–1755
mail@diagnosysllc.com
http://www.diagnosysllc.com/home/

ELECTROPHYSIOLOGY SUPPLIES

Spectra 360 Electrode Gel
Grass Technologies EC2 cream
Silvon ECG Electrode REF 03510
Diagnosys DTL plus electrode No. D141

INTRAVITREAL MEDICATIONS AND COMPOUNDING PHARMACIES

Ranibizumab

Curascript
2297 Southwest Blvd Ste D
Grove City, OH 43123
Tel: (800) 348–5578
Lucentis Direct (Genentech)
1 DNA Way
South San Francisco, CA 94080
Tel: (800) 963–1778

Intravitreal Bevacizumab and Trimacinolone

Leiter's Rx Ophthalmic Compounding
1700 Park Ave., Suite 30
San Jose, CA 95126
Tel: (408) 292–6772, (800) 292–6773, (877) EYE-DROP
Fax: (408) 288–8252
The Apothecary Shop
1144 E. McDowell Rd.
#402
Phoenix, AZ 85006
Tel: (602) 257–1133
Fax: (602) 257–1134
The Apothecary Shop
262 Neil Ave., #130
Columbus, OH 43215
Tel: (614) 360–2800
Fax: (614) 360–2801

SUPPLIES

PSS World Medical, Incorporated

4345 Southpoint Boulevard
Jacksonville, FL 32216
Tel: (904) 332–3000

Akorn

1925 West Field Court
Suite 300
Lake Forest, IL 60045
Tel: (800) 932–5676
Fax: (800) 943–3694
customer.service@akorn.com

INFORMATIONAL WEB SITES

American Diabetes Association: www.diabetes.org
American Association of Clinical Endocrinologists: www.aace.com
American Heart Association: www.americanheart.org
Diabetic Retinopathy Clinical Research Network: www.drcr.net
National Eye Institute: www.nei.nih.gov
National Institutes of Health: www.nih.gov

PATIENT EDUCATION MATERIALS

Eli Lilly and Company: www.lilly.com
Patient education guides about diabetes and diabetes care
Novartis: www.novartis.com
Patient education guides and online resources for patient education

APPENDIX C

Diabetic Recipes

CHICKEN

1. **Spicy marinated chicken breast**

   Ingredients

   4 oz chicken breast without skin

   ¼ tsp pepper

   1 Tbsp chopped fresh ginger or substitute ¼ tsp ginger powder

   1 Tbsp soy sauce

   1 small lemon wedge (for last minute garnish after cooking)

   Rub seasoning over chicken breast, let it stand at in the refrigerator for 30 minutes.

   Bake at 350°F for 35 to 40 minutes.

   Squeeze lemon over chicken.

   Prep time: 5 minutes

   Cooking time: 35 minutes

   Serve with ¼ cup rice.

   Use iceberg lettuce salad with lemon juice and pepper as dressing. Add fresh scallions for taste if desired.

   Serves 1

2. **Naked chicken breast salad**

   Ingredients

   ½ pound of skinless, boneless chicken breast

   1 tsp tarragon

   1 lemon, cut in wedges to give garnish to salad

   Bake at 375°F for 40 minutes.

   Perfect for slicing for soup or to serve with a garnish of soy sauce mixed with scallions

   Prep time: less than 1 minute

   Cooking time: 40 minutes

   Thinly slice and serve on a bed of shredded lettuce, sprinkled with tarragon and lemon juice.

   Serves 2

3. **Crispy chicken chips**

   Take the chicken breast above (recipe 2), slice thin, and broil for 2 minutes. They will curl and you can sprinkle as a topping over ¼ cup of brown rice.

   Choice of Garnishes

   A sprinkle of low- sodium soy sauce

   Lemon juice with sliced fresh ginger (½ tsp)—optional

   ⅛ tsp cinnamon and half a packet of saccharine

   Sea salt

   Chopped fresh basil mixed with chopped cilantro and garlic salt

   Prep time: 2 minutes

Cooking time: 2 minutes
Serve with iceberg lettuce cups. Side dish could be ¼ cup of brown rice.

4. **Ginger soy chicken**
Ingredients
½ lb chicken breast fillets
⅓ cup low- sodium chicken broth
⅓ cup soy sauce
1 Tbsp finely chopped ginger
3 cloves of garlic, finely chopped
3 packets of saccharine
Marinate the chicken breast overnight in ⅓ cup low sodium chicken broth, ⅓ cup soy,
3 packets of saccharine, ginger, and garlic.
Bake at 375°F 40 to 45 minutes.
Slice thinly to top rice, or use in salad.
Prep time: 5 minutes
Cooking time: 40 to 45 minutes
Serve with toasted pita bread. Lettuce and Radicchio leaves for salad. Endives serve as a substitute for the Radicchio leaves. Use 1 Tbsp lemon juice mixed with ½ packet of saccharine for salad dressing, sprinkle on top of lettuce salad.
Serves 2

5. **Orange flavored chicken**
Ingredients
½ lb chicken breast, minus the skin
3 Tbsp low fat, dietetic orange marmalade (find in the dieter's section or weight watchers section. Smucker's Low Sugar Sweet Orange marmalade, SKU 51500–02174; Smucker's, 336 N. Cassady Ave., Columbus, OH 43209–1022)
3 Tbsp soy sauce
2 cloves of garlic, chopped
1 in. of fresh ginger, chopped
Marinate chicken and the ingredients overnight.
The next day, bake at 375°F for 40 minutes.
Serve with boiled brown rice. Cook the rice as you are cooking the chicken.
Prep time: 5 minutes
Cooking time: 40 minutes

6. **Asian chicken skewers**
Ingredients
½ lb boneless, skinless chicken breast, cut into 1 ½-in. pieces
1 small zucchini, cut into 1-in. slices
4 mushrooms, fresh and large
½ cup chopped bell peppers (red, yellow, or green)
2 Tbsp low sodium soy sauce
2 medium ginger, chopped
2 medium garlic cloves, minced
2 fresh, green onions, cut into 1-in. pieces
Place cut chicken, zucchini, mushrooms, and bell peppers into a resealable plastic bag.
In a small bowl, combine soy sauce, ginger, and garlic. Mix.
Pour mixture into the plastic bag with the chicken and vegetables.
Allow bag to marinade in the refrigerator for at least 30 minutes and up to 4 hours.
Place 4 (12 in.) skewers in water to cover and let soak for 20 minutes.
Remove chicken and vegetables from the bag.
Thread chicken and vegetables alternately with onions onto skewers.
Place skewers on the rack of the broiler pan.

Place skewers 5 to 6 in. from the heat and broil for 5 minutes.
Turn over skewers and broil the other side for 5 minutes.
Broil skewers for an additional 10 minutes to ensure chicken is cooked all the way through.

Prep time: 30 minutes
Cooking time: 20 minutes
Serves 2

7. **Basil chicken and vegetables**

Ingredients
1 boneless , skinless chicken breasts, cut into 1-in. strips
½ large, red bell peppers, thinly sliced
½ small sliced zucchini
⅓ cup sliced carrots
¼ cup fresh basil, shredded, tightly packed
¼ tsp freshly grounded black pepper
1 Tbsp chicken broth
¼ cup grated low-fat parmesan cheese
PAM cooking spray (ConAgra Foods, 1 Conagra Dr Omahe, NE 68102–5001)
Tear off 4 (12-in.) lengths of heavy-duty aluminum foil; fold each piece of foil in half, shiny sides together. Place on a baking sheet, and open out flat, shiny side up. Coat with cooking spray.
Arrange one fourth of chicken strips on half of each aluminum foil square, near the crease.
Spoon vegetables evenly over the chicken; sprinkle with basil and ground pepper.
Fold aluminum foil over chicken and vegetables, bringing edges together; fold edges over to seal securely. Pleat and crimp edges to make an airtight seal. Bake at 375°F for 30 minutes.
Remove chicken mixture from packets, and transfer to individual serving plates. Or, if you like, place packets on individual serving plates; cut an opening in the top of each packet, and fold aluminum foil back.
Sprinkle each serving with 1 Tbsp Parmesan cheese. Serve immediately.

8. **Asian chicken salad**

Ingredients
1 Tbsp rice vinegar (Japanese style)
1 tsp dry chicken broth (packet)
1 Tbsp lemon juice
1 Tbsp fresh ginger, grated
1 medium garlic cloves, minced
¼ tsp hot, red pepper flakes
1 lb Lettuce, green leaf, fresh, shredded (or mixed greens)
1 cup fresh bean sprouts
½ lb cooked chicken breast, diced, shredded
1 medium carrot, shredded
2 scallions, thinly sliced
Preheat oven to 375°F.
Put ½ lb. chicken breast (no skin, no bones) into the oven for 40 minutes, slice at the end.
Remove and set aside.
Combine in a large bowl the vinegar, lemon juice, ginger, garlic, and red-pepper flakes and whisk until blended.
Add the greens, sprouts, chicken, carrot, and scallions. Toss gently to mix and serve immediately.

Prep time: 15 minutes
Cooking time: 0
Serves 2

FISH

9. **Steamed flounder in the microwave**

Ingredients

4 oz of flounder
Chopped green onions
1 Tbsp soy sauce
1 tsp chopped fresh ginger
1 tsp freshly chopped garlic
In a square microwave dish with cover, place the 4 oz of flounder.
Sprinkle ginger and garlic. Cover dish. Heat on high for 30 seconds.
Then turn the dish 90°F in the microwave oven. Heat high for 30 or 45 seconds (depending on your oven).
Then, the flounder is done. Add the chopped scallions and soy sauce and serve.

Prep time: 5 minutes
Cooking time: 1.5 minutes

Serve with ¼ cup of brown rice.
Celery sticks
Serves 1

10. **Roasted halibut**

Ingredients

5 oz of halibut or cod
2 tsp of soy sauce
1 tsp or 1 packet of saccharine
Preheat oven to 450°F. Add the soy sauce to saccharine. Add to halibut.

Prep time: 5 minutes
Cooking time: 7 to 8 minutes.

Use large leaves of iceberg lettuce to roll this halibut. Use a colored toothpick to hold this lettuce taco together.
Serve on a plate with raw carrots and celery on the perimeter and the lettuce taco in the center.
Serves 2

11. **Salmon aluminum packet with Spanish flavors**

Ingredients

5 oz salmon fillets
Salt and pepper
2 to 3 thin lemon slices
Spanish olives
⅛ tsp thyme
⅛ tsp oregano
Preheat oven to 500°F.
Tear off 12 in. square of aluminum foil with shiny side facing down on the counter. Place salmon fillets in the center. Add the salt and pepper and the spices and olives. Then, bring together the long edges of foil and fold over several times, crimping tightly to prevent leakage but leaving enough room inside the packet for heat circulation. Fold each remaining edge of the aluminum foil in a similar manner.
Put this in the center of the cookie sheet.

Prep time: 5 minutes
Cooking time: 12 minutes.

Transfer to dinner plate.
Serve with shredded cabbage, ground up carrots for color. Sprinkle with chopped, fresh coriander.
Serves 2

12. Microwave flounder (Look Ma, no oil)

Ingredients

½ lb flounder
1 tsp low-sodium soy sauce
1 Tbsp Ginger, julienned in thin strips,
5 scallions, chopped fine
½ lb of flounder fillets, place on microwave dish with a cover.
Place on top of the flounder, sliced ginger and scallions with soy sauce.
Cook for 40 seconds high on microwave oven. Turn dish 90°F and repeat 30 seconds on high setting in microwave.

Prep time: 5 minutes
Cooking time: 2 minutes
Serves 2

13. Fish marinade

Ingredients

3 Tbsp lemon juice
¼ cup reconstituted dried low-fat chicken broth
1 tsp salt
⅛ tsp pepper
½ tsp turmeric
½ tsp powdered ginger
1 clove of garlic, pressed
½ tsp grated lemon rind
Marinate fish overnight for 24 hours.
Broil fish for 5 minutes (2.5 minutes each side)

Prep time: 10 minutes
Cooking time: 5 minutes
Marinade is enough for 1 lb of fish.

14. Red snapper

Ingredients

4 scallions, chopped
1 tsp white pepper
2 Tbsp lemon juice
1 Tbsp Dijon mustard
1 clove of garlic minced
½ cup chopped leaf, parsley
4 to 5 oz of red snapper
Place spices on top of the fish. Place the fish into the microwave dish with a covering lid, heat one high for 1 minute, turn the dish, 90°F, and then heat again for 1 minute in the microwave oven. Repeat until done.

Prep time: 5 minutes
Cooking time: total of 4 minutes
Serves 2

VEGETARIAN

15. Grilled tofu

Ingredients

1 package of 8 oz of tofu
1 packet of artificial sweetener
1 Tbsp soy sauce
Mix the soy sauce with sweetener.
Then pour on top of the block of tofu
Broil for 5 minutes. The top will be crusty and brown. Serve hot or at room temperature after cooling.

Slice it in slabs.
Prep time: 3 minutes
Cooking time: 3 minutes
To be served with ¼ cup of brown rice or with dietetic bread sticks.
Vegetable: salad
Serves 1 to 2

16. Flavored mashed potatoes
Ingredients
1 large or two small red-skinned potatoes (peeled and washed)
½ tsp of salt
1 tsp of dried chicken bouillon
3 Tbsp of skim milk
1 scallion chopped
Black pepper to taste
Divide the potatoes into quarters, place in a pot, and add enough water to cover the potatoes. Add ½ tsp of salt, and bring to boil. Reduce heat, simmer covered. Drain. Take the hot potato and use potato masher to break into small chunks. Add the 3 Tbsp of skim milk. Over low heat, continue to break up the potato into smaller chunks. Add scallions and add salt and pepper to taste, at the end.
Prep time: 5 minutes
Cooking time: 15 minutes
Serves 2

17. Veggie stir fry
Morningstar Meal Starters Veggie Crumbles (distributed by Kellogg Sales, Battle Creek, Michigan, 49016)
⅔ cup is one serving
80 cal ADA exchange is 1.5 lean meat
Ingredients
⅔ cup Morningstar Meal Starters veggie crumbles, from the freezer
PAM spray oil
2 Tbsp soy sauce
2 cloves of fresh garlic, chopped and minced
1 Tbsp fresh ginger, finely chopped
Using a Teflon pan, you can spray PAM onto the surface. Heat the pan, and add the garlic and ginger. Once the garlic and ginger are brown, add the ⅔ cup of veggie crumbles. Add the soy sauce. The frozen veggie crumbles with its ice particles will melt and add moisture to the mix. It takes about 5 minutes to cook.
Prep time: 5 minutes
Cooking time: 7 minutes
Serve with ¼ cup of brown rice per person. For vegetable, serve celery sticks with carrot sticks on the side.
Serves 2

18. Low fat Morningstar veggie chili sauce
Ingredients
Morningstar Veggie Crumbles
½ bottle of commercial spaghetti sauce
2 Tbsp fresh basil, chopped
1 cloves of garlic, minced and chopped finely
In a saucepan, combine with ½ bottle of spaghetti sauce (no oil, no PAM)
Prep time: 5 minutes
Cooking time: 5 minutes
Serve on top of a slice of whole wheat toast cut in half. Or, serve with Boston lettuce cups or iceberg lettuce cups.
Or, serve with ¼ cup of brown rice.
Serves 2

19. Tofu hommus

Ingredients

½ package of 8 oz of firm tofu
¼ tsp cumin
½ tsp chopped garlic
¼ tsp salt to taste

Optional: parsley sprigs to top each serving

Drain excess water from the rectangular slab of tofu, press with paper towels to absorb excess water. Repeat about 6 times. Use 6 sheets of paper towels, one at a time to press on tofu to drain the water. Then, set tofu in food processor. Put on high to make the tofu soft and velvety in texture. Throw in spices as the food processor is working on tofu.

Prep time: 10 minutes

Cooking time: 0

Serve with pita bread triangles, toasted or lettuce cups. Sprinkle chopped parsley on top for coloring. Black olives can serve as a garnish and for coloring.

Serves 2

20. Low fat Morningstar veggie "tacos"

Ingredients

Iceberg lettuce, use one 1 leaf at a time
1 small plum tomato: chopped fresh tomato
½ tsp garlic salt
½ tsp fresh ginger, finely chopped

Using PAM on frying pan, add the veggie crumbles and all the ingredients at once. It takes about 2 minutes to stir fry.

Prep time: 5 minutes

Cooking time: 2 minutes

Using lettuce leaf as a taco wrap, this can be served for lunch or dinner for 2 people.

21. Cold tofu Japanese style

Ingredients

½ package of 8 oz of firm tofu
Sliced scallions (about 4)
2 Tbsp soy sauce

Cold tofu, get rid of excess water, see recipe 6

Slice it and leave the brick of tofu in place. Then slice again perpendicularly so the final brick of tofu looks like graph paper.

Serve with salad: watercress mixed with chopped chives. Use ¼ small avocado, mashed and serve as a relish. Sprinkle few lemon drops on top of avocado for taste and for keeping the avocado fresh looking when serving.

Prep time: 5 minutes

Cooking time: 0

Serves 2

22. Caviar sauce and salad

Ingredients

½ cup low-fat sour cream (sour cream made with skim milk)
½ tsp shallot juice (substitute: onion juice)
1 tsp capers
¼ cup of red caviar

Serve with baby spinach leaves, Boston lettuce, radicchio, and julienned carrots

Prep time: 5 minutes

Cooking time: 0

Serves 2

23. Curry dressing for fruit salad

Ingredients

1 Tbsp mild vinegar
½ Tbsp lemon juice
¼ tsp curry
½ tsp of saccharine
½ non fat vanilla yoghurt
Add to 2 small peeled and sliced apples.

Prep time: 5 minutes
Cooking time: 0

About ½ cup of dressing
Serves 2

24. Shitake delight

Ingredients

5 large, fresh shitake mushrooms (3 in. in diameter), sliced thinly
1 cup of reconstituted dried chicken broth
2 boiled eggs
5 baby carrots
½ cup raw baby spinach
¼ cup raw bean sprouts
(If you use dried shitake mushrooms, you should leave them in water overnight in the refrigerator or a cool place.)
In a saucepan, add ½ cup of water to chicken broth, and add the sliced mushrooms. Boil mushrooms, and set aside.
Boiled egg white is separated from egg yolk. Discard egg yolks. Use the egg whites only. Chop up and mix with shitake mushrooms.
Food processor, finely minced 5 baby carrots (for color)
Raw spinach leaves
Bean sprouts
Roll in large lettuce leaves, ice berg or Boston lettuce (soft and light green)
Dipping sauce
1 Tbsp soy sauce mixed with ½ tsp saccharine
1 Tbsp cilantro chopped
½ tsp finely chopped ginger
2 to 3 tsp of chicken broth from the bouillon cube

Prep time: 7 minutes
Cooking time: 3 minutes

Serves 2

25. Carrot cocktail

Ingredients

½ cup carrots
1 tomato, deseeded, chopped coarsely
1 Tbsp lemon juice
4 celery stalks, trimmed and sliced
4 scallions trimmed and coarsely chopped
Scant ⅓ cup fresh parsley
Scant ⅓ cup fresh mint
1 cup ice
Put carrots, tomatoes, and lemon juice in the food processor and process gently until combined.
Pour the mixture into glasses and garnish with celery stalks.

Prep time: 2 minutes
Cooking time: 0

Serves 2

26. Gazpacho

Ingredients

5 medium, ripe tomatoes
½ cucumber (about 3 in. piece)
½ red bell pepper
1 cloves of garlic
1 Tbsp of low-fat, low-sodium, dried chicken bouillon powder
⅛ cayenne (optional)
Put into the blender.

Prep time: 5 minutes
Cooking time: 0

Serves 2

Optional Garnishes
2 Tbsp chopped green onion or chives
¼ cup chopped parsley

27. Flavored couscous

Ingredients

½ cup boiling water
½ cup couscous
1/16 tsp cinnamon
½ packet of dried chicken bouillon powder or ½ of a bouillon cube
Top with 5 yellow raisins

In a saucepan, boil ¾ cup water, pour off excess so that you only have ½ cup of boiling water. When boiling, add couscous and all the dried ingredients, except raisins. Shut off the stove. Watch couscous rise. Then add raisins. Cover for 5 minutes. Then serve.

Prep time: less than 2 minutes
Cooking time: 5 minutes

Serve with low-fat plain yogurt as a sauce. Or, serve with tofu (recipe 15) or raw green smoothie.
Couscous serves 2.

28. Coca Cola marinated tofu

Ingredients

¾ cup diet coke (can be flat or fresh)
4 oz of firm tofu
1 clove of chopped garlic
Bake for 10 minutes
Serve with sliced green peppers or thinly sliced green tomatoes (unripened).

Prep time: less than 2 minutes
Cooking time: 15 minutes

Serves 1

Comments: The recipe was given to my by one of my Southern, Atlanta Georgia, diabetic friends. The diet coke acts as a good marinade. We have tried this on chicken and other meats. For meats, the cola acts as a meat tenderizer. The flavor is great. Sounds crazy, but it tastes good and meets the diabetic diet requirements.

29. Grilled green tomatoes

Ingredients

1 to 2 Green unripened tomatoes, sliced
½ tsp pepper
Place the slices on the cookie sheet with a foil on the bottom. Sprinkle the pepper on top. Salt is optional.
Broil 3 minutes

Prep time: 2 minutes

Cooking time: 3 minutes
Serves 1 if you use 1 tomato
Serves 2 if you use 2 tomatoes
Comments: This is great as a vegetable dish. Popular in areas where tomatoes are plentiful during the summer. Great for your non diabetic family members as well. Really flavorful.

30. Green tomato chutney
Ingredients
1 green tomato cut into wedges
1 Tbsp vinegar,
½ tsp salt
1 tsp saccharine (1 package)
1 Tbsp chopped scallions
¼ tsp basil powder
¼ tsp cilantro powder
5 raisins
Toss and serve.
Prep time: 5 minutes
Cooking time: 0

31. Ersatz egg salad
Ingredients
⅓ cup low-fat plain yogurt
4 eggs, boiled, discard egg yolks, use egg whites only
⅛ tsp white pepper
½ Tbsp finely chopped scallions (1 scallion)
Chop up egg whites.
Place in a small bowl and mix.
Using lettuce leaves, roll up and put a toothpick to hold in place.
Serve with whole wheat toast, cut into squares or triangles.
Prep time: 5 minutes
Cooking time: 0 (if you already have the boiled eggs prepared)
20 minutes if you need to boil the eggs. (boil water on high heat. Add the eggs, shut off heat, and cover for 20 minutes on low heat. Eggs will be perfectly boiled without the green coloring from excess boiling).
This makes a great protein for lettuce wraps.
Serves 2

32. Egg salad
Ingredients
2 boiled eggs
1 tsp low-fat mayonnaise
½ pickle
⅛ tsp saccharine
¼ small onion, chopped up
Add to mixture, toss
Prep time: 5 minutes
Cooking time: 0 (if eggs are boiled already), 20 minutes if you need to boil the eggs.
This makes a nice spread. Serve with green smoothie or fruit smoothie.
Serves 2

33. Vegetarian bulgogi
Ingredients A
1 cup of Harvest crumbles (Morningstar Veggie Crumbles, distributed by Kellogg Sales, Battle Creek, Michigan)
1 tsp saccharine
⅓ cup soy sauce

3 cloves of garlic, minced, chopped
¼ tsp salt
1 Tbsp sesame seeds toasted in toaster oven
1 cup green onions, cut into little round cylinders, so they form little green circles
1 Tbsp chopped fresh ginger

Ingredients B

1 Tbsp low-fat chicken broth
1 red bell pepper, cubed
1 medium onion, halved and sliced

Use PAM, cooking spray oil, on the Teflon frying pan. Throw in Ingredients A. As the ingredients start cooking and starts sizzling, (this is after 2 minutes of high heat), add Ingredients B. Cook for another 2 minutes.

Serve with whole wheat toast or brown rice.

Prep time: 20 minutes
Cooking time: 4 minutes for dish
Serves 2

34. Dill salad

Ingredients

½ head iceberg lettuce
For the salad dressing

Ingredients

¼ cup fresh dill, cut up, no stems
⅓ cup low-fat plain yogurt
⅛ tsp white pepper

Toss together and pour over iceberg lettuce.

Prep time: 5 minutes
Cooking time: 0
Serve as a vegetable.,
Serves 2

35. Grilled eggplant

Ingredients

½ lb eggplant
1 tsp chopped fresh ginger
2 Tbsp diet coke

Slice eggplant lengthwise (long oval).

Marinate with the ginger and diet coke for about 15 minutes or until the liquid penetrates the flesh of the eggplant.

Broil for 3 minutes until brown.

Then serve immediately as a vegetable/starch dish.

36. White chili

Ingredients

¼ lb northern beans, rinsed
2 cup of low-fat chicken bouillon stock (2 cubes)
1 clove of garlic chopped
1 medium onion chopped
1 Tbsp cilantro chopped
1 Tbsp flat-leaf parsley
1 bay leaf
½ tsp of crushed oregano, dried
½ tsp thyme
½ Tbsp cumin
1 Tbsp fresh mint (or ½ teaspoon of dried mint)
1 small fresh jalapeno chilled to taste (no seeds, chopped)

½ lb boneless, skinless chicken breast
Condiments
Chopped red onion
Chopped canned green chilies
Plain nonfat yogurt
Boil water, add the beans to rapid boiling water, and boil for 2 minutes. Let sit, covered for 1 hour.
Drain beans. Put 2 cups of chicken broth in pot and all of the spices. Boil then simmer for 2 hours.
In another pan, poach chicken breasts in 2 cups of water. This will take about 15 minutes. Then, cut the chicken into cubes. When beans are tender, add the chicken to the bean mixture. Cook for 15 more minutes. Chili should be thick.
Prep time: 20 minutes
Cooking time: 2 hours
Serves 2

37. Carrot and red pepper raw soup
Ingredients
1 red pepper diced
2 cup diced onion
½ pound carrots, sliced thin
Salt and ground pepper
2 Tbsp chopped parsley
1 Tbsp fresh dill
Juice from one lemon
2 cubes of low-fat, low-sodium chicken bouillon
1 cup ice
Blend under on high, 3 minutes
Prep time: 5 minutes
Cooking time: 0
Serves 2

38. Baked tofu
Ingredients
4 oz of firm tofu (½ packet of 8 oz container of tofu)
Slice tofu into about half in. slices. Place on nonstick baking tray so that they are pretty crowded. Then, pour over them the soy sauce marinade (see Rrecipe 48 , below).
Bake for about 15 to 20 minutes at 400°F. The tofu becomes crunchy on the outside and soft on the inside and delicious.
Prep time: 5 minutes
Cooking time: 20 minutes
Serves 2

39. Yummy soy sauce marinade
Ingredients
3 Tbsp soy sauce
1 packet of saccharine
½ tsp balsamic vinegar (regular vinegar is ok)
1 Tbsp grated fresh ginger
1 tsp minced garlic
1 Tbsp of orange zest (peel of orange, sliced and chopped)

40. Tofu with black beans
Ingredients
½ cup chicken broth (half bouillon of low-sodium chicken broth powder)
½ cup water

½ container of 8 oz of firm tofu, cut into cubes
10 grains of fermented salted black beans (found in Asian grocery stores)
1 tsp soy sauce
Heat the chicken broth and water together, add the tofu and beans. Let it boil once and then, simmer for 5 minutes or until tofu cubes become light brown, matching the color of the soy sauce.
Serve with iceberg lettuce leaves.
Make into a vegetable taco with the tofu as filling.
Prep time: 5 minutes
Cooking time: 20 minutes
Serves 2

41. Stir fried broccoli without oil (Teflon pan needed)
Ingredients
Morningstar veggie crumbles ½ bag (see recipe 11 for ordering the crumbles)
4 Tbsp soy sauce
4 Tbsp water
1 clove of garlic chopped
1 tsp finely chopped ginger
4 scallions finely chopped.
⅛ tsp white pepper
Broccoli, cut into florets
Spray PAM onto Teflon pan, and heat under high temperature.
Add white pepper to taste. Cook for about 5 minutes.
Prep time: 10 minutes
Cooking time: 5 minutes
Serves 2

42. Grilled summer squash medallions
Ingredients
¼ lb summer squash
1/16 tsp salt
1/16 tsp pepper
1/16 tsp garlic powder
Slice squash into round pieces, like medallions.
Place onto a cookie sheet, lined with aluminum foil.
Put the salt, pepper, and garlic powder on top of the sliced squash.
Broil for 2 minutes.
Prep time: 5 minutes
Cooking time: 2 minutes
Serves 2

43. Raw zucchini fettuccine
Ingredients A
2 medium zucchini, peeled into fettuccine
Ingredients B
2 apples cored, diced
Sugar-free applesauce
2 Tbsp plain low-fat yogurt
¼ cup mint leaves chopped
Put ingredients B into the blender, Ingredients B. Once this is prepared, thisit becomes the sauce for the vegetarian fettuccine. Then, pour sauce over fettuccine.
Prep time: 5 minutes
Cooking time: 0
Serves 2

44. Ginger carrot soup

Ingredients

1 medium carrot, peeled and chopped
1 celery stalk, chopped
2 tsp ginger, chopped
½ tsp of salt
¼ tsp pepper
¼ cup leftover brown rice
Add 1 cup of chicken broth from a fat-free bouillon cube
Toss in ingredients. Bring to boil. Add leftover rice. Let it cool. Then, pour into the blender and blend. This can be served hot or cold.

Prep time: 5 minutes
Cooking time: 3 minutes
Serves 1 to 2

45. Shrimp in ginger celery broth

Ingredients

3 medium frozen shrimp, washed
1 tsp soy sauce
¼ cup celery sliced thinly
1 low-fat chicken bouillon cube
5 snow peas (5 string beans is an acceptable substitute)
1 Tbsp chopped scallions
1 Tbsp chopped ginger
1 cup water
Place all ingredients into the saucepan and boil infor 3 minutes. Ready to serve. (Instead of using the stovetop, you can microwave in a glass container with a cover—microwave on high for 3 minutes.).
Serve with ¼ cup of hot brown rice.

Prep time: 5 minutes
Cooking time: 3 to 5 minutes
Serves 1 to 2 (Can serve two if there are other dishes to complement this soup.)

46. Couscous with chicken broth flavoring

Ingredients

½ cup of couscous
½ cup boiling water
1 bouillon cube, low fat, low sugar
Add bouillon cube to boiling water. Then, add couscous. Shut off heat, cover and watch couscous puff up in 1 minute.

Prep time: 3 minutes
Cooking time: 3 minutes
Serves 1

47. Eggplant delight

Ingredients:

1 medium eggplant, cut into ¼- in. slices, sprinkled with salt
1 large potato, sliced thin
1 small red pepper, chopped
1.5 small zucchini sliced
2 cloves of garlic, minced
1 large tomato, skinned, seeded, and chopped
Pinch of saccharine
Spray PAM into the Teflon pan. Fry potato slices. Add red pepper, zucchini, and eggplant.
When browned, add the tomato last. Sprinkle saccharine. Broil for 5 minutes.

Prep time: 10 minutes
Cooking time: 10 minutes
Serves 2

SMOOTHIES

48. Kiwi smoothie (needs 750-W blender)

Ingredients

3 kiwi fruits, peeled, cut up into chunks,
20 blueberries
20 blackberries berries
½ banana, cut up
6 Tbsp fat-free yogurt
1 cup skim milk
1 apple, cut and peeled
Use a blender. Add all ingredients and blend until smooth.

Prep time: 10 minutes
Cooking time: 0
For diabetics: this can serve as a lunch or breakfast.
Serves 2

49. Green smoothie for breakfast (needs 750-W blender)

Ingredients

½ cup of spinach/kale (a handful)
1 stalk of celery
½ banana (previously frozen) cut into chunks
½ apple (peeled)
3 to 5 strawberries
1 cup of water
3 to 4 ice cubes
High-speed blender (750-W motor needed) for 30 to 50 seconds

Prep time: 3 minutes
Cooking time: 0
Serves 2

50. Pomegranate smoothie (needs 750-W blender)

Ingredients

⅔ cup of pomegranate seeds
20 raspberries (to balance the pomegranate taste)
3 strawberries
1 apple
1 banana
1 cup fat-free plain yogurt
1 tsp saccharine

Prep time: 3 minutes
Cooking time: 0
Serves 2

51. Raw- food smoothie (needs 750-W blender)

Ingredients

5 to 6 leaves of dark green kale
A handful of parsley
Handful of baby spinach
½ lemon or lime
1 in. fresh ginger
2 stalks of celery

1 small apple
1 cup of ice
Blend until smooth. (in a 750-W Blender) for 30 to 50 seconds.
Prep time: 3 minutes or less
Cooking time: 0
Serves 1 to 2

52. Green tea smoothie (needs 750-W blender)
Ingredients
1 green tea bag with Eastern spice (available at grocery stores in the organic section)
1–¼ cups of boiling water
1 Tbsp diet sweetener
¼ cup of ripe yellow plums, halved and pitted
Put tea bag in tea pot or pitcher and pour over boiling water. Let infuse for 7 minutes.
Remove and discard the tea bag. Let chill.
Poor chilled tea in the food processor, and add sweetener and plums and process until smooth.
Prep time: 7 minutes (but there is the 1 to 2 hours of chill time in refrigerator)
Cooking time: 0
Serves 1

53. Raw bitter melon smoothie (needs 750-W blender)
Bitter melon is found in Asian grocery stores. It is light green and in the shape of a cucumber, but its outer surface is rough with bumps and indentations. Inside is a yellow pulp with large seeds. You can discard the seeds or put the entire melon through the blender. It has a slightly sour taste but has a "kick" for a smoothie.
Ingredients
¼ lb of bitter melon (about ½ of the melon)
A handful of fresh coriander (substitute parsley)
½ lemon or lime
1 in. fresh ginger
2 stalks of celery
1 quarter of an apple
1 cup of ice
Blend until smooth (in 750-W Blender) for 30 to 50 seconds.
Prep time: 3 minutes or less
Cooking time: 0
Serves 2

54. Red delicious apple and watermelon rind smoothie (needs 750-W blender)
Ingredients
1 small red delicious apple, cored
½ lb watermelon rinds or two cups
¼ tsp cinnamon
½ lemon
1 tsp saccharine
1 cup ice
Blend until smooth.
Red color from the red delicious apple peel gives it the color.
Prep time: 5 minutes
Cooking time: 0
Serves 2

55. Avocado smoothie (needs 750-W blender)

Ingredients

¼ avocado
½ cup grated cucumber
½ tsp chopped ginger
½ cup ice
Juice of one lemon
Salt and pepper
Blend for about 3 minutes and serve.

Prep time: 5 minutes
Cooking time: 0
Serves 1

Optional garnishes

1 Tbsp fresh chives, chopped
1 Tbsp fresh, chopped coriander

56. Raw Green veggie lunch/snack smoothie (needs 750-W blender)

Ingredients

1 fresh tomato
½ cup fresh spinach
Two slices of onion
⅛ tsp garlic salt
⅛ tsp pepper
¼ tsp balsamic vinegar
½ cup ice
1 sprig of parsley for garnish—optional
Use a food processor to blend this. Then, serve in a cup with a sprig of parsley.

Prep time: 5 minutes
Cooking time: 0
Serve with 2 slices of low- fat cheese for protein or ½ cup low-fat plain yogurt
Serves 1

57. Lipton tea smoothie (needs 750-W blender)

Ingredients

Lipton tea nor any black tea in a tea bag
1 –¼ cups of boiling water
1 tsp diet sweetener (1 packet)
1/16 tsp cinnamon powder
¼ cup of ripe apple chunks, no seeds
1 cup of ice
Put tea bag in tea pot or pitcher and pour over boiling water. Let infuse for 7 minutes.
Remove and discard tea bag. Let chill.
Poour chilled tea in food processor, add sweetener, ice, and apple, and process until smooth

Prep time: 3 minutes
Cooking time: 0
Serves 1

58. Mexican tomato smoothie (needs 750-W blender)

Ingredients

½ cup frozen chopped onion
1 minced clove of garlic
1 jalapeno chili pepper, seeded and minced
2 tomatoes (peeled, cut into chunks, deseeded)
Blend until smooth. At end, add the basil.

Prep time: 5 minutes
Cooking time: 0
Serves 2

59. Cinnamon carrot smoothie (needs 750-W blender)

Ingredients

1 large carrot
½ tsp cinnamon
½ tsp saccharine (½ packet)
½ tsp ginger, chopped
¼ cup chives, chopped
½ cup scallions, chopped
1 cup ice
Blend all together.

Prep time: 10 minutes
Cooking time: 0
Serves 2

60. Raw carrot smoothie sauce (needs 750-W blender)

Ingredients

1 large carrot, shredded
A handful of cilantro, chopped
4 green onions, diced
1 tomatoes, diced
¼ cup of fresh lime juice
2 cloves of garlic
Blend until smooth.

Prep time: 10 minutes
Cooking time: 0
Serve with ¼ cup of brown rice per person.
Serves 2

61. Apple and celery smoothie (needs 750-W blender)

Ingredients

2 small apples, washed and cored
1 to 2 celery stalks
1 packet of saccharine or 1 tsp of saccharine
1 cup ice
Blend with 750-W blender. Stir and serve.

Prep time: 3 minutes
Cooking time: 0
Serves 2

62. Ginger carrot celery smoothie (needs 750-W blender)

Ingredients

1 medium carrot, peeled and chopped
1 celery stalk, chopped
2 tsp ginger, chopped
½ tsp of salt
¼ tsp pepper
½ cup ice
Blend on high (with a 750-W Blender) until smooth. Serve on a hot summer day.

Prep time: 5 minutes
Cooking time: 0
Serves 1 to 2

63. Ginger ice (needs 750-W blender)

Ingredients

3 Tbsp ginger cut up
Handful of mint leaves
Handful of spinach
1 tsp or 1 package of saccharine
1 cup of ice
Blend until smooth, about 1 minute.
Lots of vitamin C

Prep time: 5 minutes
Cooking time: 0 minutes
Serves 1

64. Tomato juice ice cubes (needs 750-W blender)

Ingredients

1 cup of dietetic tomato juice, low sodium and low sugar
2 celery stalks for garnish
Pour tomato juice into ice cube tray.

Prep time: 2 hours of freezer time. During this time, you can wash celery stalks and prepare the glasses for this treat.
Cooking time: 0
Serves 2

65. Strawberry smoothie (needs 750-W blender)

Ingredients

1 cup of low-fat plain yogurt
1 tsp or 1 package of saccharine (optional)
3 whole strawberries
½ banana
Add all ingredients to blender and blend until smooth, about 1 minute.

Prep time: 5 minutes
Cooking time: 0 minutes
Serves 1

66. Raw broccoli smoothie (needs 750-W blender)

Ingredients

1 head of broccoli florets
1 Tbsp chopped ginger
1 Tbsp tarragon
1 Tbsp chives
½ carrot
1 cup ice
Add all ingredients to blender and blend until smooth, about 1 minute.

Prep time: 5 minutes
Cooking time: 0 minutes
Serves 1

RICE

67. Unflavored brown rice

Ingredients

1 cup water

½ cup brown rice.

Wash rice with cool water. Repeat once more. Put the water and rice into a saucepan. Cook over medium heat in a small pot for 40 minutes. Or, microwave in glass dish with cover for 40 minutes. Or, use a rice cooker, set on "brown rice setting" which takes about 40 minutes.

Prep time: 3 minutes

Cooking time: 40 minutes

Serves 2

68. Flavored brown rice

Ingredients

1 cup water

½ cup brown rice

½ packet of low-sodium chicken bouillon

⅛ tsp garlic powder

¼ tsp ground cilantro

In a saucepan, put in the ingredients, put under medium heat for 20 minutes, low-medium heat for an additional 20 minutes. Total time is 40 minutes.

Prep time: 1 minute

Cooking time: 40 minutes

Serves 2 to 3

Optional ways of making boiled rice:

Basic Ingredients

1 cup water

½ cup brown rice

½ packet of low-sodium chicken bouillon

Option 1

⅛ tsp cinnamon

1 Tbsp chopped walnuts or almonds

Option 2

⅛ tsp ginger

¼ tsp saccharine

¼ tsp saffron

Option 3

Ingredients

½ cup water

½ cup skim milk

½ cup brown rice

½ packet of low-sodium chicken bouillon

¼ tsp cinnamon

½ tsp basil powder

1 tsp fresh, finely chopped ginger

Add pinch of oregano (less than ⅛ tsp).

Cook in saucepan, under medium heat for 40 minutes.

INDEX

Page numbers in *italics* denote figures; those followed by a "t" denote tables.